Pharmaceutical Technology II

Pharmaceutical Technology

II

Gaurav Agarwal MPharm (BITS-Pilani) PhD
Dean, Faculty of Pharmacy
RP Educational Trust
Karnal, Haryana

Atul Kaushik MPharm (BITS-Pilani) PhD
Principal Scientist
Glenmark Research Laboratories
Mumbai

CBSPD

CBS Publishers & Distributors Pvt Ltd

New Delhi • Bengaluru • Chennai • Kochi • Kolkata • Lucknow • Mumbai
Hyderabad • Jharkhand • Nagpur • Patna • Pune • Uttarakhand

Pharmaceutical Technology II

ISBN: 978-81-239-2031-3

Copyright © Authors and Publishers

First Edition: 2012

Reprint: 2017, 2019, 2022

Published by Satish Kumar Jain and produced by Varun Jain for

CBS Publishers & Distributors Pvt Ltd

4819/XI Prahlad Street, 24 Ansari Road, Daryaganj, New Delhi 110 002, India
Ph: 011-23289259, 23266861, 23266867   Website: www.cbspd.com
Fax: 011-23243014   e-mail: delhi@cbspd.com; cbspubs@airtelmail.in
Corporate Office: 204 FIE, Industrial Area, Patparganj, Delhi 110 092

Ph: 011-4934 4934   Fax: 011-4934 4935   e-mail: publishing@cbspd.com; publicity@cbspd.com

Branches

- **Bengaluru:** Seema House 2975, 17th Cross, K.R. Road, Banasankari 2nd Stage, Bengaluru 560 070, Karnataka, India
  Ph: +91-80-26771678/79   Fax: +91-80-26771680   e-mail: bangalore@cbspd.com
- **Chennai:** 7, Subbaraya Street, Shenoy Nagar, Chennai 600 030, Tamil Nadu, India
  Ph: +91-44-26680620, 26681266   Fax: +91-44-42032115   e-mail: chennai@cbspd.com
- **Kochi:** 42/1325, 1326, Power House Road, Opp. KSEB, Power House, Ernakulam 682018, Kochi, Kerala, India
  Ph: +91-484-4059061-65   Fax: +91-484-4059065   e-mail: kochi@cbspd.com
- **Kolkata:** 147, Hind Ceramics Compound, 1st Floor, Nilgunj Road, Belghoria, Kolkata-700056, West Bengal, India
  Ph: 033-25633055, 033-25633056   e-mail: kolkata@cbspd.com
- **Lucknow:** Basement, Khushnuma Complex, 7, Meerabai Marg (Behind Jawahar Bhawan), Lucknow 226001 (UP), India
  Ph: 0522-4000032   e-mail: tiwari.lucknow@cbspd.com
- **Mumbai:** PWD Shed, Gala No. 25/26, Ramchandra Bhatt Marg, Next to JJ Hospital, Gate No. 2, Opp. Union Bank of India, Noorbaug, Mumbai 400009 Maharashtra, India
  Ph: +91-22-66661880/89   e-mail: mumbai@cbspd.com

Representatives

- **Hyderabad** 0-9885175004
- **Jharkhand** 0-9811541605
- **Nagpur** 0-9421945513
- **Patna** 0-9334159340
- **Pune** 0-9623451994
- **Uttarakhand** 0-9716462459

Printed at Neekunj Print Process, Haryana, India

to
_____
angels
Shreya and Danya

Foreword

It is privilege to write a few words about the textbook *Pharmaceutical Technology II* written by Dr Gaurav Agarwal and Dr Atul Kaushik which is a ready-reckoner for B Pharmacy students.

Efforts have been made mainly to focus on the primary aspects for students of pharmacy undergoing degree and diploma courses of various degree/diploma awarding bodies. It seems to be one of the finest efforts of its own kind to offer a wide range of fundamentals in the field of pharmaceutics ranging from the very traditional to the modern trends of sciences and present-day cutting edge technologies. Pharmaceutics, being an interdisciplinary subject, now covers a wide range of interests among the students as well as the teaching communities. We compliment the authors for simple and explicit presentation. Surely, this book is going to become popular and sought-after by pharmacy students. We wish the authors success in their present venture and urge them to continue this good and noble work by publishing more books for the benefit of pharmacy students.

Dr Agarwal and Dr Kaushik have put in tremendous amount of effort in compiling this useful work for budding pharmacy technocrats. The book admirably fills up various gaps between the pharmacy students and the basic knowledge required for specialised training of the subject. Authors have distilled their vast experience of teaching and research for pharmacy students in this compact and concise text for students and teachers of pharmacy.

Presently, Dr Agarwal is working with RP Educational Trust Institute, an institution par excellence, which has reached unflinching success in its strides for imparting quality education as it is the largest integrated, hi-tech, state-of-art facilitated private campus in Northern India located at Karnal, Haryana. The Institute is presently offering various technical and professional courses like BTech, BArch, BPharmacy, MBA and PGDBM affiliated to Kurukshetra University and Pt BD Sharma University of Health Sciences, Haryana. The main objective of the Institute is to train the students in such a manner that they can consider every problem as a challenge, transform every challenge into opportunity, seize every opportunity, and ensure growth in every aspect of life by utilizing all the technical skills imbibed.

Dr Rajiv Singal

MD MS (orthopaedics)

Vice Chairman
RP Educational Trust Group of Institutions,
Karnal (Haryana)

Dr Nidhi Singal

MD MS (gynaecology)

Preface

Pharmaceutical Technology II is expected to be one of the its kind to span a wide gamut of basic of pharmaceutics from the very traditional to what is cutting-edge today. It contains a comprehensive description and an overview of existing knowledge of pharmaceutics making it appropriate for introductory and institutional purposes.

Being an interdisciplinary subject, it now covers a wide range of interests both among the students and teaching communities. Taking this increasing interest into account, this book gives a comprehensive introduction to the subject. The book is primarily intended as text for students of pharmacy for degree and diploma courses.

The book contains numerous specimens, vivid illustrations, tables, diagrams and flow diagrams to present the ideas. The distinguishing feature is an ample question bank at the end of the book.

In spite of good care, there might be some mistakes and deficiencies. We will be grateful to the readers for giving suggestions to make further improvements. So please go through the text and do mail us your observations, comments and suggestions at *gbitsian@rediffmail.com*. Because you share that spirit, the book is dedicated to you.

Gaurav Agarwal
Atul Kaushik

Acknowledgments

It is a moment of great pleasure and immense satisfaction to express deep gratitude and gratefulness to Prof. AN Naggapa, President, ACPI, Manipal University, for inspiring me to bring out this book.

I am specially thankful to Mr RP Singal, Chairman, RP Educational Trust, for his all time support and encouragement.

My special thanks to Er. Bharat Singal, Secretary, RP Educational Trust, for inspiring me to bring out this book.

I am indebted to Dr SC Gupta, Director, RPIIT; Dr SK Srivastav, Director, RPET; Dr RK Chaudhary, Dean, RPET; Prof. Sanjay Gupta, Dean (Architecture), and Dr Anjana Srivastav, Dean (Management), for their motivation.

Special thanks to my peers Rajesh, Sandeep, Nitika, Harshwardhan, Kiran, Jasvinder, Sandeep, Jagjit Singh and Hemant Joshi for their moral support.

I wish to place on record my appreciation and thanks to Ms Arti Sharma who helped in typing work, at the same time she gained access to the pharmacy subject also.

I wish to thank my numerous students, whom I cannot possibly name individually, for their class interaction which has been the guiding spirit in selection of the subject matter and its logical arrangement.

I express my gratefulness to Mr YN Arjuna, Senior Director— Publishing, Editorial and Publicity, and special thanks to Mr SK Jain, Managing Director, CBS Publishers & Distributors, for their sincere efforts.

I am indebted to my parents for their virtues, patience, perseverance and positive thinking.

Last but not least, I express my love to my wife Shilpi for her all time inspiration and dedication. She is the major driving force in this achievement.

Gaurav Agarwal

My parents receive my deepest gratitude and love for their unflagging belief and love for me. I am indebted to them for inculcating in me the confidence and discipline to do whatever I undertake well.

I would like to acknowledge the help given by my colleagues and relatives. My father-in-law was supportive from the beginning and encouraged me to write my first book. I hope students of pharmacy courses will appreciate the end product.

All the way, critical eyes and view points were invaluable. From friends like Ravindra, Alok, Vikram, Pratit, Manoj, Amrinder, Subas, Alpa, Modak and Munish, who read rough drafts and kept me on the correct path. Colleagues like Haripriya Puthoori spent a good deal of time with me typing the text of a few chapters in the book. Mr Praveen Raheja, Mr Rakesh Kumar Bhasin and Dr V Venkateswar have always been an inspiration. Dr Gaurav Agarwal has helped me a lot in making my first bookwriting venture possible. He is smart, astute, and did not mind telling me a thing or two during the editing process.

This book is dedicated to all the students whom I have taught in IFTM, Moradabad, and ITS, Ghaziabad.

I would like to pay my gratitude to my wife Herina. Her support made the writing of the text possible. At last, I would like to thank the Almighty with a quote from GK Chesterton.

When we were children we were grateful to those
who filled our stockings at Christmas time.
Why are we not grateful to God for
filling our stockings with legs?

Atul Kaushik

Contents

Foreword   vii
Preface   xi

1. CAPSULES   1

Introduction 1
Hard gelatin capsules 2
Raw materials used 3
Angle of repose 6
Capsule filling devices 13
Liquids in hard gelatin capsules 15
Difficulties in filling capsules 16

Soft-gelatin capsules 17
Materials to be filled 20
Large-scale manufacture 23
Seamless gelatin capsules 23
Ingredients used in formulation
  of soft-gelatin capsules 24
Quality control of capsules 25

2. MICROENCAPSULATION   44

Definition 44
Core material 44
Coating material 44
Application of microencapsulation
  in pharmacy 45
Microencapsulation
  techniques 46

Chemical methods 47
Physicochemical methods 49
Mechanism of microcapsule
  formation 49
Complex coacervation—general
  outline 55

3. TABLETS   71

Advantages of the tablet 72
Disadvantages of tablet 72
Different types of tablets 73
Tablets ingested orally 73
Tablets used in oral cavity 74
Tablets administered by other
  route 75
Tablets used to prepare
  solution 76
Tablet excipients 77
Diluents 77
Classification of diluents 79
Binders 81
Disintegrant 85

Miscellaneous excipients 92
Tablet manufacturing 97
Tablet manufacturing
  methods 102
Slugging process 108
Roller compaction 109
Formulation for dry granulation 109
Direct compression 109
Manufacturing steps for direct
  compression 111
Advancement in granulations 114
Steam granulation 114
Melt granulation (thermoplastic
  granulation) 114

Moisture activated dry granulation (MADG) 114
Thermal adhesion granulation process (TAGP) 115
Foam granulation 115
Problems in tablet manufacturing 115
Tablet testing 123
General appearance 124
Size and shape 124
Organoleptic properties 125
Assay 125
Content uniformity test 125
Hardness or crushing strength 127
Tablet disintegration 127
Friability test 130
Dissolution 132
Procedure 134

4. TABLET COATING 144

Advantages of tablet coating 144
Type of tablet coating process 145
  1. Sugar coating 145
  2. Film coating 147
Materials used in film coating 148
Solvents 151
Plasticizers 151
Colourants 152
Opacifier 152
Miscellaneous coating solution component 153
  3. Enteric coating 153
  4. Specialized coating 155
Factors affecting coating 156
Conventional pan system 157
Immersion sword 158
Immersion tube 158
Accela-cota and driacoater systems 159
Fluidized bed dryer (FBD) 160
Principle of operation 160
Bottom spray coating (continuous fluid bed) 162
Tangential spray coating (rotor pellet coating) 162
Problems in tablet coating 163
Evaluation of coated tablets 168
Isolated key points 169
Coating problems and remedy 170

5. SUSTAINED AND CONTROLLED RELEASE DOSAGE FORMS 174

Definition 174
Classification 174
Physicochemical properties of drug 177
Biological properties 182
Pharmacokinetics 182
Pharmacodynamic characteristics 182
Oral controlled release systems 185
Dissolution controlled release systems 186
Matrix dissolution controlled systems 186
Coating dissolution controlled systems 187
Diffusion controlled release systems 187
Matrix diffusion controlled systems 187
Dissolution and diffusion controlled release systems 189
Ion exchange resin-drug complexes 189

6. OPHTHALMIC PRODUCTS 220

Physiology of eye 221
Ideal ophthalmic
    formulations 222
Important characteristics
    required for ophthalmic
    preparation 222
Various types of ophthalmic
    products 224
Eye drops 224
Formulation of eye drops 224
Excipients used in eye drops 225
Precaution used in handling eye
    drops 226
Eye-lotions 226
Formulation of eye-lotion 226
Eye ointments 227
Formulation of eye ointments 227
Contact lens solutions 228

Soft contact lens liquid 229
Enhancement in controlled
    drug-delivery 231
1. In situ forming gels 231
2. Oil in water emulsions 232
3. Colloidal particles 232
4. Liposomes 232
5. Nanoparticles 234
6. Micro particulates 234
7. Inserts 235
8. Implantable systems 235
9. Minidisc 236
10. Soft contact lenses 236
11. Niosomes 236
12. Pharmacosomes 236
13. Collagen shields 236
Recent advances 237

7. NASAL PRODUCTS 250

Advantages 250
Disadvantages 251
Limitations 251
Drug concentration, dose
    and dose volume 254

Formulation pH 255
Buffer capacity 255
Osmolarity 255
Formulation ingredients 256

8. OTIC (EAR) PRODUCTS 279

Anatomy of ear 279
External or outer ear 279
Middle ear (tympanic cavity) 280
Inner ear 280
Applications 284
Drawbacks 284
Microcatheter injection 284

Osmotic pump 287
Reciprocating perfusion
    system 287
Drawbacks 287
Evaluation of otic products 287
Particle size determination 287

9. PARENTERAL PRODUCTS 298

Definition 289
Classifications 299
Classification of injections on the
    basis of injection volumes 303
Preformulation studies of
    parenteral formulation 304

Components of parenteral
    formulation 306
Vehicles 306
Container types 316
Plastic 316
Glass 317

Closure 319
Rubber closure 319
Criteria for selecting closure 320
Rubber closures compendial
test series 327
Elastomeric closure/plunger test
series 327
Compendial drug product
testing 322
Plastics test series 323
Pharmaceutical container
testing 323
Container closure integrity
testing methodologies 324
Helium leak testing 324
Method of preparing parenteral
suspension and solution 329

Method 1 330
Method 2 330
Important unit operations
involved during parenteral
preparation 331
Ampoule filling 335
Features of ampoule filling
machines 335
Sealing 335
Sealing of vials and bottles 337
Lyophilization 340
Methods of sample frozen 341
Characteristics of the finished
product 346
Contamination of the
lyophilizer 346
Clean room area for sterile
products 349

10. PACKAGING OF PHARMACEUTICALS 362

Packaging types 362
Functions of packaging 363
Desirable qualities of good
containers 365
Types of containers 365
Materials used for containers 366

Glass 366
Types of glass used for pharma-
ceutical packaging 370
Paper and board 375
Package validation 376

Appendices
   Appendix 1: List of some commonly used additives   *383*
   Appendix 2: Units and conversion factors   *388*
Glossary   *391*
Index   *403*

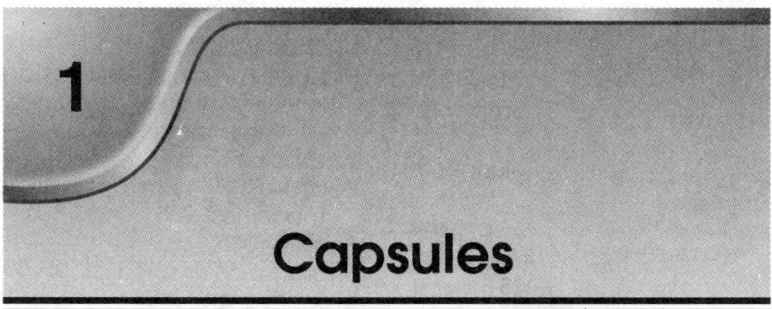

Capsules

INTRODUCTION

The word *capsule* is derived from the Latin word capsule meaning "small box". In pharmacy capsule is described as an edible package made from gelatin or other suitable material which is filled with medicines to be produced a unit dosage form mainly for oral use.

or

"The capsule may be consider a container drug delivery system that provide a tasteless and odorless dosage form without need for a secondary coating steps as may be required for tablets."

There are two types of capsules, "hard" and "soft". The hard capsule is also called "two piece" as it consists of two pieces in the form of small cylinders closed at one end, the shorter piece is called the "cap" which fits over the open end of the longer piece, called the "body". The soft gelatin capsule is also called as "one piece". Capsules are available in many sizes to provide dosing flexibility. Unpleasant drug tastes and odors can be masked by the tasteless gelatin shell. The administration of liquid and solid drugs enclosed in hard gelatin capsules is one of the most frequently utilized dosage forms.

Advantages of Capsules

    i. Capsules mask the taste and odor of unpleasant drugs and can be easily administered.

    ii. They are attractive in appearance.

    iii. They are slippery when moist and, hence, easy to swallow with water.

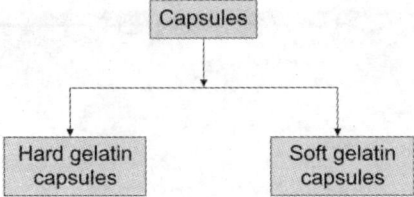

iv. As compared to tablets less excipient are required.
v. The shells are physiologically inert and get easily and quickly digested in the gastrointestinal tract.
vi. They are economical and easily available.
vii. They are easy to handle and carry.
viii. The shells can be opacified (with titanium dioxide) or colored, to give protection from light.
ix. They have better shelf life and bioavailability as compared to tablets.

Disadvantages of Capsules

i. The drugs which are hygroscopic absorb water from the capsule shell making it brittle and hence are not suitable for filling into capsules.
ii. The concentrated solutions which require previous dilution are unsuitable for capsules because if administered as such lead to irritation of stomach.

Hard Gelatin Capsules

Hard gelatin capsule shells are used to manufacture most of the commercially available medicated capsules. They are also commonly employed in clinical drugs trials to compares the effects of investigations of drugs also. They are made from a mixture of gelatin sugar and water as they are clear and colorless and essentially tasteless. They may be colored with various FD and C and ID and C dyes and may be made opaque by adding agents such as titanium dioxide.

Advantages

1. Hard gelatin capsules have better bioavailability than tablets.
2. They are easier to formulate.

3. Modern filling equipment makes possible the multiple ingredients or drug filling in the same capsule which offers the possibilities to overcome incompatibility by separating the ingredients with in the same capsule.
4. Hard gelatin capsules are uniquely suitable for the blinding clinical tests and are widely used in the preliminary drug studies.

Disadvantages

1. Filling equipment is slower than tabletting process.
2. More costly as compared to tablet formulation.
3. Not suitable for administration of extremely soluble material such as KCl, KBr. Since the sudden release of such compounds in the stomach could result in gastric irritation.
4. Not suitable for encapsulated for highly influorescent or deliquescent material. If fluorescent material may cause the capsules to soften whereas deliquescent materials may dry the capsule shell to excessive brittleness.

Raw Materials Used

The raw materials used in the manufacture of both hard and soft gelatin capsules are similar. Both contain gelatin, water, colorants as main ingredient and other pharmaceutical aids.

1. *Gelatin:* Gelatin is the major component of the capsules and is the raw material of choice because of ability of its solution to form a gel solid at a temperature just above ambient temperate conditions, which enables a homogeneous film to be formed rapidly on a mould pin. Gelatin is a translucent brittle solid substance, colorless or slightly yellow, nearly tasteless and odorless, which is created by prolonged boiling of animal skin connective tissues or bones. There are two types of gelatin:

Type A: It produced by acid hydrolysis and is manufacture mainly from pork skin.

Type B: It produced by alkaline hydrolysis is manufacture from animal bones.

Type A gelatin is derived from an acid-treated precursor and exhibits an isoelectric point in the region of pH 9, whereas type B gelatin is from an alkali-treated precursor and has its isoelectric zone in the region of pH 4.7. Capsules may be made from either type of gelatin, but mostly a mixture of both types is used considering availability and cost. Blends of bone and pork skin gelatins of relatively high strength are normally used for hard capsule production. The bone gelatin produces a tough, firm film, but tends to be hazy and brittle. The pork skin gelatin contributes plasticity and clarity to the blend there by reducing haze or cloudiness in the finished capsule. Gelatin is used because of following characteristics.

- It is non-toxic, widely used in foodstuffs and acceptable worldwide.
- It is readily soluble in biological fluids at body temperature.
- The gelatin films are homogeneous in structure, which gives them strength.
- It is good film forming material producing a strong flexible film.
- The wall thickness of a hard gelatin capsule is about 100 micrometer.
- Solution of higher concentration 40% w/v are mobile at 50°C.

The major disadvantages of gelatin for hard capsules is that it undergo cross-linking due to high moisture content, although moisture is required which is essential for its plasticizing property under guidelines of international conference on harmonization of technical requirements for registration of pharmaceuticals for human use (ICH) conditions and for accelerated storage testing.

Production of gelatin: On a commercial scale, gelatin is made from by-products of the meat and leather industry, mainly pork skins, pork and cattle bones, or split cattle hides. Contrary to popular belief, horns and hooves are not commonly used. The raw materials are prepared by different curing, acid, and alkali processes which are employed to extract the dried collagen hydrolysate. The entire process takes several weeks. The flow chart for gelatin production has been shown in Fig. 1.1.

2. *Colorants:* Color is used principally to identify a product in all stages of its manufacture and use. The colorants that can be used in capsules are of two types.

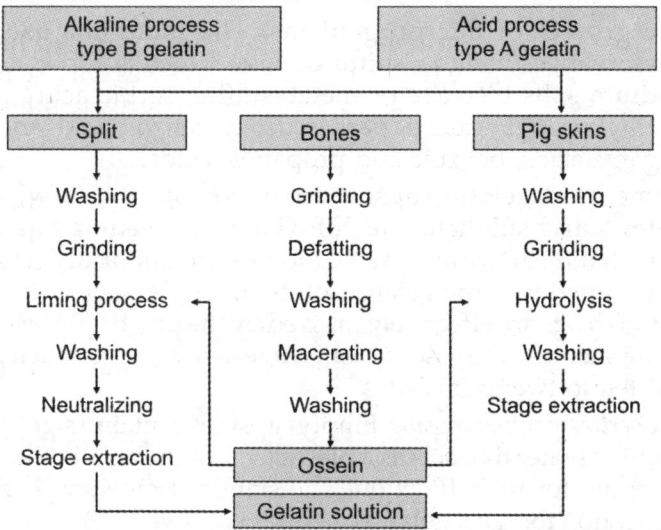

Fig. 1.1: Gelatin production process

1. Water soluble dyes
2. Insoluble dyes, the dyes used are mostly synthetic in origin and can be sub divided as:

   a. Azo dyes

   b. Non-azo dyes, most dyes used currently are the non-azo class and the three wildly used are:

   - Erythrosine (E-127)
   - Indigo (E-132)
   - Quinolin yellow (E-104)

   To make a range of colors dyes and pigments are mixed together as solutions or suspensions. The two types of pigments used are iron oxides-black, red and yellow and titanium dioxide which are white and used to make the capsule opaque. Capsules are colored by the addition of colorants to the gelatin solution during the manufacturing stage.

3. *Pharmaceutical aids:* Preservatives and surfactants are added to the gelatin solution during capsule manufacture to aid in processing. Gelatin solutions are an ideal medium for bacterial growth at temperatures below 55°C. Preservatives are added to the gelatin and colorant solutions to reduce

the growth of microorganisms. The materials used as preservatives include: sulfur dioxide which is added as the sodium salts bisulfite or metabisulfite, sorbic acid or the methyl propyl esters of para hydroxy-benzoic acid, and the organic acids, benzoic and propanoic acids.

Some hard gelatin capsules may contain 0.15% w/w of sodium lauryl sulphate which functions as wetting agent, to ensure that the lubricated metal moulds are uniformly covered when dipped into the gelatin solution. Unpleasant tastes and odors of drugs are effectively masked by the practically tasteless capsule shell which dissolves or is digested in the stomach after about ten to twenty minutes.

Properties of empty capsule: Empty capsules contain a significant amount of water that acts as a plasticizer for the gelatin film and is essential for their function. The standard moisture content specification for hard gelatin capsules is between 13% and 16% w/w. This value can vary depending upon the conditions to which they are exposed that is at low humidity's they will lose moisture and become brittle, and at high humidity's they will gain moisture and soften. The moisture content can be maintained within the correct specification by storing them in sealed containers at controlled temperature.

Capsules are readily soluble in water at 37°C. When the temperature falls below this, their rate of solubility decreases. At below about 30°C they are insoluble and simply absorb water, swell and distort. This is an important factor to take into account during disintegration and dissolution testing. Because of this most Pharmacopoeia have set a limit of 37°C ± 1°C for the media for carrying out these tests. Capsules made from have different solubility profile, being soluble at temperatures as low as 10°C.

Types of materials for filling into hard gelatin capsules:
Dry solids: Powders, pellets, granules or tablets
Semisolids: Suspensions or pastes
Liquids: Non-aqueous liquids

Angle of Repose

Angle of repose (Φ) is the maximum angle between the surface of a pile of powder and horizontal plane. The maximum angle which is formed between the surface of a pile of powder and horizontal surface of a pile of powder and horizontal surface is called the "angle of repose". An angle of repose is defined by the equation.

$$\Phi = \tan^{-1}(h/r)$$

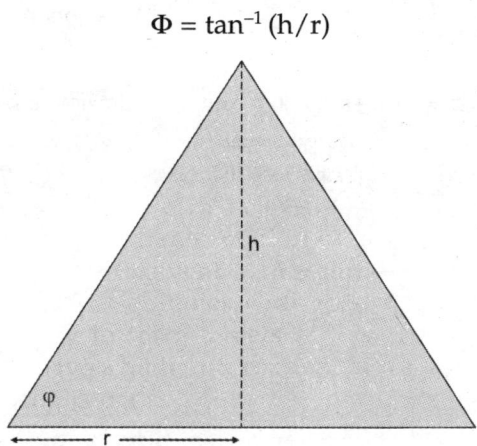

Where, h = height of heap of pile r = radius of base of pile

The angle of repose is not effected by the charge on the particles, but it depends on the shape of the particles. The angle of repose is quite high in case of the particles of a powder which are rough and have an irregular surface. Lubricants decrease the angle of repose to a certain extent but the excess quantity of the lubricant increase the angle of repose. The angle of repose depends upon the cohesive forces of the particles. The powder flows smoothly, if the angle of repose is 25°. The powder does not flow properly, if the angle of repose is more than 50°. List of angle of repose and flow properties is in Table 1.1.

Capsule Sizes

The empty capsules are available in various sizes. They are numbered according to the capacity of the capsules. The number starts from 000 and goes up to 5. The approximate capacity of a capsule with respect to its number is given in the following table and the various sizes are shown in Table 1.2 and Fig. 1.2.

Table 1.1: Angle of repose (Φ)

Angle of repose	Type of flow
<25	Excellent
25–30	Good
30–40	Passable
>40	Very poor

Table 1.2: Capsules number and its approximate capacity

Capsule number	Approximate capacity in mg	Actual volume in ml
000	950	1.37
00	650	0.95
0	450	0.68
1	300	0.50
2	250	0.37
3	200	0.30
4	150	0.21
5	100	0.13

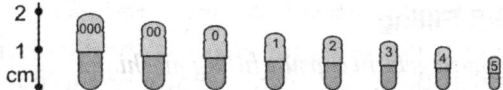

Fig. 1.2: Size of hard gelatin capsules

Excipients used in the Filling of Capsules

While filling solid medicaments in power from into the body of a hard gelatin capsules, the following additives are also included in the formulation:

1. *Diluents:* The diluent is needed in certain cases where the quantity of the medicament is too small in bulk to get it filled in the smallest available capsule size. In such cases, diluent is added to bring the medicament up to the desired bulk. The commonly used diluents are lactose, mannitol, sorbitol, starch, etc. The quantity of the diluent to be incorporated depends on the medicament and the capsule size.

2. *Absorbents:* Sometimes the medicaments are physically incompatible with each other, e.g. eutectic substance or

hygroscopic substances. In such cases, absorbents, such as oxides and carbonates of magnesium and calcium and kaolin are added to the powered drug. These inert material acts as a protective absorbent.

3. *Glidants:* To ensure a regular flow of power into the automatic capsule machine glidants are mixed with the medicaments. The various glidants used for the purpose are talc, magnesium stearate and calcium stearate.

4. *Antidusting compounds:* During the filling of capsules by an automatic filling machine, a lot of dust comes out of the machines. The dust is inhaled by the operator of the machine. It can pose a serious health hazard especially when the dust of the potent drugs is inhaled by the workers. To avoid this, some antidusting components, like edible oils, are added to the formulation.

5. *Wetting agents:* Which improve water penetration for poorly soluble drugs, e.g. sodium lauryl sulfate.

6. *Disintegrants:* Which produce disruption of the powder mass, e.g. crospovidone, sodium starch glycolate.

Capsule Shell Filling

Hand operated hard gelatin capsule filling machines: Hand operated and electrically operated machines are in practice for filling the capsules but for small and quick dispensing hand operated machines are quite economical.

A hand operated gelatin capsule filling machine consists of the following parts and is shown in Fig. 1.3.

1. A bed with 200–300 holes.
2. A capsule loading tray.
3. A powder tray.
4. A pin plate having 200 or 300 pins corresponding to the number of holes in the bed and capsule loading tray.
5. A lever.
6. A handle.
7. A plate fitted with rubber top.

All parts of the machine are made up of stainless steel. The machines are generally supplied with additional loading trays, beds, and pin plates with various diameters of holes so as to

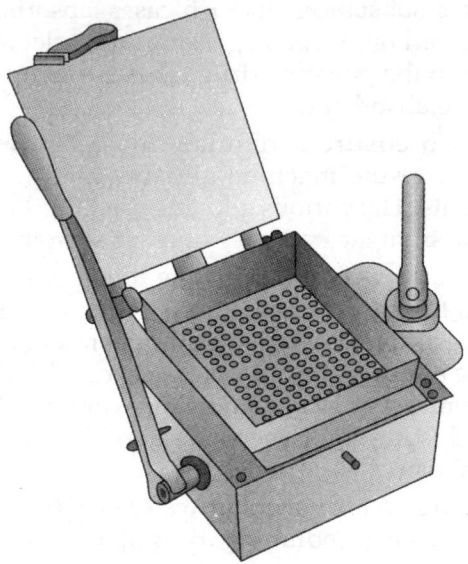

Fig. 1.3: Hand operated hard gelatin capsule filling machine

fill the desired size of the capsules. These machines are very simple to operate, can be easily dismantled and reassembled.

Working: The empty capsules are filled into the loading tray which is then placed over the bed. By opening the handle, the bodies of the capsules are locked and caps separated in the loading tray itself which is then removed by operating the liver. The weighed amount of the drug to be filled in the capsules is placed in powder tray already kept in position over the bed. The powder is spread with the help of a powder spreader so as to fill the bodies of the capsules uniformly. Collect excess of the powder on the platform of the powder tray. Lower the pin plate and move it downward so as to press the powder in the bodies. Remove the powder tray and place the caps holding tray in position. Press the caps with the help of plate with rubber top and operate the lever to unlock the cap and body of the capsules. Remove the loading tray and collect the filled capsules in a tray. With 200 hole machine about 5000 capsules can be filled per hour and with 300 hole machine 7500 capsules can be filled per hour.

On large-scale manufacturing various types of semi-automatic and automatic machines are used. They operate on the same principle as manual filling, namely the caps are removed, powder filled in the bodies, caps replaced and filled capsules are ejected out. With automatic capsule filling machines powders or granulated products can be filled into hard gelatin capsules. With accessory equipment, pellets or tablets along with powders can be filled into the capsules.

Shell Manufacture

Completely automatic machines are used for the production of hard gelatin capsules shells. The manufacturing machines having two parts:

1. On one half the capsule cap is made.
2. On the other capsule body is made.
3. The thickness of the gelatin walls must be strictly controlled.
4. The caps are slightly larger in diameter than the bodies.

The moulds commonly referred to pins are made of stainless steel and mounted on metal strips called bars. The small the capsule the higher is the output. The sequence of manufacturing process is as follows:

Dipping → Rotation → Drying → Stripping → Trimming → Joining → Sorting → Painting

Dipping

- Pairs of stainless steel pins lubricated, are dipped into the dipping solution to form caps and bodies simultaneously.
- The pins are at ambient temperature, 22°C whereas the dipping solution is at 50°C in heated jacketed heating pan.
- The dipping time to cast the film is about 12 seconds.

Rotation

- After dipping, the pins are withdrawn from dipping solution. They are elevated and rotated until they are facing upward.
- This helps distribution of the gelatin over the pins uniformly and to avoid the formation of bead at the capsule ends.
- After rotation they are given a blast of cool air to set the film

Drying

- The racks of gelatin coated pins then pass into a series of four drying ovens
- Drying is mainly done by dehumidification by passing large volumes of dry air over the pins
- Temperature elevation of few degrees are permissible to prevent film melting
- Drying also must be too rapid to prevent case hardening
- Under drying leave film sticky for subsequent operations
- Over drying must be avoided as this could cause the films to split on the pins due to shrinkage or at least make them brittle for later trimming step.

Stripping

A series of bronze jaws strip the cap and body portions of the capsules from the pins.

Trimming

- The stripped caps and bodies are delivered to collects in which they are firmly held
- As the collects rotate the knives are brought against the shells to trim them to the required length.

Joining

- The cap and body portions are aligned concentrically in channels, and the two portions are slowly pushed together
- The entire cycle takes about 45 minutes, about two-thirds of which is required for the drying step alone.

Sorting

- The moisture content of capsules as they are ejected from machine will be in the range of 15–18% w/w
- During sorting, the capsules passing on a lighted moving conveyor are observed visually by inspector
- Any defective capsules spotted are thus manually removed.

Painting

- In general, capsules are printed prior to filling as they are easy to handle

- Generally printing is done on offset rotary presses having through capabilities as high as ¾ million capsules per hour
- Available equipment can print axially along the length or radially around the circumference of capsules.

CAPSULE FILLING DEVICES

A number of different manually operated capsule filling devices are commercially available for filling up to 50 or 100 capsules at a time. The method of using these machines requires a careful determination of the capsule formulation. The powder is blended as previously discussed. Empty gelatin capsules are placed into the device and, oriented so that the cap is on top. The machine is worked to separate the base from the cap and the portion of the machine holding the caps is removed and set aside.

The capsule bases are allowed to "drop" into place so that the tops are flush with the working surface. The powder mix is spread over the working surface. A plastic spatula can be used carefully to spread the powder uniformly and evenly into the capsule bases or the machine can be "tapped" to spread the powder and drop it down into the capsule bases. A small device consisting of several "pegs" on a handle can be used to tamp the powder into the capsule bases gently and evenly. Any remaining powder then is spread evenly over and into the capsule bases and tamped. These procedures are repeated until all of the powder is in the capsules. The capsule caps are then fitted over the machine, fixed in place, and the filled capsules removed, dusted using a clean cloth, and packaged. A process flow diagram for automated capsule filling is shown in Fig. 1.4.

Filling capsules with a semisolid mass: If the material to be placed into hard gelatin capsules is a semisolid, it can be encapsulated by either forming a pipe or pouring a melt (Fig. 1.5).

1. *Pipe:* If the material is sufficiently plastic, it can be rolled into a pipe with a diameter slightly less than that of the inner diameter of the capsule in which it will be enclosed. The desired quantity of material is cut using a spatula or knife, the length determining the weight of the material enclosed. The pieces may be dusted with corn starch (check patient allergies) prior to individual insertion into the capsules. If a material is too fluid to be worked as described, it may be

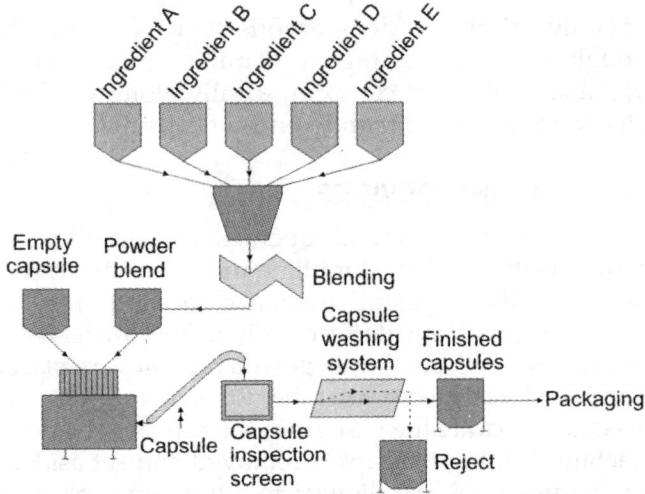

Fig. 1.4: Process flow diagram for automated capsule filling

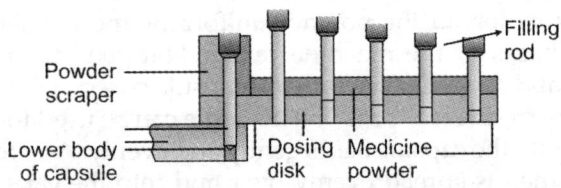

Fig. 1.5: Diagram for capsule filling

necessary to add cornstarch or some similar material to yield a more firm consistency. The quantity to be added can be determined empirically.

2. *Semisolid pour:* If the material is too firm to roll into a pipe but its melting point is satisfactory, it can be melted and poured into the capsule bases, cooled, and the caps replaced. A stand to hold the capsule bodies may be fashioned from a block of wood into which a series of holes the diameter of the capsule caps is drilled. When capsule caps are glued into these holes, capsule bases may be inserted for filling without scratching or marking by the wood. This method also can be used to enhance the bioavailability of drugs, which are poorly soluble and exhibit bioavailability problems. For this purpose, the drug is added to a melt of a material such as

polyethylene glycol (PEG). The mixture is heated and stirred until the powder is either melted or thoroughly mixed in the PEG. The melt is cooled to just above the melting point of the PEG and poured into the capsule shells as described. When this method is used, the desired quantities can be measured using a pipet, syringe, or calibrated dropper to deliver the volume to the individual capsules.

Liquids in Hard Gelatin Capsules

Liquids can be prepared in hard gelatin capsules if the gelatin is not soluble in the liquid to be encapsulated; alcoholic solutions and fixed and volatile oils work well. It may be necessary to determine the solubility of gelatin in the liquid by experimentation. The liquid can be measured accurately using a pipette (micropipette) or a calibrated dropper and dropped into the gelatin base, taking care not to touch the opening. The gelatin caps can be touched, open end down, on a moist towel to soften the gelatin at the opening of the caps or a cotton swab dipped in warm water can be rubbed around the edge of the capsule cap to soften. The cap is placed over the base containing the liquid with a slight twist and the softened edge of the cap should form a seal with the base to prevent leakage. Prior to packaging, these capsules should be placed on a clean, dry sheet of paper and observed for leakage. Another method of sealing makes use of a warm gelatin solution that is painted around the capsules and the inside of the caps prior to placing on the base.

Industrial scale filling: The machines for industrial-scale filling of hard gelatin capsules come in great variety of shapes and sizes, varying from semi-to fully automatic and ranging in output from 5000 to 15000 per hour. Automatic machines can be either continuous in motion, like a rotary tablet press, or intermittent, where the machine stops to perform a function and then indexes round to the next position to repeat the operation on a further set of capsules. The capsule filling process is illustrated in Fig. 1.6.

The dosing systems can be divided into two groups:

Dependent: Dosing systems that use the capsule body directly to measure the powder. Uniformity of fill weight can only be achieved if the capsule is filled completely, e.g. auger filling.

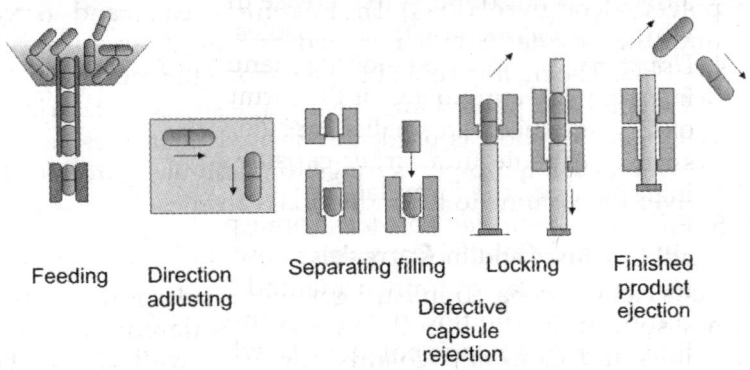

Feeding   Direction   Separating filling   Locking   Finished
         adjusting   Defective   product
                                     capsule   ejection
                                     rejection

Fig. 1.6: Diagram showing capsule filling process

Independent: Dosing systems where the powder is measured independently of the body in a special measuring device. Weight uniformity is not dependent on filling the body completely. With this system the capsules can be part filled, e.g. dosator.

Difficulties in Filling Capsules

1. *Deliquescent or hygroscopic powders:* A gelatin capsule contain water which is extracted or taken up by a hygroscopic drug and renders the capsule very brittle which leads to cracking of the capsule. The addition of an adsorbent like magnesium carbonate, heavy magnesium oxide or light magnesium oxide overcomes this difficulty provided the capsules are packed in tightly closed glass capsule vials.

2. *Eutectic mixtures:* Certain substances when mixed together tend to liquefy and form a pasty mass due to the formation of a mixture which has a lower melting point than room temperature. For filling these types of substances each troublesome ingredient is mixed with an absorbent separately then mixed together and filled in capsules. The absorbents used are magnesium oxide and kaolin. Another method in dealing with such type of difficulty is that the substances are mixed together so as to form a eutectic mixture, then an absorbent like magnesium carbonate or kaolin is added.

3. *Addition of inert powders:* When the quantity of the drug to be filled in capsules is very small and it is not possible to fill this much small amount in capsules then inert substance or

a diluent is added so as to increase the bulk of the powder, which can be filled easily in capsules.

4. *Use of two capsules:* Some of the manufacturers separate the incompatible ingredients of the formulation by placing one of the ingredients in smaller capsule, and then placing this smaller capsule in a larger capsule containing the other ingredients of the formulation.

5. *Filling of granular powder:* Some powders which lack adhesiveness and most granular powders are difficult to fill in the capsules by punch method because they are not compressible and flow out of the capsule as soon as they are lifted from the pile of powder into which they are punched. To overcome this difficulty the non-adhesive powders should be moistened with alcohol and the granular powders should be reduced to powder before filling into capsules.

Alternative Material for Hard-shell Capsules

Several materials have been examined as a substitute for the gelatin in two-piece hard capsules. Hydroxypropylmethyl cellulose (HPMC) has become a successful alternative material for two-piece capsules and is actually on the market in the world. HPMC capsules have been developed for both pharmaceutical products and dietary supplements. QUALI-V, developed by Shionogi qualicaps, is the first HPMC capsule developed for eventual use in pharmaceutical products.

SOFT-GELATIN CAPSULES

A soft gel (a soft-gelatin capsule) is a solid capsule (outer shell) surrounding a liquid or semi-solid center (inner fill). An active ingredient can be incorporated into the outer shell, the inner fill, or both. The formulation of drugs into soft-gelatin capsules has gained popularity throughout the past decade due to the many advantages of this dosage form. The bioavailability of hydrophobic drugs can be significantly increased when formulated into soft-gelatin capsules. Many problems associated with tabletting, including poor compaction and lack of content or weight uniformity, can be eliminated when a drug is incorporated into this dosage form. Improved stability of drugs that are highly susceptible to oxidation can be achieved when formulated into a soft gelatin capsule. Gelatin soft capsules are made from gelatin and water but with the addition of a polyhydric alcohol, such as glycerol or sorbitol, to make them flexible. Sorbitol is less hygroscopic than glycerol. They usually contain a preservative, such as beta-naphthol. They are available in variety of shapes and sizes as shown in Figs 1.7 a and b. They are most suitable for liquids and semisolids and are widely used, in spherical and ovoid forms for vitamin preparations such as cod-liver oil, vitamins A and D and multiple vitamins.

- Spherical-0.05–5 ml
- Ovoid-0.05–7 ml
- Cylindrical-0.15–25 ml
- Tubes-0.5–0 ml
- Pear shaped-0.3–5 ml

Soft Gel Capsules

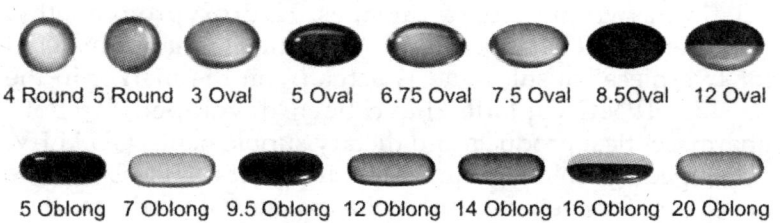

4 Round 5 Round 3 Oval 5 Oval 6.75 Oval 7.5 Oval 8.5Oval 12 Oval

5 Oblong 7 Oblong 9.5 Oblong 12 Oblong 14 Oblong 16 Oblong 20 Oblong

Fig. 1.7a: Diagram showing soft gel capsules

Soft Gel Tubes

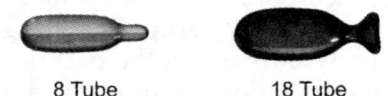

8 Tube   18 Tube

Fig. 1.7b: Diagram showing soft gel tubes

Advantages

1. Ease of use – easy to swallow, no taste, unit dose delivery, temper proof.
2. Versatile.

- Accommodates a wide variety of compounds filled as a semisolid, liquid, gel or paste.
- Wide variety of colors, shapes and sizes.
- Immediate or delayed drug delivery-can be used to improve bioavailability by delivering drug in solution or other absorption enhancing media.

Disadvantages

1. Requires special manufacturing equipment.
2. Stability concerns with highly water soluble compounds, and compounds susceptible to hydrolysis.
3. Limited choices of excipients/carriers compatible with the gelatin.

Content of a soft gel capsule is a liquid, or a combination of miscible liquids, a solution of a solid (s) in a liquid (s) or a suspension of a solid (s) in a liquid (s). Liquids are an essential part of the capsule content. Only those liquids that are both water miscible and volatile cannot be included as major constituents of the capsule content since they can migrate into the hydrophilic gelatin shell and volatilize from its surface. Water, ethyl alcohol and emulsions fall into this category.

There are a large number of liquids that do not fall into the above category and thus can function as active ingredients, solvents or vehicles for suspension type formulations. These liquids include aromatic and aliphatic hydrocarbons, high molecular weight alcohols, esters or organic acids. The mostly widely used liquids for human use are oily active ingredients such as vegetable oils (soy bean oil), mineral oil, non-ionic surface active agents (polysorbate 80) and PEG (400 and 600) either alone or in combination. There are three primary types of inner fill materials:

1. Neat substances, especially oily liquids, e.g. cod-liver oil capsules.
2. *Solution fills:* Actives dissolved in a carrier.
   - Oils such as soybean oil and miglyol 812 (neutral oil, triglycerides of medium chain fatty acids).
   - Polyethylene glycols: especially PEG 400–600.

Other solvents: Any other solvent, which does not degrade or solubilize the gelatin shell, i.e. dimethyl isosorbide, surfactants, diethylene glycol monoethyl ether.

Optional ingredients for solution fills are mentioned below:
- *Water or alcohol:* Up to 10% w/w (if needed for solubility).
- *Glycerin:* 1 to 4% w/w (to retard the migration of the glycerin out of the shell into the fill).
- *Polyvinylpyrrolidone:* Up to 10% w/w used in combination with PEG (can increase drug solubility, and also improve stability by inhibiting drug recrystallization).

3 *Suspension fills:* Active dispersed in a carrier.
- Suspensions can accommodate about 30% solids before viscosity and filling become a problem.
- Suspensions can be heated up to 35°C to decrease viscosity during the filling process.
- Suspended solids must be smaller than 80 mesh–mill or homogenize before filling to prevent needles from clogging during filling.

Materials to be Filled

As stated earlier, it is possible to fill liquids, semi-solids as well as solids into soft gelatin capsules. The liquids that are packaged are generally of the following kinds:

1. Vegetable or aromatic oils, hydrocarbons, ethers, esters, alcoholos and organic acids which are water immiscible.
2. Polyethylene glycols and non-ionic surfactants which are water miscible.
3. Water miscible and relatively non-volatile compounds such as glycerin, propylene glycol (up to 5–10% of total liquid), isopropyl glycol, etc.

The liquid combinations for encapsulation in soft-gelatin capsules must be able to flow by gravity at about 35°C or less. In general, liquids ranging in viscosity from 0.2 to 3000 CPS. at 25°C, can be encapsulated without any difficulty, except in few cases like glycerin, where due to lack of tack, the blinding of slide valves and pumps may be caused. The liquids to be filled in soft capsules generally call for no formulation and can be right away filled. Liquids which cannot be capsulated are water (more than 5%), alcohols, ketones, acids, amines, esters, etc. which can leak through the capsule shell. Liquids with pH below 2.5 or above 7.5 should also be avoided since acidic liquids cause hydrolysis of the shell and alkaline ones cause tanning affecting solubility characteristics of the shells.

Solids that are not sufficiently soluble in liquids or in combinations of liquids are capsulated as suspensions. Most organic and inorganic solids or compounds may be capsulated. Such materials must be 80 mesh or finer in particle size, owing to certain close tolerances of the capsulation equipment and for the maximum homogeneity of the suspension. Many compounds cannot be capsulated, owing to their solubility in water and thus their ability to affect the gelatin shell, unless they are minor constituents of a formula or are combined with a type of carrier (liquid or solid) that reduces their effect on the shell. Examples of such solids are strong acids (citric), strong alkalies (sodium salts of weak acids), salts of strong acids and bases (sodium chloride) and ammonium salts. Also, any substance that is unstable in the presence of moisture (e.g. aspirin) would not exhibit satisfactory chemical stability in soft gelatin capsules.

Base adsorption of solids to be suspended in soft gelatin capsules: Base adsorption is expressed as the number of grams of liquid base required to produce a capsulatable mixture when mixed with one gram of solid (s). The base adsorption of a solid is influenced by such factors such as the solids particle size and shape, its physical state (fibrous, amorphous, or crystalline), its density, its moisture content, and its lipophilic or hydrophilic nature.

In the determination of base adsorption, the solid (s) must be completely wetted by the liquid base. For glycol and nonionic type bases, the addition of a wetting agent is seldom required, but for vegetable oil bases, complete wetting of the solid (s) is not achieved without an additive. Soy lecithin, at a concentration of 2 to 3% by weight of the oil, serves excellently for this purpose, and being a natural product, is universally accepted for good drug use. Increasing the concentration above 3% appears to have no added advantage.

A practical procedure for determining base adsorption and for judging the adequate fluidity of a mixture is as follows. Weigh a define amount of the solid (40 g is convenient) into a 150 ml teared beaker. In a separate 150 ml beaker tared beaker, place about 100 g of the solid base. Add small increments of the liquid base to the solid, and using a spatula, stir the base into the solid after each addition until the solid is thoroughly wetted and uniformly coated with the base. This should produce a mixture that has a soft ointment like consistency. Continue to add liquid and stir until the mixture flows steadily from the spatula blade when held at a 45-degree angle above the mixture. The base adsorption is obtained by means of the following formula.

Weight of the base/weight of the solid = Base adsorption

The base adsorption is used to determine the "minim per gram" factor (M/g) of the solid (s). The minim per gram factor is the volume in minims that is occupied by one gram (S) of the solid plus the weight of the liquid base (BA) required making a capsulatable mixture. The minim per gram factor is calculated by dividing the weight of the base plus the gram of solid base (BA + S) by the weight of the mixture (W) per cubic centimeter or 16.23 minims (V). A better formula is.

$$(BA + S) \times V/W = M/g$$

Thus lower the base adsorption of the solid (s) and higher the density of the mixture, the smaller the capsule will be. This also indicates the importance of establishing specifications for the control of those physical properties of a solid mentioned previously that can affect its base adsorption. The final formulation of a suspension invariably requires a suspending agent to prevent the settling of the solids and to maintain homogeneity prior to, during, and after capsulation. The nature and the concentration of the suspending agent vary. In all instances the suspending agent used is melted in a suitable portion of the liquid base, and the hot melt is added slowly, with stirring, into the bulk portion of the base, which has been pre-heated to 40 degrees prior to the addition of any solids. The solids are then added, one by one, with sufficient mixing between additions to ensure complete wetting. Incompatible solids are added as far apart as possible in the mixing order to prevent interaction prior to complete wetting by the base.

Example of suspension fills include drug suspended in the following carriers:

1. *Oily mixtures:*
   a. Soybean oil with beeswax (4–10% w/w) and lecithin (2–4% w/w). The lecithin improves material flow, and

imparts some lubrication during filling. Add enough beeswax to get a good suspension, but avoid creating a non-dispersible plug.

  b. Gelified oil (e.g. gel oil SC), a ready to use system composed of soybean oil, a suspending agent, and a wetting agent.

2 Polyethylene glycol
  • PEG 800–1000 for semi-solid fills
  • PEG 10,000–100,000 for solid fills
  • Or mixtures of the above. (Heat up to 35°C to make fluid enough for filling)

3. Optional ingredients that can be added in the suspension fill
  • *Surfactant:* Sorbitan derivatives such as polysorbate 80 or lecithin.
  • For hydrophobic drugs dissolved or dispersed in an oily matrix, a surfactant of HLB 10 will increase the dispersibility of the product in aqueous fluids and also may improve bioavailability.

LARGE-SCALE MANUFACTURE

Rotary capsule machine: This machine has two, side-by-side cylinders in each of which half-moulds are cut. These cylinders, like the rollers of a mangle, rotate in contrary direction and as they are mirror images the moulds come together precisely during rotation. Two ribbons of gelatin are fed between the rollers and, just before the opposing rollers meet, jets of medicament press the gelatin ribbon into the moulds, filling each half.

The moment of pressure follows, immediately sealing the two halves together to form a capsule. These rotary machines are capable of producing between 25000 and 30000 capsules an hour with an accuracy of dosage of approximately ± 1 percent. An automated soft-gelatin encapsulation machine is shown in Fig. 1.8.

Seamless Gelatin Capsules

Another method of making soft capsules takes advantage of the phenomenon of drop formation. The essential part of the

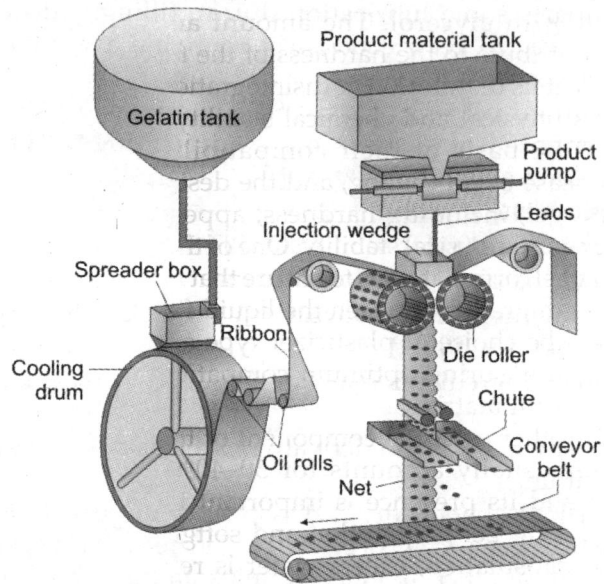

Product material tank

Gelatin tank

Product pump

Leads

Injection wedge

Spreader box

Cooling drum

Ribbon

Die roller

Chute

Conveyor belt

Oil rolls

Net

Fig. 1.8: Automatic soft gelatin encapsulation machine

apparatus consists of two concentric tubes. Through the inner tube flows the medicament and, through the surrounding outer tube, the gelatin solution. The medicament, therefore, issues from the tube surrounded by gelatin and forming a spherical drop. This is ensured by allowing the drop to form in liquid paraffin in which the gelatin is insoluble. Regular induced pulsations cause drops of the correct size to be formed, and a temperature of C ensures that the gelatin shell is rapidly congealed. The capsules are then subsequently decreased and dried.

Ingredients Used in Formulation of Soft-Gelatin Capsules

Gelatin shell formulation: Typical soft gels are made-up of gelatin, plasticizer, and materials that impart the desired appearance (colorants and/or opacifiers), and sometimes flavors.

Plasticizers: These are used to make the softgel shell elastic and pliable. They usually account for 20–30%. The most common plasticizers used in softgels is glycerol, although sorbitol and propylene glycol are used frequently often in combination with glycerol. The amount and choice of the plasticizer contribute to the hardness of the final product and may even affect its dissolution or disintegration characteristics, as well as its physical and chemical stability. Plasticizers are selected on the basis of their compatibility with the fill formulation, ease of processing, and the desired properties of the final soft gel, including hardness, appearance, handling characteristics and physical stability. One of the most important aspects of softgel formulation is to ensure that there is minimum interaction or migration between the liquid fill matrix and the softgel shell. The choice of plasticizer type and concentration is important in ensuring optimum compatibility of the shell with the liquid fill matrix.

Water: The other essential component of the softgel shell is water. Water usually accounts for 30–40% of the wet gel formulation and its presence is important to ensure proper processing during gel preparation and softgel encapsulation. Following encapsulation, excess water is removed from the softgels through controlled drying. In dry gels the equilibrium water content is typically in the range 5–8% w/w, which represents the proportion of water that is bound to the gelatin in the soft gel shell. This level of water is important for good physical stability, because in harsh storage conditions softgels will become either too soft and fuse together, or too hard and embrittled.

Colorants/opacifiers: Colorants (soluble dyes, or insoluble pigments or lakes) and opacifiers are typically used in the wet gel formulation. Colorants can be either synthetic or natural, and are used to impart the desired shell color for product identification. An opacifier, usually titanium dioxide may be added to produce an opaque shell when the fill formulation is a suspension, or to prevent photodegradation of light-sensitive fill ingredients. Titanium dioxide can either be used alone to produce a white opaque shell or in combination with pigments to produce a colored opaque shell (Table 1.3).

Quality Control of Capsules

Whether capsules are produced on a small scale or large scale all of them are required to pass not only the disintegration test, weight variation test and percentage of medicament test

Table 1.3: Difference between hard gelatin and soft gelatin capsules

Hard-gelatin capsules	Soft-gelatin capsules
1. The hard gelatin capsules shell consists of two parts a. Body b. Cap	1. The soft gelatin capsule shall becomes a single unit after sealing the two halve of the capsules.
2. They are cylindrical in shape.	2. They available in round, oval and tube like shapes.
3. The contents of a hard gelatin capsule usually consist of the medicament or mixture of medicaments in the form of powder, beads or granules.	3. The contents of soft gelatin capsules usually consist of liquids or solids dis-solved or dispersed in suitable excipients to give a paste -like consistency.
4. These are prepared from gelatin titanium dioxide, colouring agent and plasticizer.	4. These are prepared from gelatin plasticizer (glycerin or sorbitol) and a preservative.
5. Capsules are sealed after they are filled to ensure that the medicaments may not come out of the capsule due to rough handling.	5. Filling and sealing of soft gelatin capsules are done in a combined operation on machines.

but a visual inspection must be made as they roll off the capsule machine onto a conveyor belt regarding uniformity in shape, size, color and filling. As the capsules moves in front of the inspectors the visibly defective or suspected of being less than the perfect are picked out. The hard and soft-gelatin capsules should be subjected to following tests for their standardization.

- Shape and size
- Color
- Thickness of capsule shell
- Leaking test for semi-solid and liquid ingredients from soft capsules
- Disintegration tests
- Weight variation test
- Percentage of medicament test.

Quality control should be carried out during all stages of manufacturing operation which is the primary requirement of good manufacturing practices as per schedule M. In official books the following quality control tests are recommended for capsules.

1. Standard for Content of Active Ingredients

This test determines the amount of active ingredient by the method in the assay. For example, assay of indomethacin capsules.

- To a quantity of the mixed contents of 20 capsules equivalent to 50 mg of indomethacin, add 10 ml of water in a volumetric flask 100 ml.
- Stand for 10 minutes, shaking occasionally.
- Add 75 ml of methanol shake well and add sufficient methanol to produce 100 ml and filter if necessary.
- To 5 ml of the filtrate, add sufficient of a mixture of equal volumes of methanol and phosphate buffer (pH 7.2) to produce 100 ml in a volumetric flask.
- Measure the absorbance of the resulting solution at λ max = 318 nm.
- Calculate the content of indomethacin, taking 0.193 as the value of E1%.
  Limit is 90–110% of the labeled amount.

Calculations

- Weight of 20 capsules = W_1
  Weight of empty shells = W_2
  Weight of contents = $W_1 - W_2 = W_3$
- Amount of drug = 20 capsule × 25 mg each → W3
  50 mg $\qquad\qquad\qquad$ → X
- Abs. = 0.452

- Concentration = $\dfrac{\text{Abs.} \times \text{volume of last flask}}{E_1\% \times 100}$

$$= \frac{0.452}{0.193} \times \frac{100}{100} = 2.34 \, \text{mg\%}$$

- Theoretical amount of indomethacin:
  50 $\longrightarrow$ 100 ml
  X $\longrightarrow$ 5 ml
  X = 2.5 mg% because we completed the volume to 100

- % of drug = $\dfrac{\text{Concentration} \times 100}{\text{Amount of indomethacin}}$

  $= \dfrac{2.34 \times 100}{2.5} = 93.6\%$

2. Empty Hard Capsules

According to Japanese pharmacopoeia, the test called 'purity' uses five capsules which are tested individually. Each is placed in a 100 ml conical flask and shaken vigorously after adding 50 ml of water at 37°C throughout the test. The capsule passes the test if it completely dissolves within 10 minutes giving odorless, neutral or slightly acidic pH.

3. Uniformity of Weight

This test applies to all types of capsules and it is to be done on 20 capsules:

- Weigh an intact capsule.
- Open the capsule without losing any part of the shell and remove the contents as completely as possible.
- Weigh the shell.
- The weight of the contents is the difference between the weighing.
- Repeat the procedure with a further 19 capsules selected at random.
- Determine the average weight.

Limit is not more than two of the individual weights deviate from the average weight by more than the percentage deviation given below, and none deviates by more than twice that percentage.

Average weight of capsule content	Percentage deviation
Less than 300 mg	10
300 mg or more	7.5

Record results

Capsule number	Weight of intact capsules (A)	Weight of empty shell (B)	Weight of contents = A − B
1			
2			
–			
–			
-up to 20			
Total weight			X

Average weight = X/20

Upper limit = average weight + (Average weight × error)

Lower limit = average weight − (Average weight × error.

4. Content Uniformity

Hard capsules containing below or less than 25 mg of the drug contents should meet content uniformity requirements. Assay 10 capsules individually and calculate the acceptance value.

The requirement is met if the acceptance value of 10 capsules is less than or equal to 15%. If acceptance value is greater than 15% or is about 25% then, test the next 20 units and calculate the acceptance value. The 30 capsules if less than or equal to 15% and no individual unit is 1−25×0.01 nor more than 1 + 25×0.01.

Calculation of Acceptance Value

(Reference value-mean of individual contents) + acceptability constant × sample standard deviation.

5. Disintegration

Disintegration is the state in which no residue except fragments of capsule shell, remains on the screen of the test apparatus or adheres to the lower surface of the disc. The disintegration test determines whether tablets or capsules disintegrate within a prescribed time when placed in a liquid medium under the prescribed experimental conditions.

The disintegration of capsules is different from those of tablets because the determination of end point is difficult owing to the adhesive nature of shell. The shell pieces after disintegration may agglomerate forming large mass of gelatin taking more time to dissolve and may adhere to the mesh thus, blocking the holes.

According to USP, place one dosage unit in each of the tubes of the basket with water or any other specified medium (depends on individual monograph) maintained at 37 + 2°C. Attach a removable wire cloth with a plain square weave of 1.8–2.2 mm of mesh aperture and a wire diameter of 0.60–0.655 mm to the surface of upper rack of the basket assembly. Observe the capsules for a time limit (specified in individual monograph), at the end of prescribed time, all of the capsules must have been disintegrated excluding the fragments from the capsule shell. If 1 or 2 capsules fail, the test should be repeated on additional of 12 capsules. Then, not fewer than 16 of the total 18 capsules tested should disintegrate completely.

According to the B.P. (for both hard and soft capsules):

- Introduce one capsule into each tube and suspend the apparatus in a beaker containing 600 ml water at 37°C.
- If hard capsules float on the surface of the water, the discs may be added.
- Operate the apparatus for 30 minutes; remove the assembly from the liquid.
- The capsules pass the test if:
  - No residue remains on the screen of the apparatus
  - If a residue remains, it consists of fragments of shell
  - Is a soft mass with no palpable core
  - If the disc is used, any residue remaining on its lower surface should only consist of fragments of shell.

6. Dissolution

Place each of the capsules in the apparatus 1, excluding air bubbles from the surface of the capsule. Operate immediately at specified rate within specified dissolution medium at 37 + 0.5°C. Aliquots should be withdrawn at specified time points mentioned in individual monograph. The requirements are met if the quantity of active ingredients dissolved conforms the following:

1. *At stage 1 (S_1):* When 6 capsules are tested, amount of each of the dissolved content should not be less than +/ − 5% of the mentioned in monograph.

2. *At stage 2 (S_2):* When 6 capsules are tested, the average of 12 (both from step 1 and 2) should be equal to or greater than 15% and no capsule should be than 15%.

3. *At stage 3 (S_3):* When 12 capsules are tested, the average of 24 capsules (all 1, 2 and 3 steps) should be equal to or greater than the amount mentioned in the monograph, not more than two units are less than 15% and no units less than 25%.

Note: 15%, 25% represent Q_1 and Q_2 unless and otherwise mentioned in the monograph.

"Quality is not the step that can be incorporated at last, it is mandatory and should be inbuilt into the products" to make this happen, apart from all these mandatory tests certain other tests can be performed-like.

7. Raw Materials

The gelatin of the capsule shells should be assayed for various physical properties like bloom strength, viscosity and its loss (by atomic force microscopy). Chemical tests like purity, microbial properties, and limits for heavy metals like arsenic, ash content should be determined. The colorants should also be checked for purity, limits for heavy metals, color properties, dye content, subsidiary dye content and color value.

8. Machine Output

The manufacturing machine's output should be monitored continuously via the dimensional correctness during each lot production. The color of the capsules should be checked against a standard strip; in case of any changes the gelatin solution should be adjusted by adding standardized dye solutions which can be ensured via thin layer chromatography.

9. Sorting of Defects

After electronic or manual inspection, they are sampled by quality control inspectors. The results should meet the inspection plan, if not the capsules should be resorted or rejected depending upon frequency of faults.

10. Printing Inspection

Quality inspectors sample the lot and are inspected for quality of print. The results will again be compared with the inspection plan and in case if it does not match then, either capsules should be resorted or rejected depending upon number of faults present.

11. Final Inspection

After the capsules are placed in final containers, samples are checked for various parameters like dimensions, physical defects and color. These samples are also subjected to various microbial tests also.

Capsule stability: Unprotected soft capsules (i.e. capsules that can breathe) rapidly reach equilibrium with the atmospheric conditions under which they are stored. General statements relative to the effects of temperature and humidity on soft-gelatin capsules must be confined to a control capsule that contains mineral oil, with a gelatin shell having a dry glycerin to dry gelatin ratio of about 0.5 to 1 and a water to dry gelatin ratio of 1 to 1, and that is dried to equilibrium with 20 to 30% RH at 21 to 24°C, the physical stability of soft-gelatin capsules is associated primarily with the pick-up or loss of water by the capsule shell. If these are prevented by proper packaging, the above control capsule should have satisfactory physical stability at temperature ranging from just above freezing to as high as 60°C, for the unprotected control capsule, low humidity's (less than 20% RH), low temperature (less than 2°C) and high temperatures (greater than 38°C) or combinations of these conditions have only transient effects. The capsule returns to normal when returned to optimum storage conditions. The total moisture content of the capsule shell, at equilibrium with any given relative humidity within a reasonable temperature range, should closely approximate the sum of the moisture content of the glycerin and the gelatin when held separately at the stated conditions. The effect of temperature and humidity on capsule shell has been illustrated in Table 1.4.

Capsules containing water-soluble or miscible liquid bases may be affected to a greater extent than oil-based capsules, owing to the residual moisture in the capsule content and to the

Table 1.4: Effect of temperature and humidity on capsule shell

Temperature	Humidity	Effect on capsule shell
21–24°C	60%	Capsules become softer, tackier and bloated More rapid and pronounced effects — unprotected capsules
Greater than 24°C	Greater than 45%	Melt and fuse together

dynamic relationship existing between capsule shell and capsule fill during the drying process. The capsule manufacturers routinely conduct accelerated physical stability tests on all new capsule products as an integral part of the product development program. The following tests have proved adequate for determining the effect of the capsule shell content on the gelatin shell. The tests are strictly relevant to the integrity of the gelatin shell and should not be confused as stability tests for the active ingredients in the capsule content. The results of such tests are used as a guide for the reformulation of the capsule content or the capsule shell, or for the selection of the proper retail package. The test conditions for such accelerated physical stability tests are shown in Table 1.5.

The capsules at these stations are observed periodically for 2 weeks. Both gross and subtle effects of the storage conditions on the capsule shell are noted and recorded. The control capsule should not be affected except at the 80% RH station, where the capsule would react as described under the effects of high humidity.

Packaging and Storage of Capsules

Capsules should be packed in a well-closed glass or plastic containers and stored in a cool place. These type of containers have advantage over cardboard boxes that they are more convenient to handle and transport and protect the capsules from moisture and dust. To prevent the capsules from rattling a tuft of cotton is placed over and under the capsules in the vials. In vials containing very hygroscopic capsules a packet-containing desiccant like silica gel or anhydrous calcium chloride may be placed to prevent the absorption of excessive

Table 1.5: Test conditions for accelerated physical stability tests for capsule dosage forms

Test conditions	Observation
80% RH at room temperature in an open container. 40°C in an open container	Capsules are observed periodically for 2 weeks, both gross and subtle effects of the storage conditions are noted and recorded.
40°C in a closed container (glass bottle with tight screw-cap).	The control capsule should not be affected except at the 80% RH condition

moisture by the capsules. Generally capsules have a longer shelf in unopened glass bottles than in strip-packs but this is reversed, once a bottle has been opened. Nowadays capsules are strip packaged which provide sanitary handling of medicines, ease in counting and identification. Empty gelatin capsules should be stored at room temperature at constant humidity. High humidity may cause softening of the capsules and low humidity may cause drying and cracking of the capsules. Storage of capsules in glass containers will provide protection not only from extreme humidity but also from dust. Storage of filled capsules is dependent on the characteristics of the drugs they contain. Semisolid filled hard gelatin capsules should be stored away from excessive heat, which may cause a softening or melting of the contents. The capsules are finally packed for shipment in moisture proof liners preferably heat sealed aluminum foil bags in cardboard cartons.

Capsule Administration

Capsules of the size number 5 to number 0 generally are not too difficult to swallow. Many patients may have difficulty swallowing the number 00 and number 000 capsules. If this occurs, the patient may be advised to place the capsule on the back of the tongue before drinking a liquid, or to place the capsule in warm water for a few seconds prior to taking to make it slide over mucous membranes easily. The pharmacist may suggest an alternative dosage form, e.g. smaller capsules or a liquid or rectal preparation.

Special Types of Hard Gelatin and Soft Gelatin Capsules

Altered release: The rate of release of capsule contents can be varied according to the nature of the drug and the capsule excipients. If the drug is water-soluble and a fast release is desired, the excipients should be hydrophilic and neutral. If a slow release of water-soluble drug is desired, hydrophobic excipients will reduce the rate of drug dissolution. If the drug is insoluble in water, hydrophilic excipients will provide a faster release; hydrophobic and neutral excipients will slow its release. A very rapid release of the capsule contents can be obtained by piercing holes in the capsule to allow faster penetration by fluids in the gastrointestinal tract, or by adding a small quantity of sodium bicarbonate and citric acid to assist in opening the capsule by the evolution of carbon dioxide. About 0.1 to 1% of sodium lauryl sulfate may be added to enhance the penetration of water into the capsule and speed dissolution. If slower release of the active drug is desired, it can be mixed with various excipients, such as cellulose polymers (methyl cellulose) or sodium alginate. In general, the rate of release is delayed as the proportion of polymer or alginate is increased relative to water soluble ingredients, such as lactose. It should be mentioned that it is difficult to predict the exact release profile for a drug and to obtain consistent results from batch to batch. Further, reliable, consistent blood levels and duration of action can only be proved with controlled bioequivalence studies. In addition, many medications exhibit narrow therapeutic indices as the toxic and therapeutic doses are very close. Therefore, extemporaneous attempts to alter release rates to this extent should be avoided.

Coating capsules: Coatings have been applied extemporaneously to enhance appearance and conceal taste, as well as to prevent release of the medication in the stomach (enteric coated products). Most coating of capsules requires considerable formulation skill and quality control equipment found in manufacturing facilities. Capsules can be coated to delay the release of the active drug until it reaches a selected portion of the gastrointestinal tract. Materials found suitable include stearic acid, shellac, casein, cellulose acetate phthalate and natural and synthetic waxes; the basis of their use is their acid insolubility but alkaline solubility. Many of the newer coating materials are time:erosion-dependent rather than acid: base-dependent, i.e. they erode over time on exposure to gastrointestinal contents rather than over a pH gradient. There are, in addition, a number of newer materials with predictable pH solubility profiles.

Enteric-coated capsules: Enteric-coated capsules resist disintegration in the stomach but break up in the intestine. They have largely been superseded by enteric-coated tablets. Types of coating used commercially include cellulose acetate phthalate and mixtures of waxes and fatty acids and/or their esters. Enteric coating may be given to following categories of drugs.

- For substances that irritate the gastric mucosa or are destroyed by the gastric juice, and for medicaments, such as amoebicides and anthelmintics that are intended to act in the intestine.
- Which interfere with digestion, e.g. tannins, silver nitrate and other salts of heavy metals.
- Which are required to produce delayed action of the drug.

    In general, the application of a coating requires skill and additional equipment. A general coating can be applied but should probably only be used in medications that would not be of a critical nature. In many cases, experience must be developed for specific formulations depending upon the requests of the physicians and the needs of the individual patients. Several coating methods may be used and are described as follows:

1. *Beaker-flask coating:* Place a very small quantity of the coating material in the flask and gently heat until it has melted. Add a few capsules, remove from the heat and rotate the flask to start application of the coating. Periodically add a few more drops of melted coating material with continued rotation. The addition of very small quantities is all that is required to keep the capsules from sticking together and clumping.

2. *Dipping:* Heat the coating material in a beaker at the lowest feasible temperature. Individual capsules can be dipped using tweezers, allowing the coating to cool and repeating the process until a sufficient layer has been developed.

3. *Spraying:* An alcoholic or ethereal solution of the coating material is prepared and placed in a small sprayer

(a model airplane paint sprayer works well). The capsules are placed on a screen in a well-ventilated area. The solution of coating material is applied in very thin coats with sufficient time allowed for drying between coats (a hair dryer may be used cautiously for this step). The process is repeated until a sufficient layer has been developed.

Sustained release capsules: The traditional method of taking a dose three or four times a day leads to periods of excess and deficiency in blood concentration of the medicament. One way of correcting this and, at the same time, reducing the number of doses per day, is to administer a capsule containing numerous coated pellets that release the drug successively over a long period. The finely powdered drug is first converted into pellets, usually by attaching it to sugar granules with an adhesive. The pellets are then treated with protective coatings that delay release of the drug, each batch receiving a different thickness. The batches are mixed thoroughly and suitable doses are filled into capsules. For example, a mixture might contain 30 percent of uncoated pellets, for immediate release of drug, 30 percent each of coated pellets that release at 4 hours and 8 hours, and 10 percent of neutral pellets, used solely to fill the capsule. Each batch may be colored differently to simplify identification and facilitate control of mixing.

Liquid Filled Hard Gelatin Capsules

It is generally accepted that many of today's NCEs (new chemical entities) are poorly water soluble and the classical methods, such as reduction in particle size are no longer adequate to achieve satisfactory drug adsorption from a solid oral dosage form. One of the most promising strategies to deliver these insoluble compounds is using dissolved systems like using lipids, liquids or semi-solids to formulate new products. Two pieces hard shell capsules are one of the most logical approaches when choosing the best dosage form to deliver these new liquid formulations. The new technology of packaging liquids in hard gelatin capsules is considered a major breakthrough. It can make a significant contribution to the development of efficacious pharmaceutical products by providing the flexibility to rapidly develop and test in-house formulations when only small quantities of drug substance is available. The process can be scaled-up and also kept in-house similar to the operations of tabletting or powder/pellet filling of hard gelatin capsules.

Rectal Capsules

Soft gelatin capsules may be used as substitutes for rectal and vaginal suppositories. Various shapes and sizes are used for this purpose. They are generally wider at one end which is inserted first; the movement of the sphincter muscles forces the capsules forward into the rectum. Liquids or solids can be filled into rectal capsules but the base in which the medicaments have been incorporated must be non-toxic, non-irritant and compatible with the capsule shell.

Capsules for Packing of Ophthalmic Ointments

It is very important that the ophthalmic ointments should be sterile and free from irritant effect. Therefore, they must be packed in such a manner that the product remains sterile until whole of it is used up. The best method to keep the preparation free from contamination during use is to pack it in single dose containers. Nowadays soft-gelatin capsules are very commonly used for filling ophthalmic ointments. These capsules are meant for single application to the eye. Just before application, the capsule is punctured with a sterile needle, the contents instilled into the eye and the shell discarded.

Recent Updates in Capsule Technology

A. New Products by Capsugel

1. Capsugel has introduced oceancaps capsules, these capsules made from all natural fish gelatin derived from farm-raised fish, they have the same characteristics as traditional gelatin capsules, including appearance, machinability, mechanical properties, hygroscopic and oxygen properties, chemical stability, and versatility. Plus, they are odorless and tasteless.
2. Licaps new 000 size capsules are ideal for maximizing liquid dosage with a fill capacity of 1000 mg to 1400 mg depending on the density of the liquid fill material. This two-piece capsules has been specially designed to be sealed for secure containment of liquids and semi-solids without banding. Available in both gelatin and HPMC (hydroxypropyl methyl

cellulose) capsules they are available in a variety of colors to meet your specific needs.

B. New Product by NATCO Pharma

1. Hyderabad-based NATCO pharma limited has launched Lukatret—a medicine used in the treatment of a rare form of leukemia. Lukatret (tretinoin—all trans retinoic acid) available in the form of 10 mg capsules (in a pack of 100 capsules) is used in the treatment of acute promyelocytic leukemia (APL). Lukatret is a treatment option for remission induction in newly diagnosed, relapsed and/or refractory, chemotherapy non-responsive patients and for patients where anthracycline based chemotherapy is contraindicated. Use of lukatret results in differentiation and clinical remission.

C. New Products by Banner Pharmacaps Inc

Banner pharmcaps has developed an enteric softgel called entericare, with enteric properties built into the shell matrix of the capsules for delivering very potent (small quantities) as well as drugs that require larger quantities and provide sustained delivery for more than an 8 to 12 hour period.

D. New Product by Shionogi Qualicaps

QUALI-V, developed by shionogi qualicaps, is the first HPMC capsule developed for eventual use in pharmaceutical products.

REVISION QUESTIONS

Answer the following questions in short

1. Define the term "Capsule".
2. Name the different ingredients used in the preparation of head gelatin capsules.
3. What are the various excipients used in the filling of head gelatin capsules?
4. What are the various ingredients used in the preparation of soft-gelatin capsules?
5. What is the approximate capacity in mg of a capsule having number 000, 00, 0, 1, 2, 3, 4, 5?

6. What is the output of a hand-operated capsule filling machine, having 200 holes and 300 holes?
7. What is the output of a rotary machine?
8. What percentage deviation in weight is allowed in the pharmacopoeia of a capsule weighting 358 mg?
9. Name the various types of glidants used along with medicaments in filling the hard gelatin capsules.
10. Name the various tests which can be carried out for the purpose of maintaining the quality control of capsules.
11. What are the materials commonly used in the enteric coating of capsules?
12. Name the various diluents which are mixed with the medicament before filling it into capsules.
13. Write the advantages and disadvantages of a capsule.
14. Described in brief a hard gelatin capsule.
15. Explain the term soft gelatin capsule.
16. How will you differentiate between a hard gelatin capsule and soft gelatin capsule?
17. Explain the packaging and storage of capsules.

Long Answer Type Questions

18. What are hard gelatin capsules? Described the construction and working of a capsule filling machine (hand operated)?
19. Write in brief about a soft gelatin capsule. Explain the construction and working of a rotary machine with the help of neat diagram?
20. What are the various tests recommended by the I.P. for evaluation of capsules?
21. Describe the various types of excipients used in filling of hand gelatin capsules?
22. Write short notes on the following:
    a. Hard gelatin capsule
    b. Soft gelatin capsule
    c. Enteric coated capsule
    d. Sustained release capsule
    e. Rectal capsule
23. What are the various sizes of hard gelatin capsules? Explain it with the help of suitable diagram.
24. Compare and contrast hard gelatin capsule and soft gelatin capsules?

Objective Type Questions

25. Micro-capsules provide the _____ form.
26. The hygroscopic/eutectic substance are filled into capsules by mixing _____ as absorbents.
27. The lubricants _____ the angle of repose but excess quantities of lubricants _____ the angle of repose.
28. In general the disintegration time of hard gelatin capsules is _____ minutes.
29. The glidants such as _____ are used to ensure a _____ of power into the automatic capsule machine.
30. Match the following.

Column I	Column II
a. Glidant	i. Required when quantity of medicament is small
b. Protective coating on drug particles	ii. Used in enteric-coated capsule
c. Soft capsule	iii. Used to fill medicament in the form of powder, beads or granules
d. Diluent	iv. Required to ensure a regular flow of powder into an automatic capsule machine
e. Cellacephate	v. Used in a sustained release capsule
f. Hard capsule	vi. Needed to fill liquid or paste

31. The word capsule is derived from the Latin word capsule meaning ……….
32. The hard capsule is also called "two-piece" as it consists of two-pieces, the shorter piece is called the …….. which fits over the open end of the longer piece, called the ……..
33. Which of the following is not true for hard gelatin capsules.
    i. Capsules mask the taste and odor of unpleasant drugs.
    ii. They are slippery when moist and, hence, easy to swallow with water.
    iii. They are suitable for hygroscopic drugs.

iv. The shells can be opacified (with titanium dioxide) or colored, to give protection from light.

34. The major component of the capsules is ....

35. Type A gelatin capsule is produced by .... and is manufacture mainly from pork skin, while type B is produced by .... and is manufacture from animal bones.

36. Match the following:

S. no.	Ingredient	Example
1.	Diluents	a Crospovidone
2.	Glidants	b lactose
3.	Wetting agents	c talc
4.	Disintegrants	d edible oils
5.	Antidusting compounds:	e SLS

37. Which of the following is not true for soft gelatin capsules.
   i. Easy to manufacture.
   ii. Accommodates a wide variety of compounds filled as a semisolid, liquid, gel or paste.
   iii. Available in wide variety of colors, shapes and sizes.
   iv. Immediate or delayed drug delivery—can be used to improve bioavailability by delivering drug in solution or other absorption enhancing media.

38. .... is expressed as the number of grams of liquid base required to produce a capsulatable mixture when mixed with one gram of solid (s).

ANSWERS

25. Sustained released dosage form,
26. Oxides and carbonates of magnesium and calcium and kaolin,
27. Decrease, increase,
28. 30
29. Talc, magnesium, stearate and calcium stearate, regular flow,
30. A (i), B (V), C (vi), D (i), E (ii), F (iii),
31. Small box,
32. Cap, body,
33. 3,

34. Gelatin,
35. Acid hydrolysis, acid hydrolysis,
36. 1-b, 2-c, 3-e, 4-a, 5-d,
37. 1,
38. Base absorption.

2

Microencapsulation

DEFINITION

As name depicts microencapsulation is a process by which solids, liquids or even gases may be enclosed or encapsulated using thin coatings of wall material in to microscopic particle. In simple terms, we can say that microencapsulation is the process of preparing microscopic particle or microcapsule having two components one is core, which can be solids, liquid or even gas and another is coat. As microcapsule has two components (i.e. core and coat) so, properties of microcapsule governed by nature of the core and coating materials.

Core Material

In general core material, defined as the specific material to be coated, is either liquid or solid in nature. The composition of the core material can be varied as the liquid core can include dispersed and/or dissolved material. The solid core can be mixture of active constituents, stabilizers, diluents, excipients and release-rate retardants or accelerators. The ability to vary the core materials composition provides definite flexibility and often allows design and development of the desired micro-capsules properties.

Coating Material

The selection of appropriate coating material decides the physical and chemical properties of the resultant micro-capsules/microspheres. While selecting a polymer the product requirements, i.e. stabilization, reduced volatility, release characteristics, environmental conditions, etc. should be taken into consideration. The polymer should be capable of forming a film that is cohesive with the core material. It should be chemically compatible, non-reactive with the core material and provide the desired coating properties such as strength, flexibility, impermeability, optical properties and stability. Generally hydrophilic polymers, hydrophobic polymers (or) a combination of both are used for the microencapsulation process. A number of coating materials have been used successfully; examples of these include gelatin, polyvinyl alcohol, ethyl cellulose, cellulose acetate phthalate and styrene maleic anhydride. The film thickness can be varied considerably depending on the surface area of the material to be coated and other physical characteristics of the system.

The microcapsules may consist of a single particle or clusters of particles. After isolation from the liquid manufacturing vehicle and drying, the material appears as a free flowing powder. The powder is suitable for formulation as compressed tablets, hard gelatin capsules, suspensions, and other dosage forms.

Application of Microencapsulation in Pharmacy

The technique of microencapsulation has gained popularity primarily because of its potential applicability in a wide variety of situations. In the pharmaceutical industry, micro- encapsulation is used for:

1. Sustained or prolonged release of drugs, e.g. aspirin.
2. Taste-masking of bitter drugs, e.g. acetyl-p-aminophenol and masking of unpleasant odors.
3. Elimination of incompatabilities, e.g. eutectic substances stabilization of drugs sensitive to oxygen, light, moisture, e.g. vitamins A and K.
4. Preparation of free-flowing powders.
5. Prevention of vaporization of volatile drugs, e.g. carbon tetra chlorides and a number of other substances have been microencapsulated to reduce their odor and volatility.
6. Modifying the physical properties of chemical entities, e.g. oils may be encapsulated to produce free-flowing powders.
7. Facilitating the dispersion of one substance in another, e.g. to stabilize emulsions.

8. Altering the rate of solubility of chemical reactants, e.g. to slow down the rate of a chemical reaction.
9. Reducing the toxicity, e.g. the handling of fumigants, insecticides, herbicides, and pesticides.
10. Many drugs have been microencapsulated to reduce gastric and other GI tract irritations, e.g. sustained release aspirin preparations have been reported to cause significantly less GI bleeding than conventional preparations.
11. Hygroscopic properties of core materials may be reduced by microencapsulation, e.g. sodium chloride.
12. Microencapsulation has been employed to provide protection to the core materials against atmospheric effects, e.g. vitamin A palmitate.

Table 2.1: Examples of some microencapsulated drugs

Drug/care material	Characteristic	Purpose of encapsulation	Final product form
Aetaminophen	Slightly water soluble solid	Taste masking	Tablet
Aspirin	Slightly water soluble solid	Taste masking, sustained release, reduced gastric irritation.	Tablet in capsule
Isosorbide dinitrate	Water soluble solid	Sustained release	Capsules
Menthol	Volatile solution	Reduction of volatility, sustained release	Lotion
Progesterone	Slightly water soluble solid	Sustained release	Varied
Potassium	Highly water soluble solid	Reduced gastric irritation	Capsule
Vitamin A palmitate	Nonvolatile liquid	Stabilization to oxidation	Dry powder

Microencapsulation Techniques

There are various techniques are available for the encapsulation of core materials. Broadly the methods are divided into three types.

1. Chemical methods

2. Physico-chemical methods
3. Physico-mechanical methods.

Table 2.2: Different techniques used for microencapsulation

Chemical processes	Physico-chemical processes	Physico-mechanical processes
Interfacial polymerization	Coacervation and phase separation	Spray drying and congealing
In situ polymerization	Sol-gel encapsulation	Fluid bed coating
Poly condensation	Supercritical CO_2 assisted microencapsulation	Pan coating solvent evaporation

The above mentioned techniques are widely used for microencapsulation of several pharmaceuticals. Among these techniques fluidized bed or air suspension method, co-acervation and phase separation, spray drying and spray congealing, pan coating, solvent evaporation methods are widely used techniques so we will discuss these techniques in details. Depending on the physical nature of the core substance to be encapsulated the technique used will be varied Table 2.3.

Chemical Methods

1. Interfacial Polymerization (IFP)

In this technique the capsule shell will be formed at or on the surface of the droplet or particle by polymerization of the reactive monomers. The substances used are multifunctional monomers. Generally used monomers include multifunctional isocyanates and multifunctional acid chlorides. These will be used either individually or in combination. The multifunctional monomer dissolved in liquid core material and it will be dispersed in aqueous phase containing dispersing agent. A coreactant multifunctional amine will be added to the mixture. This results in rapid polymerization at interface and generation of capsule shell takes place. A polyurea shell will be formed when isocyanate reacts with amine, polynylon or polyamide shell will be formed when acid chloride reacts with amine.

Table 2.3: Microencapsulation processes and their applicabilities

S. no.	Method	Applicable material	Particle size	Production scale	Process reproducibility and consistency	Time required	Cost	Operation skill
1.	Air suspension	Solids	35–5000	Pilot scale	Moderate	High	High	High
2.	Coacervation and phase separation	Solids and liquids	2–5000	Lab scale	Good	Less	Less	Less
3.	Multi-orifice centrifugal	Solids and Liquids	1–5000	Pilot scale	Moderate	High	High	High
4.	Pan coating	Solids	600–5000	Pilot scale	Moderate	High	High	High
5.	Solvent evaporation	Solids and liquids	5–5000	Lab scale	Good	Less	Less	High
6.	Spray drying and spray congealing	Solids and liquids	600	Pilot scale	Moderate	High	High	High

Note: The 5000 μm size is not a particle size limitation. The Methods are also applicable for macrocoating Chemical methods

When isocyanate reacts with hydroxyl containing monomer produces polyurethane shell, e.g. diammonium hydrogen phosphate (DAHP) encapsulated by polyurethane-urea membrane using an interfacial polymerization method.

2. In Situ Polymerization

Like interfacial polymerization (IFP) the capsule shell formation occurs because of polymerization monomers added to the encapsulation reactor. In this process no reactive agents are added to the core material, polymerization occurs exclusively in the continuous phase and on the continuous phase side of the interface formed by the dispersed core material and continuous phase. Initially a low molecular weight prepolymer will be formed, as time goes on the prepolymer grows in size, it deposits on the surface of the dispersed core material there by generating solid capsule shell, e.g. encapsulation of various water immiscible liquids with shells formed by the reaction at acidic pH of urea with formaldehyde in aqueous media.

Physico-chemical Methods

1. Coacervation and Phase Separation

The term originated from the Latin (acervus), in Latin acervus means heap, coacervation then means literally "heaping together." This was the first reported process to be adapted for the industrial production of microcapsules. Coacervation is a colloidal phenomenon. Currently, two methods for coacervation are available.

1. Simple.
2. Complex processes.

The mechanism of microcapsule formation for both processes is identical, except for the way in which the phase separation is carried out. In simple coacervation a desolvation agent is added for phase separation, whereas complex coacervation involves complexation between two oppositely charged polymers (Table 2.4).

Mechanism of Microcapsule Formation

Three basic steps in coacervation:

i. Formation of three immiscible phases.

Table 2.4: Difference between simple coacervation and complex coacervation

S. no.	Simple coacervation	Complex coacervation
1.	Simple coacervation is concerned with the non-ionized groups in the macromolecule. It can be brought about by a reduction in the solubility of the macromolecule and the associations deriving from it.	Complex coacervation is concerned with the charges and consequently with the formation of salt bonds associated with the macromolecules.
2.	Generally, simple coacervation usually deals with systems containing only one colloidal solute.	Complex coacervation almost always deals with systems containing more than one colloid.

ii. Deposition of the coating

iii. Rigidization of the coating.

First step-formation of three immiscible phases: Liquid manufacturing vehicle, core material, coating material. The core material is dispersed in a solution of the coating polymer. The coating material phase, an immiscible polymer in liquid state is formed by:

i. Changing temperature of polymer solution, e.g. ethyl cellulose in cyclohexane (N-acetyl P-amino phenol as core).

ii. Addition of salt, e.g. addition of sodium sulphate solution to gelatin solution in vitamin encapsulation.

iii. Addition of nonsolvent, e.g. addition of isopropyl ether to methyl ethyl ketone solution of cellulose acetate butyrate (methylscopalamine hydrobromide is core).

iv. Addition of incompatible polymer to the polymer solution, e.g. addition of polybutadiene to the solution of ethylcellulose in toluene (methylene blue as core material).

v. *Inducing polymer:* Polymer interaction, e.g. interaction of gum arabic and gelatin at their isoelectric point.

Second step, includes deposition of liquid polymer upon the core material.

Finally, the prepared microcapsules are stabilized by cross-linking, desolvation or thermal treatment (Fig. 2.1).

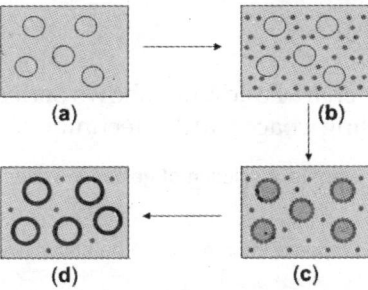

Figs 2.1 a to d: Schematic representation of coacervation process. (a) Core material dispersion in solution of shell polymer, (b) Separation of coacervate from solution, (c) Coating of core material by microdroplets of coacervate, (d) Coalescence of coacervate to form continuous shell around core particles

Simple Coacervation

Simple coacervation is concerned with the non-ionized group in the macromolecule. Simple coacervation can be induced in a dispersion of a less concentrated single colloid by the addition of a strongly hydrophilic substance such as alcohol or sodium sulfate. The addition of a hydrophilic substance causes two phases to be formed, one rich and the other poor in colloidal materials. Simple coacervation depends primarily on the degree of hydration produced and it is possible to redisperse the aggregated colloidal droplets by addition of water. The principle requirement here is the creation of an insufficiency of water in a part of the total system. The most commonly employed simple coacervation procedures utilize gelatin as the wall-forming material. In a system consisting of gelatin and water, coacervation is brought about by the addition of a third component which may be any one of the following:

1. Alcohol
2. Sodium sulfate
3. Ammonium sulfate
4. Macromolecules, e.g. starch
5. Phenol
6. Diphenols, e.g. catechol, resorcinol, hydroquinone
7. Triphenols, e.g. pyrogallol, phloroglucinol
8. Digalloyl glucose

9. Chebulic acid

10. Tannic acid

Folliwng flow chart Following shows series of activities for encapsulation using coacervation technique.

Prepare a solution of gelatin in water

↓

Disperse the material to be encapsulated

↓

Add slowly and uniformly saturated solution of sodium sulfate

↓

Above procedure conducted at a high enough temperature to prevent gelation

↓

Pour mixture in cold solution of sodium sulfate

↓

Filter and wash with cold water

↓

Harden with formaldehyde

↓

Filter and remove residual formaldehyde by washing with water

↓

Dry

Examples of simple coacervation:

Example 1: Ternary diagram for the system gelatin-water-alcohol

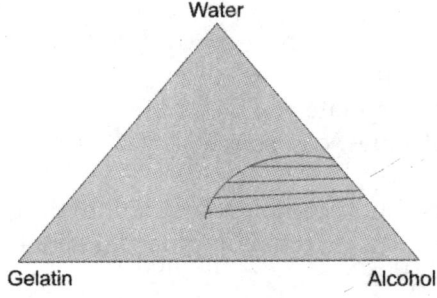

Example 2: Ternary diagram for the system gelatin-water-sodium sulphate

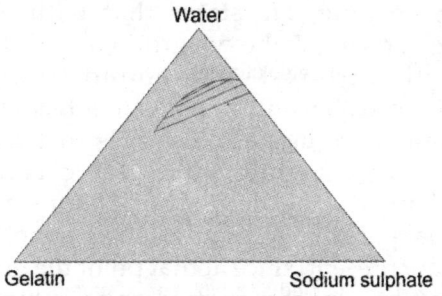

Example 3: Ternary diagram for the system gelatin-water-resorcinol

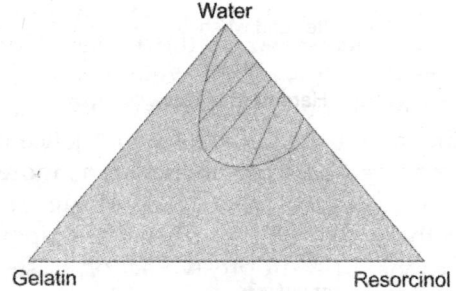

Complex Coacervation

Complex coacervation has a number of characteristic features, but depends primarily on pH. It can be induced in systems having two dispersed hydrophilic colloids of opposite electrical charges. Bungenberg de Jong studied phase separation in colloids by mixing aqueous solutions of gum arabic and gelatin. One important point to be noted that phase separation was produced at pH values below the isoelectric point of gelatin, but not above this pH. Phase separation also occurred in other systems containing two dispersed colloids, one of which was ampholytic. In either case, one phase contained most of the two polymers combined with a small amount of solvent, and the other phase was often a very dilute solution of one or both the polymers. The process of complex coacervation using gelatin and acacia has been explained by Bungenberg de Jong. He states that with gum arabic, a carbohydrate carrying carboxyl' group, and gelatin, a protein carrying both carboxyl and amino groups, complex coacervation is possible only at pH values below the isoelectric point of gelatin since it is at those pHs that gelatin becomes positively charged, while gum arabic continues to be negatively charged. The optimum pH for complex coacervation was that pH at which equivalents of oppositely charged molecules were present, since at that point the greatest possible number of salt bonds were formed and the highest degree of coacervation occurred. In such a system, therefore, the pH is adjusted so that the gelatin particles are positive, while the gum arabic particles remain negative. Lowering the pH beyond this can suppress the dissociation of the carboxyl groups of gum arabic. The tendency towards coacervation was found to be decreased in the presence of electrolytes, since the charged groups on the colloids are screened by the formation of dense ionic atmosphere around each charge, thereby diminishing the interactions and hence the attractions between the charged groups. This effect is more pronounced in the presence of electrolytes or ions of higher valency. It is obvious that this effect will be dependent upon the valency of the added ions. The suppresive action is seen to increase with the valency of the added ions and the suppression of coacervation by salts, therefore, should follow a Schulze-Hardy rule both with respect to the cations and to the anions.

$4 - 1 > 3 - 1 > 2 - 1 > 1 - 1$: valency rule of the cations, and
$1 - 4 > 1 - 3 > 1 - 2 > 1 - 1$: valency rule of the anions.

General outline of coacervation process by mixing aqueous solutions of gum arabic and gelatin:
- Solution of the shell material (coacervate) in water. Example: Copolymer coating
- Gum arabic solution 20–30%
- Gelatin solution 20%
  1. *Preparation:* The core material will be added to the solution. The core material should not react or dissolve in water (maximum solubility 2%).

2. *Dispersion:* The core material is dispersed in the solution. The particle size will be defined by dispersion parameter, as stirring speed, stirrer shape, surface tension and viscosity. Size range 2–1200 mm.

3. *Coacervation:*
   - Coacervation starts with a change of the pH value of the dispersion, e.g. by adding H_2SO_4, HCl or organic acids. The result is a reduction of the solubility of the dispersed phases (shell material).
   - The shell material (coacervate) starts to precipitate from the solution.
   - The shell material forms a continuous coating around the core droplets.

4. *Cooling and hardening phase:*
   - The shell material is cooled down to harden and forms the final capsule.
   - Hardening agents like formaldehyde can be added to the process.
   - The microcapsules are now stable in the suspension and ready to be dried.

5. *Drying phase:*
   - The suspension is dried in a spray dryer or in a fluidized bed drier.
   - Spray drying is a suitable method for heat sensitive Products.
   - The atomized particles assume a spherical shape. The rapid the coating material keeps the core material below 100°C, even if the temperature in the drying chamber is much greater.
   - Microencapsulation makes the spray drying process easier for sticky products like fruit pulp or juice, with a high content of invert sugar.

Complex Coacervation—General Outline

Prepare a first solution of water and a hydrophilic colloid which becomes ionized in water

↓

Disperse the material to be encapsulated

↓

Prepare a second solution of water and a hydrophilic colloid which becomes
ionized in water with an electrical charge opposite to that of the first sol

↓

Mix

↓

Adjust pH to induce coacervation

↓

Add formaldehyde solution

↓

Above procedure conducted at a high enough temperature to prevent gelation

↓

Lower the temperature to 10°C

↓

Filter and dry the product

↓

Recovery of the product

Microencapsulation by Coacervation—Dilution with Water

Prepare a first solution of water and a hydrophilic colloid which becomes
ionized in water

↓

Disperse the material to be encapsulated

↓

Prepare a second solution of water and a hydrophilic colloid which
becomes ionized in water with an electrical charge opposite to
that of the first sol

↓

Mix

↓

Add water slowly and with constant agitation

↓

Above procedure conducted at a high enough temperature to
prevent gelation

↓

Pour into water at 0°C, agitate, and let stand for one hour at
less than 25°C

↓

Hardening of the microcapsules

↓

Dry the product

↓

Recover the product

Microencapsulation by Coacervation-pH Control

Prepare a first solution of water and a hydrophilic colloid which ionized in water

↓

Disperse the material to be encapsulated

Prepare a second solution of water and a hydrophilic becomes colloid which becomes ionized in water with an electrical charge opposite to that of the first solution.

Mix
↓
Adjust pH to induce coacervation
↓
Add formaldehyde solution
↓
Above procedures conducted at a high enough temperature to prevent gelation
↓
Lower the temperature to 10°C
↓
Filter and dry the product
↓
Recovery of the product

Non-aqueous Phase Separation

The foregoing discussion has been restricted to the coacervation process involving microencapsulation of water insoluble substances. This has been referred to as for aqueous. Phase separation. When the substance to be encapsulated is water-soluble, the technique of non-aqueous phase separation" is employed. In this technique the continuous wall-containing phase is organic or hydrophobic in nature and a suitable combination of organic solvents or polymers are used to induce phase separation. In order to effect non-aqueous phase separation, an emulsion consisting of the aqueous dispersed phase containing the material to be encapsulated is prepared in the organic continuous phase containing the organic polymeric wall material.

Microencapsulation of the aqueous phase is achieved by inducing phase separation from the organic phase. This may be achieved by the addition of a suitable second organic solvent which must be miscible with the first organic solvent but must be a non-solvent for the polymer. Thus, due to the decreased solubility of the polymeric wall material in the new solvent system, the wall material is forced to phase out and forms a film around the aqueous droplets.

Polymer Encapsulation by Rapid Expansion of Supercritical Fluids

Supercritical fluids are highly compressed gasses that possess several advantageous properties of both liquids and gases. The most widely used being supercritical carbon dioxide (CO_2), alkanes (C_2 to C_4), and nitrous oxide (N_2O). A small change in temperature or pressure causes a large change in the density of supercritical fluids near the critical point. Supercritical CO_2 is widely used for its low critical temperature value, in addition to its nontoxic, non-flammable properties; it is also readily available, highly pure and cost-effective. This technology is also applicable to prepare nanoparticles.

The most widely used methods are as follows:

- Rapid expansion of supercritical solution (RESS)
- Gas anti-solvent (GAS)
- Particles from gas-saturated solution (PGSS).

Rapid Expansion of Supercritical Solution

In this process, supercritical fluid containing the active ingredient and the shell material are maintained at high pressure and then released at atmospheric pressure through a small nozzle. The sudden drop in pressure causes desolvation of the shell material, which is then deposited around the active ingredient (core) and forms a coating layer. The disadvantage of this process is that both the active ingredient and the shell material must be very soluble in supercritical fluids. In general, very few polymers with low cohesive energy densities (e.g. polydimethylsiloxanes, polymethacrylates) are soluble in supercritical fluids such as CO_2. The solubility of polymers can be enhanced by using co-solvents. In some cases nonsolvents are used; this increases the solubility in supercritical fluids, but the shell materials do not dissolve at atmospheric pressure. Kiyoshi et al. had very recently carried out microencapsulation of TiO_2 nanoparticles with polymer by RESS using ethanol as a nonsolvent for the polymer shell such as polyethylene glycol (PEG), poly (styrene)-b-poly (methylmethacrylate)-copoly (glycidal methacrylate) copolymer (PS-b-(PMMA-co-PGMA) and poly (methylmethacrylate) Fig. 2.2.

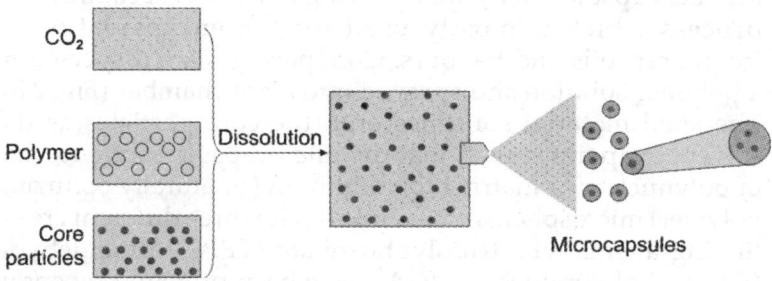

Fig. 2.2: Microencapsulation by rapid expansion of supercritical solutions (RESS)

Gas Anti-solvent (GAS) Process

This process is also called supercritical fluid anti-solvent (SAS). Here, supercritical fluid is added to a solution of shell material and the active ingredients and maintained at high pressure. This leads to a volume expansion of the solution that causes super saturation such that precipitation of the solute occurs. Thus, the solute must be soluble in the liquid solvent, but should not dissolve in the mixture of solvent and supercritical fluid. On the other hand, the liquid solvent must be miscible with the supercritical fluid. This process is unsuitable for the encapsulation of water-soluble ingredients as water has low solubility in supercritical fluids. It is also possible to produce submicron particles using this method.

Particles from a Gas-saturated Solution (PGSS)

This process is carried out by mixing core and shell materials in supercritical fluid at high pressure. During this process supercritical fluid penetrates the shell material, causing swelling. When the mixture is heated above the glass transition temperature (Tg), the polymer liquefies. Upon releasing the pressure, the shell material is allowed to deposit onto the active ingredient. In this process, the core and shell materials may not be soluble in the supercritical fluid.

Physico-mechanical Process

Spray Drying and Congealing

Microencapsulation by spray-drying is a low-cost commercial process which is mostly used for the encapsulation of fragrances, oils and flavours. Core particles are dispersed in a polymer solution and sprayed into a hot chamber (Fig. 2.3). The shell material solidifies onto the core particles as the solvent evaporates such that the microcapsules obtained are of polynuclear or matrix type. Chitosan (a naturally occurring polymer) microspheres cross-linked with three different cross-linking agents, viz. tripolyphosphate (TPP), formaldehyde (FA) and gluteraldehyde (GA) have been prepared by spray drying technique. The influence of these cross-linking agents on the properties of spray dried chitosan microspheres was extensively investigated. The particle size and encapsulation efficiencies of thus prepared chitosan microspheres ranged mainly between 4.1–4.7 μm and 95.12–99.17%, respectively. Surface morphology, % erosion, % water uptake and drug release properties of the spray dried chitosan microspheres was remarkably influenced by the type (chemical or ionic) and extent (1 or 2% w/w) of cross-linking agents. Spray dried chitosan microspheres cross-linked with TPP exhibited higher swelling capacity, % water uptake, % erosion and drug release rate at both the cross-linking extent (1 and 2% w/w) when compared to those cross-linked with FA and GA. The sphericity and surface smoothness of the spray dried chitosan microspheres was lost when the cross-linking extent was increased from 1 to 2% w/w. Release rate of the drug from spray dried chitosan microspheres decreased when the cross-linking extent was increased from 1 to 2% w/w. The physical state of the drug in chitosan-TPP, chitosan-FA and chitosan-GA matrices was confirmed by the X-ray diffraction (XRD) study and found that the drug remains in a crystalline state even after its encapsulation. Release of the drug from chitosan-TPP, chitosan-FA and chitosan-GA matrices followed Fick's law of diffusion.

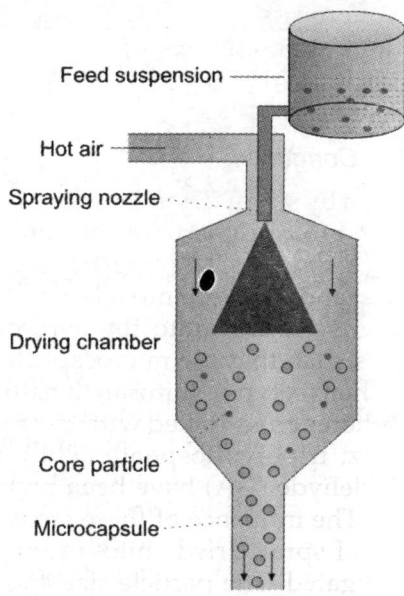

Feed suspension

Hot air

Spraying nozzle

Drying chamber

Core particle

Microcapsule

Fig. 2.3: Schematic illustrating the process of microencapsulation by spray-drying

Spray congealing can be done by spray drying equipment where protective coating will be applied as a melt. Core material is dispersed in a coating material melt rather than a coating solution. Coating solidification is accomplished by spraying the hot mixture into cool air stream. Waxes, fatty acids, and alcohols, polymers which are solids at room temperature but meltable at reasonable temperature are applicable to spray congealing. Albertini B et al. prepared mucoadhesive micro particles and to designed an innovative vaginal delivery systems for econazole nitrate (ECN) to enhance the drug antifungal activity.

Fluidized-bed Technology

The liquid coating is sprayed onto the particles and the rapid evaporation helps in the formation of an outer layer on the particles. The thickness and formulations of the coating can be obtained as desired. Different types of fluid-bed coaters include top spray, bottom spray, and tangential spray (Fig. 2.4).

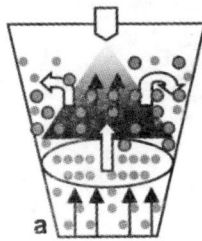 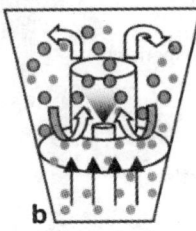 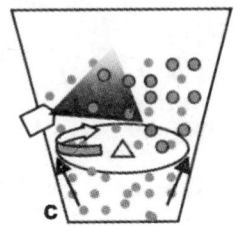

Figs 2.4a to c: Schematics of a fluid-bed coater. (a) Top spray, (b) Bottom spray, (c) Tangential spray

In the top spray system the coating material is sprayed downwards onto the fluid bed such that as the solid or porous particles move to the coating region they become encapsulated. Increased encapsulation efficiency and the prevention of cluster formation is achieved by opposing flows of the coating materials and the particles. Dripping of the coated particles depends on the formulation of the coating material. Top spray fluid-bed coaters produce higher yields of encapsulated particles than either bottom or tangential sprays.

The bottom spray is also known as "Wurster's coater" in recognition of its development by Prof. D.E. Wurster. This technique uses a coating chamber that has a cylindrical nozzle and a perforated bottom plate. The cylindrical nozzle is used for spraying the coating material. As the particles move upwards through the perforated bottom plate and pass the nozzle area, they are encapsulated by the coating material. The coating material adheres to the particle surface by evaporation of the solvent or cooling of the encapsulated particle. This process is continued until the desired thickness and weight is obtained. Although it is a time-consuming process, the multilayer coating procedure helps in reducing particle defects.

The tangential spray consists of a rotating disc at the bottom of the coating chamber, with the same diameter as the chamber. During the process the disc is raised to create a gap between the edge of the chamber and the disc. The tangential nozzle is placed above the rotating disc through which the coating material is released. The particles move through the gap into the spraying zone and are encapsulated. As they travel a minimum distance there is a higher yield of encapsulated particles.

Solvent Evaporation

The coating material is dissolved in a volatile solvent, which is immiscible with the liquid manufacturing vehicle phase. A core material to be encapsulated to be dissolved or dispersed in the coating polymer solution. This mixture is added to the liquid manufacturing vehicle phase with agitation, the mixture is heated to evaporate the solvent for polymer. Here, the coat material shrinks around the core material and encapsulate the core, e.g. Microspheres of 5-fluorouracil and pseudoephedrine HCl prepared by solvent evaporation is mentioned in literature.

Pan Coating

The pan coating process, widely used in the pharmaceutical industry, is among the oldest industrial procedures for forming small, coated particles or tablets. The particles are tumbled in a pan or other device while the coating material is applied slowly. The pan coating process, widely used in the pharmaceutical industry, is among the oldest industrial procedures for forming small, coated particles or tablets. The particles are tumbled in a pan or other device while the coating material is applied slowly with respect to microencapsulation, solid particles greater than 600 microns in size are generally considered essential for effective coating, and the process has been extensively employed for the preparation of controlled—release beads. Medicaments are usually coated onto various spherical substrates such as nonpareil sugar seeds, and then coated with protective layers of various polymers (Fig. 2.5).

In practice, the coating is applied as a solution, or as an atomized spray, to the desired solid core material in the coating pans. Usually, to remove the coating solvent, warm air is passed

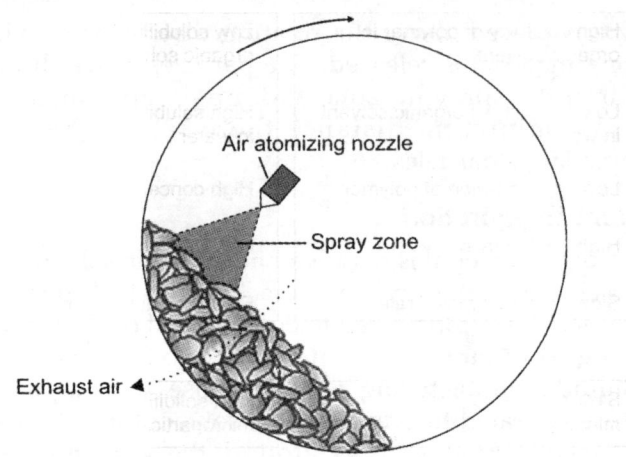

Fig. 2.5: Representation of a typical pan coating

over the coated materials as the coatings are being applied in the coating pans. In some cases, final solvent removal is accomplished in a drying oven.

Coating Process

Pan/ tablet-related parameters	Spray-related parameters
Pan diameter	Spray rate
Pan speed	Inlet airflow
Pan depth	Inlet temperature
Pan brim volume	Air properties
Pan load	Exhaust temperature
Core shape	Atomizing air
Core size	Solution properties
Baffle efficiency	Gun-to-bed distance
Number of guns	Nozzle type and size coating time
Acc. due to gravity	

Fig. 2.6: List of variables affecting pan coating process

Factors Influencing Encapsulation Efficiency

The encapsulation efficiency of the microparticle or microcapsule or microsphere will be affected by different parameters, various factors influencing encapsulation efficiency Fig. 2.7.

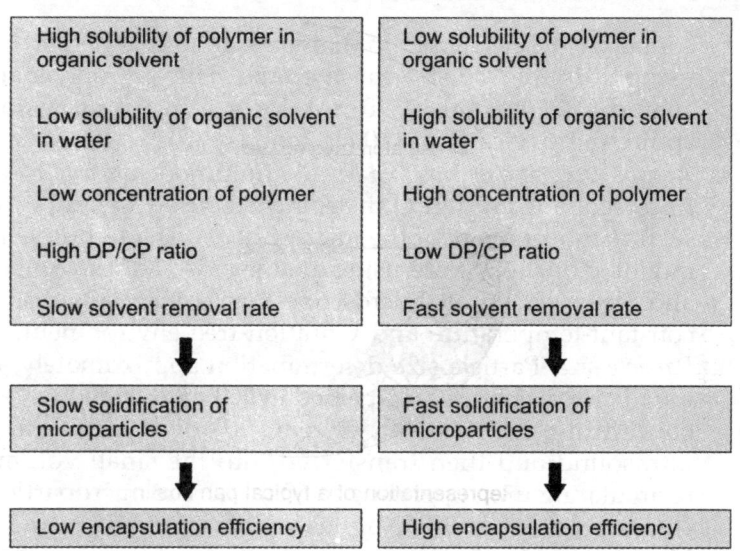

High solubility of polymer in organic solvent	Low solubility of polymer in organic solvent
Low solubility of organic solvent in water	High solubility of organic solvent in water
Low concentration of polymer	High concentration of polymer
High DP/CP ratio	Low DP/CP ratio
Slow solvent removal rate	Fast solvent removal rate
↓	↓
Slow solidification of microparticles	Fast solidification of microparticles
↓	↓
Low encapsulation efficiency	High encapsulation efficiency

Fig. 2.7: Factors influencing encapsulation efficiency

Physico-chemical Evaluation of Microcapsules

1. *Characterization:* The characterization of the microparticulate carrier is an important phenomenon, which helps to design a suitable carrier for the proteins, drug or antigen delivery. These microspheres have different microstructures. These microstructures determine the release and the stability of the carrier.

2. *Sieve analysis:* Separation of the microspheres into various size fractions can be determined by using a mechanical sieve shaker (sieving machine, retsch, Germany). A series of five standard stainless steel sieves (20, 30, 45, 60 and 80 mesh) are arranged in the order of decreasing aperture size. Five grams of drug loaded microspheres are placed on the uppermost sieve. The sieves are shaken for a period of about 10 min, and then the particles on the screen are weighed.

3. *Morphology of microspheres:* The surface morphologies of microspheres are examined by a scanning electron microscope (XL 30 SEM Philips, Eindhoven, and The Netherlands). The microspheres are mounted onto a

copper cylinder (10 mm in diameter, 10 mm in height) by using a double-sided adhesive tape. The specimens are coated at a current of 10 mA for 4 min using an ion sputtering device (JFC-1100 E, Jeol, Japan).

4. *Atomic force microscopy (AFM):* A multimode atomic force microscope from digital instrument is used to study the surface morphology of the microspheres. The samples are mounted on metal slabs using double-sided adhesive tapes and observed under microscope that is maintained in a constant-temperature and vibration-free environment.

5. *Particle size:* Particle size determination approximately 30 mg microparticles is redispersed in 2–3 ml distilled water, containing 0.1% (m/m) Tween 20 for 3 min, using ultrasound and then transferred into the small volume recirculating unit, operating at 60 ml/s. The microparticle size can be determined by laser diffractometry using a Malvern Mastersizer X.

6. *Polymer solubility in the solvents:* Subjected to the determination of active constituents as per monograph requirement. The percent encapsulation efficiency is calculated using following equation:

% Entrapment = Actual content/theoretical content × 100

7. *Angle of contact:* The angle of contact is measured to determine the wetting property of a microparticulate carrier. It determines the nature of microspheres in terms of hydrophilicity or hydrophobicity. This thermodynamic property is specific to solid and affected by the presence of the adsorbed component.

The angle of contact is measured at the solid/air/water interface. The advancing and receding angle of contact are measured by placing a droplet in a circular cell mounted above objective of inverted microscope. Contact angle is measured at 20°C within a minute of deposition of microspheres.

8. *In vitro methods:* There is a need for experimental methods which allow the release characteristics and permeability of a drug through membrane to be determined. For this purpose, a number of in vitro and in vivo techniques have been reported. In vitro drug release studies have been

employed as a quality control procedure in pharmaceutical production, in product development, etc. sensitive and reproducible release data derived from physico-chemically and hydro-dynamically defined conditions are necessary. The influence of technologically defined conditions and difficulty in simulating in vivo conditions has led to development of a number of in vitro release methods for buccal formulations; however no standard in vitro method has yet been developed. Different workers have used apparatus of varying designs and under varying conditions, depending on the shape and application of the dosage form developed.

9. *Beaker method:* The dosage form in this method is made to adhere at the bottom of the beaker containing the medium and stirred uniformly using over head stirrer. Volume of the medium used in the literature for the studies varies from 50–500 ml and the stirrer speed form 60–300 rpm.

10. *Dissolution apparatus:* Standard USP or BP dissolution apparatus have been used to study in vitro release profiles using both rotating elements, paddle. Dissolution medium used for the study varied from 100–900 ml and speed of rotation from 50–100 rpm.

ISOLATED KEY POINTS

1. Microencapsulation is the process of preparing microscopic particle or microcapsule having two components one is core, which can be solids, liquid or even gas and another is coat.

2. In the pharmaceutical industry, microcapsulation is used for sustained or prolonged release of drugs, taste-masking of bitter drugs, elimination of incompatibilities, preparation of free-flowing powders, prevention of vaporization of volatile drugs, modifying the physical properties of chemical entities, faciliating the dispersion of one substance in another, altering the rate of solubility chemical reactants, reducing the toxicity, many drugs have been microencapsulated to reduce gastric and other GI tract irritations, microencapsulation has been employed to provide protection to the core materials against atmospheric effects.

3. There are various techniques are available for the encapsulation of core materials. Broadly the methods are

divided into three types—chemical methods, physico-chemical methods and physico-mechanical methods.

Chemical processes	Physico-chemical processes	Physico-mechanical processes
Interfacial polymerization	Coacervation and phase separation	Spray drying and congealing
In situ polymerization	Sol-gel encapsulation	Fluid bed coating
Poly condensation	Supercritical CO_2 assisted micro-encapsulation	Pan coating solvent evaporation

4. Coacervation term originated from the Latin >acervus<, in Latin acervus means heap, coacervation then means literally "heaping!! it can be categorized into two categories—simple coacervation and complex coacervation.

5. The encapsulation efficiency of the microparticle or microcapsule or microsphere will be affected by following parameters.

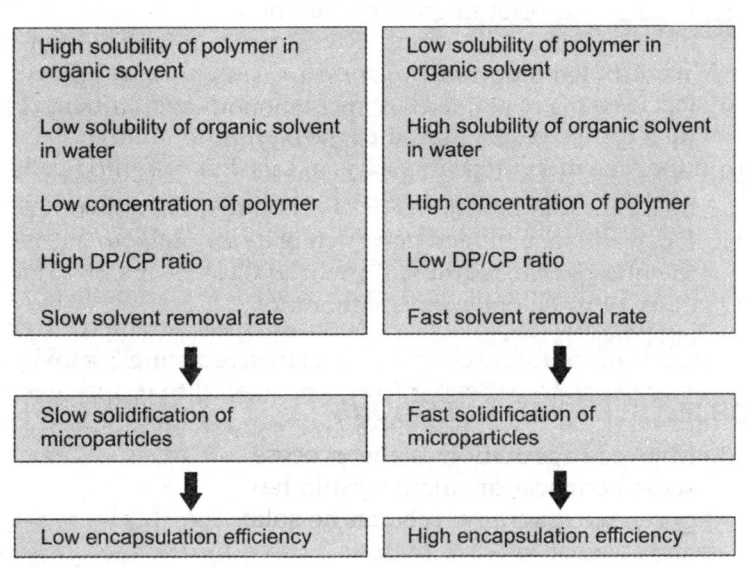

6. Microencapsules can be evaluated by seive analysis, morphology, atomic force microscopy, particle size, polymer solubility, angle of contact, in vitro methods, beaker method and dissolution.

PRACTICE QUESTIONS

1. What do you mean by the term microencapsulation? Discuss in brief about core and coating material used for microencapsulation.
2. Write in detail about application of microencapsulation in pharmacy. Give some examples.
3. Discuss in brief about various microencapsulation techniques. Give there applications.
4. Differentiate between chemical and physico-chemical methods of microencapsulation.
5. Give various mechanism of microencapsulation formation.
6. Differentiate between simple and complex coacervation techniques of microencapsulation.
7. Write short notes on various microencapsulation systems
   a. Gelatin-water-sodium sulphate system
   b. Gelatin-water-sodium resorcinol system
8. Describe in brief microencapsulation by rapid expansion of supercritical solutions (RESS) with the help of a neat and labeled diagram.
9. Describe in detail microencapsulation by spray drying with the help of a neat and labeled diagram.
10. What is FBD? Give various methods of FBD used for microencapsulation.
11. Differentiate between pan coating and spray coating used for microencapsulation.
12. Give physico-chemical methods of evaluation of micro-capsules.

OBJECTIVE TYPE QUESTIONS

13. Microencapsulation is the process of preparing microscopic particle or microcapsule having two components one is .... which can be solids, liquid or even gas and another is ....

14. The core material, defined as the specific material to be coated, is either .... in nature.

15. .... is the technique in which the capsule shell will be formed at or on the surface of the droplet or particle by polymerization of the reactive monomers.

16. In the pharmaceutical industry microencapsulation is used for:
    - Sustained or prolonged release of drugs
    - Taste-masking of bitter drugs
    - Immediate release of drug
    - Preparation of free-flowing powders

17. Match the following microencapsulation technique and particle size.

S. no.	Method		Particle size
1.	Air suspension	a	600
2.	Pan coating	b	35–5000
3.	Solvent evaporation	c	5–5000
4.	Spray drying and spray congealing	d	600–5000

18. Match the following:

S. no.	Drug/core material		Purpose of encapsulation
1.	Actaminophen	a	Reduced gastric irritation
2.	Isosorbide dinitrate	b	Stabilization to oxidation
3.	Potassium	c	Sustained release
4.	Vitamin A palmitate	d	Taste masking

ANSWERS

13. Core, coat
14. Liquid or solid
15. Interfacial polymerization (IFP)
16. 5
17. 1-b, 2-d, 3-c, 4-a
18. 1-d, 2-c, 3-a, 4-b

3

Tablets

Tablets and capsules, on the other hand, currently account for well over two-thirds of the total number and cost of medicines produced all over the world. Tablet is defined as a compressed solid dosage form containing medicaments with or without excipients. According to the Indian pharmacopoeia pharmaceutical tablets are solid, flat or biconvex dishes, unit dosage form, prepared by compressing a drugs or a mixture of drugs, with or without diluents. They vary in shape and differ greatly in size and weight, depending on amount of medicinal substances and the intended mode of administration. It is the most popular dosage form and 70% of the total medicines are dispensed in the form of tablet. All medicaments are available in the tablet form except where it is difficult to formulate or administer.

General properties of tablet: A well-prepared tablet should possess the following qualities:
1. It should, within permitted limits, contain the stated dose of drug.
2. It should deliver its dose of drug at the site and at the speed required.
3. Its size, taste, and appearance should not detract from its acceptability by the patient.
4. A tablet should have elegant product identity while free of defects like chips, cracks, discoloration, and contamination.
5. Should have sufficient strength to withstand mechanical shock during its production packaging, shipping and dispensing.

6. Should have the chemical and physical stability to maintain its physical attributes over time.
7. The tablet must be able to release the medicinal agents in a predictable and reproducible manner.
8. Must have a chemical stability over time so as not to follow alteration of the medicinal agents.

Advantages of the Tablet

1. They are unit dosage form and offer the greatest capabilities of all oral dosage form for the greatest dose precision and the least content variability.
2. Cost is lowest of all oral dosage form.
3. Lighter and compact.
4. Easiest and cheapest to package and strip.
5. Easy to swallowing with least tendency for hang-up.
6. Sustained release product is possible by enteric coating.
7. Objectionable odour and bitter taste can be masked by coating technique.
8. Suitable for large scale production.
9. Greatest chemical and microbial stability overall oral dosage form.
10. Product identification is easy and rapid requiring no additional steps when employing an embossed and/or monogrammed punch face.

Disadvantages of Tablet

1. Difficult to swallow in case of children and unconscious patients.
2. Some drugs resist compression into dense compacts, owing to amorphous nature, low density character.
3. Drugs with poor wetting, slow dissolution properties, optimum absorption high in GIT may be difficult to formulate or manufacture as a tablet that will still provide adequate or full drug bioavailability.
4. Bitter testing drugs, drugs with an objectionable odor or drugs that are sensitive to oxygen may require encapsulation or coating. In such cases, capsule may offer the best and lowest cost.

5. Slow onset of action as compared to parenterals, liquid orals and capsules.
6. Patients undergoing radiotherapy cannot swallow tablet.

DIFFERENT TYPES OF TABLETS

Tablets Ingested Orally

These tablets are meant to be swallowed intact along with a sufficient quantity of drinking water. Exception is chewable tablet. This is the most popular type of tablet dosage form and over 90% of the tablets manufactured today are ingested orally. The different types of tablet ingested orally are mentioned below.

1. Compressed tablet, e.g. paracetamol tablet
2. Multiple compressed tablet
3. Repeat action tablet
4. Delayed release tablet, e.g. enteric coated bisacodyl tablet
5. Sugar coated tablet, e.g. multivitamin tablet
6. Film coated tablet, e.g. metronidazole tablet
7. Chewable tablet, e.g. antacid tablet

Compressed tablets (CT): These tablets are uncoated and made by compression of granules. These tablets are usually intended to provide repaid disintegration and drug release. These tablets contain water soluble drugs which after swallowing get disintegrated in the stomach and its drug contents are absorbed in the gastrointestinal tract and distribute in the whole body.

Multiple compressed tablets (MCT): These tablets are prepared on separate physically or chemically incompatible ingredients or to produce repeat-action or prolonged action products. To avoid incompatibility , the ingredients to the formulation except the incompatible material are compressed into core tablet and then incompatible substance along with necessary excipients are compressed over the previously compressed core tablets. A special type of tablet making machine is used which provides two compressions.

Multilayered tablets these tablets consist of two or more layers of materials compressed successively in the same tablets. The colour of each layer may be the same or different. The tablets having layers of different colours are known as "multicoloured tablets". These tablets are prepared to separate incompatible ingredients physically.

Sustained action tablets: These tablets are used to get a sustained action of medicament. These tablets when taken orally release the medicament in a sufficient quantity as and when required to maintain the maximum effective concentration of the drug in the blood throughout the period of treatment. Controlled release of drug helps in getting the desired degree of action. These tablets are gaining popularity these days.

Enteric coated tablets: These are compressed tablets meant for administration by swallowing and are designed to bypass the stomach and get disintegrated in the intestines only. These tablets are made to release the drug undiluted and in the highest concentration possible within the intestine, e.g. tablets elegant and it also safeguards the drug from atmospheric effects.

Sugar coated tablets: The compressed tablets having a sugar coating are called "sugar coated tablets". Sugar coating is done to mark the bitter and unpleasant odour and the taste of the medicament. The sugar coating makes the tablet elegant and it also safe guards the drug from atmospheric effects.

Film coated tablets: The compressed tablets having a film coating of some polymer substance, such as hydroxypropyl cellulose, hydroxy propylment cellulose and ethyl cellulose. The film coating protects the medicament from atmospheric effects. Film coated tablets are generally tasteless , having little increase in the tablet weight and have less elegance than that of sugar coated tablets.

Chewable tablets: These tablets are chewed in the mouth and broken into smaller pieces. In this way, the disintegration time is reduced and the rate of absorption of the medicament is increased, e.g. aluminum hydroxide tablets and phenol-phthalein tablets.

Tablets Used in Oral Cavity

These tablets released the drug in oral cavity and gives localize action. These tablets bypass first-pass metabolism, decomposition in gastric environment and gives rapid onset of action. The different types of tablet used in oral cavity are mentioned below.

1. Buccal tablet, e.g. vitamin C tablet

2. Sublingual tablet, e.g. vicks menthol tablet
3. Troches or lozenges
4. Dental cone

Buccal tablets: These tablets are to be placed in the buccal pouch or between the gums and lips or cheek where they dissolve or disintegrate and are absorbed directly without passing into the alimentary cannel, e.g. tablets of ethisterone.

Sub lingual tablets: These tablets are to be placed under the tongue where they dissolve or disintegrate quickly and are absorbed directly without passing into GIT, e.g. tablets of glyceryl trinitrite.

Lozenge tablets and troches: These tablets are designed to exert a local throat. These tablets are commonly used to treat sore throat or to control coughing in common cold. They may contain local anaesthetics antiseptic, antibacterial agents, astringents and antitussives, They are prepared by compression at a high pressure or by the moulding process and generally contain a sweetening agent, a flavouring agent and a substance which produces a cooling effect along with medicaments.

Dental cones: These are relatively minor compressed tablets meant for placing them in the empty sockets after tooth extraction. They prevent the multiplication of bacteria in the socket following such extraction by using slow-releasing antibacterial compounds or to reduce bleeding by containing the astringent. These tablets contain an excipient like lactose, sodium bicarbonate and sodium chloride, etc. These cones generally get dissolve in 20 to 40 minutes time.

Tablets Administered by other Route

These tablets are administered by other route, hence the drugs are avoided from passing through gastrointestinal tract. These tablets may be inserted into other body cavities or directly placed below the skin to be absorbed into systemic circulation from the site of application. The different types of tablet administered by other routes are mentioned below.

1. Implantation tablet
2. Vaginal tablet, e.g. clotrimazole tablet

Implantation tablets: These tablets are placed under the skin or inserted subcutaneously by means of minor surgical operation and are slowly absorbed. These may be made by heavy compression but are normally made by fusion. The implants must be sterile and should be packed individually in sterile condition. Implements are mainly used for administration of hormones such as testosterone and deoxycorticosterone.

Vaginal tablets: These tablets are meant to dissolve slowly in the vaginal cavity. The tablets are typically ovoid or pear shaped to facilitate retention in the vagina. This tablet from is used to release steroids, antibacterial agents antiseptics or astringents to treat vaginal infections. The tablets are often buffered to promote a pH Favourable to the action of a specified antiseptic agent. They contain excipients, such as, lactose or sodium bicarbonate.

Tablets Used to Prepare Solution

These types of tablets get dissolved first in water or other solvents before administration or application. This solution may be for ingestion or parenteral application or for topical use depending upon type of medicament used. The different types of tablet used to prepare solution are mentioned below.

1. Effervescent tablet, e.g. dispirin tablet (Aspirin)
2. Dispensing tablet, e.g. enzyme tablet (Digiplex)
3. Hypodermic tablet
4. Tablet triturates, e.g. enzyme tablet (Digiplex).

Effervescent tablets: These tablets when added in water produce effervescence. So they dissolved rapidly in water due to the chemical reaction which takes place between alkali bicarbonate and citric acid or tartaric acid or combination of both. These tablets are to be protected from atmospheric moisture during storage. So these tablets should be stored in well-closed airtight containers.

Dispensing tablets: This type of tablets is intended to be added to a given volume of water to produce a solution of a given concentration. The medicaments commonly incorporated in dispensing these tablets include mild silver proteinate, bichloride of mercury merbromin and quaternary ammonium compounds. These tablets contain excipient which gets dissolved quickly to from a clear solution. These tablets are highly toxic if taken orally by mistake. So, great care must be taken in the packaging and labeling of such tablets in order to prevent their misuse.

Hypodermic tablets: These are compressed tablets which are composed of one or more drugs with readily water soluble ingredients. These tablets are dissolved in sterile water or water for injection and administered by parental route. So, special precautions are needed to be taken during their preparation. These tablets however are not preferred nowadays as there are chances that the solution preferred from hypodermic tablets may be a non-sterile.

TABLET EXCIPIENTS

Excipient means any component other than the active pharmaceutical ingredient (s) intentionally added to the formulation of a dosage form. Many guidelines exist to aid in selection of non-toxic excipients such as IIG (Inactive Ingredient Guide), GRAS (Generally Regarded as Safe), Handbook of Pharmaceutical Excipients and others. Excipients play an important role in formulating the dosage form, determining its quality and bioavailability. Excipients perform a variety of functions like:

i. They act as binders, glidants, lubricants, etc.
ii. They increase patient compliance acceptance by adding flavoring and colouring agents.
iii. They optimize and modifying drug release by adding disintegrants, wetting agents and polymers.
iv. For enhancing stability by adding antioxidant and UV absorbers (Table 3.1).

Diluents

In order to formulate an adequate size and shape and have content uniformity, the tablet size should be kept above 2–3 mm and weight of tablet should be above 50 mg. Many potent drugs have low dose (for, e.g. diazepam, clonidine hydrochloride) in such cases diluents provide the required bulk of the tablet. Generally diluents vary from 5–80%, they are also called as fillers. Diluents provide better tablet properties like:

i. Improved cohesion.
ii. Facilitate direct compression.
iii. Increase flow of powders.
iv. To adjust weight of tablet as per die capacity.

Table 3.1: Excipients and their functions

Excipients	Functions
Diluents or fillers	To increase the required bulk of the tablet when the active drug is less to produce tablets of adequate weight and size.
Binders or granulating agents or adhesives	Binders are added to tablet formulations to add cohesiveness to powders, thus providing the necessary bonding to form granules.
Disintegrants	A disintegrant is added to give bursting effect or breakup of the tablet when placed in an aqueous environment.
Lubricants	Lubricants are added to reduce the friction during tablet ejection from die cavity.
Antiadherents	Antiadherents are added to reduce sticking or adhesion of tablet granulation or powder to the faces of the punches or to the die wall.
Glidants	Glidants are intended to increase the flow of tablet granulation or powder mixture from hopper to the die cavity by reducing friction between the particles.
Dissolution retardants	Dissolution retardants retards the dissolution of active pharmaceutical ingredient (s).
Dissolution enhancers	Dissolution enhancers enhance the dissolution rate of active pharmaceutical ingredient (s).
Adsorbents	Adsorbents are capable of retaining large quantities of liquids without becoming wet; this helps many oils, fluid extracts and eutectic melts to be added into tablets.
Buffers	Buffers are added to maintain the pH to get improved stability and bioavailability.
Antioxidants	Antioxidants are added to maintain product stability and shelf life of the product.

Contd.

Table 3.1: Excipients and their functions (Contd.)

Excipients	Functions
Preservatives	Preservatives are added to prevent the growth of microorganisms.
Colours	Colours are added to mask the colour of drugs and impart better colour.
Flavours	Flavours are added to make them palatable enough in case of chewable tablet by improving the taste.
Sweeteners	Sweeteners are added to tablet formulation to improve the taste of chewable tablets especially in case of bitter tasting drugs.
Wetting agents	Wetting agents are added to help in water absorption during disintegration and assist in drug dissolution.

An ideal diluent should have following properties:

i. Should not react with the drug substance.
ii. Should not have any therapeutic pharmacological activity.
iii. Should be easily reduced in size to match the particle size distribution of the active pharmaceutical ingredient.
iv. Should neither support microbiological growth.
v. Should not interfere with the bioavailability of active pharmaceutical ingredient.
vi. Should not impart any colour to the formulation.

Classification of Diluents

Tablet diluents or fillers can be divided into following categories:

i. Organic materials—Carbohydrate and modified carbo-hydrates.
ii. Inorganic materials—Calcium phosphates and others.
iii. Co-processed diluents.

Tablet diluent or filler may also be classified on the basis of their solubility in water as soluble and insoluble. Selection of diluent should be done after considering properties of diluent, such as compactibility, flowability, solubility, disintegration qualities, hygroscopicity, lubricity and stability.

Table 3.2: Tablet diluents

S. no.	Diluents	Comment
1.	Calcium carbonate	Insoluble in water
2.	Calcium phosphate, dibasic	Insoluble in water, good flow properties.
3.	Calcium phosphate, tribasic	Insoluble in water
4.	Calcium sulfate	Insoluble in water
5.	Cellulose, microcrystalline	Good compression properties, also act as disintegrant.
6.	Cellulose, microcrystalline silicified	Combination of microcrystalline cellulose and silica.
7.	Dextrose	Hygroscopic, reducing sugar
8.	Mannitol	Freely soluble in water, noncarcinogenic
9.	Sodium chloride	Freely soluble in water, used in solution tablets.
10.	Xylitol	Good taste
11.	Lactose monohydrate	The most commonly used diluent, inexpensive takes part in maillard reaction.
12.	Starch	Also acts as disintegrating agent, may give soft tablets.
13.	Starch, pregelatinized	Also acts as disintegrating agent.
14.	Sucrose	Freely soluble in water, sweet taste, hygroscopic

Table 3.3: Direct compressible tablet diluents

S. no.	Diluent	Porprietary name	Comment
1.	Calcium phosphate, dibasic	Ecompress, Di-tab	Good flow properties, high density, insoluble in water.
2.	Calcium phosphate, tribasic	Tri-tab	Insoluble in water
3.	Calcium sulfate	Compactrol	Insoluble in water
4.	Cellulose, microcrystalline	Avicel, emcocel, vivacel	Highly compressible

Contd.

Table 3.2: Direct compressible tablet diluents

S. no.	Diluent	Porprietary name	Comment
5.	Cellulose, powdered	Elcema	
6.	Dextrates	Emdex	
7.	Maltodextrin	Lycatab, matrin	Fairly soluble in water, slight lubricant effect.
8.	Mannitol	Pearlitol	Freely soluble in water, negative heat of solution.
9.	Sorbitol	Neosorb	
10.	Starch, pregelatinized starch	Starch 1500, Strax 1500	Disintegrant
11.	Sucrose-maltodextrin coprecipitate	Des-tab, dipac, Nu-tab	Good flow properties, moisture sensitive.
12.	Xylitol	Xylitab	Freely soluble in water, negative heat solution.

Binders

Binder is one of an important excipient to be added in tablet formulation. In simpler words, binders or adhesives are the substances that promote cohesiveness. It is utilized for converting powder into granules through a process known as granulation.

Table 3.4: Types of binders

Sugars	Natural binders	Synthetic/semisynthetic polymer
Sucrose	Acacia	Methyl cellulose
Liquid glucose	Tragacanth	Ethyl cellulose
	Gelatin	Hydroxy propyl methyl cellulose (HPMC)
	Starch paste	Hydroxy propyl cellulose
	Pregelatinized starch	Sodium carboxymethyl cellulose
	Alginic acid	Polyvinylpyrrolidone (PVP)
	Cellulose	Polyethylene glycol (PEG)

Table 3.5: Binders used in the wet granulation process

S. no.	Binder	Concentration (% w/v)
1.	Acacia mucilage	Up to 20
2.	Algnic acid	1–5
3.	Carbomer	5–10
4.	Carboxymethyl cellulose calcium	5–15
5.	Carboxymethyl cellulose sodium	5–15
6.	Polyethylene oxide	5
7.	Povidone	0.5–5
8.	Sodium alginate	1–3
9.	Starch paste	5–25
10.	Starch, pregelatinized	5–10
11.	Sucrose (syrup)	Up to 70
12.	Hydroxyethyl cellulose	2–6
13.	Hydroxypropyl cellulose-low substitute	5–25
14.	Hydroxypropylmethyl cellulose	2–5
15.	Magnesium aluminum silicate	2–10
16.	Maltodextrin	2–10
17.	Methyl cellulose	1–5

Direct Compression Binders

Due to ease of manufacture, product stability and high efficiency, the use of direct compression for tabletting has increased. For direct compression, directly compressible binders are required which should exhibit adequate powder compressibility and flowability. Direct compression binders should be selected on the basis of compression behavior, volume reduction under applied pressure and flow behavior in order to have optimum binding performance. The choice and selection of binders is extremely critical for direct compression (Tables 3.6 and 3.7).

Following factors influence the final tablet dosage form.

Particle Size and Particle Size Distribution

The particle size of granules affect the average tablet weight, tablet weight variation, disintegration time, granule friability,

Table 3.6: Commonly used directly compressible binders

DC binder	Class
Avicel (PH 101)	Microcrystalline cellulose
SMCC (50)	Silicified microcrystalline cellulose
UNI-pure (DW)	Partially pregelatinized starch
UNI-pure (LD)	Low density starch
DC Lactose	DC lactose anhydrous
DI tab	Dibasic calcium phosphate dihydrate

Table 3.7: Characteristics of DC binders

Flow behavior	DI TAB > SMCC (50) > DC lactose, UNI pure (DW) > Avicel (PH 101) > UNI pure (LD)
Compressibility	UNI pure (LD) > SMCC (50), Avicel (PH 101) > UNI pure (DW), DC lactose > DI tab
Crushing strength	UNI pure (LD) > SMCC (50) > UNI pure (DW) > Avicel (PH 101) > DC lactose and gt DITAB

granulation flowability and the drying rate kinetics of wet granulations. Therefore, the effects of granule size and size distribution on the quality of tablet should be determined by formulator. The methods usually adopted for measurement of particle size and particle size distribution includes microscopy, sieving.

Surface Area

Surface area of the drug effects upon dissolution rate especially in cases where drug have limited water solubility. The two most common methods for surface area determination are gas adsorption and air permeability.

Density

Granule density, true density, bulk density may influence compressibility, tablet porosity, flow property, dissolution and other properties. Higher compression load is required in case of dense and hard granules which in turn increases the tablet disintegration and drug dissolution times. Density is usually determined by pycnometer.

% Compressibility

Compressibility is the ability of powder to decrease in volume under pressure. Compressibility is a measure that is obtained from density determinations.

% Compressibility = (Tapped density – Bulk density/tapped density) × 100

Compressibility measures gives idea about flow property of the granules as per Carr's index which is as follows:

Table 3.8: Carr's index

% Compressibility	Flow description
5–15	Excellent
12–16	Good
18–21	Fair
23–28	Poor
28–35	Poor
35–38	Very poor
>40	Extremely poor

Flow Properties

It is very important parameter to be measured since it affects the mass of uniformity of the dose. It is usually predicted from hausner ratio and angle of repose measurement.

Hausner ratio = Tapped density/bulk density

Table 3.9: Hausner ratio and type of flow

Hausner ratio	Type of flow
Less than 1.25	Good flow
1.25–1.5	Moderate
More than 1.5	Poor flow

Angle of repose (Φ) is the maximum angle between the surface of a pile of powder and horizontal plane. It is usually determined by fixed funnel method and is the measure of the flowability of powder/granules.

$\Phi = \tan^{-1}(h/r)$ where, h = height of heap of pile
r = radius of base of pile

Table 3.10: Angle of repose (Φ) and type of flow

Angle of repose	Type of flow
<25	Excellent
25–30	Good
30–40	Passable
>40	Very poor

Friability

Friability is important since it affects in particle size distribution of granules affecting compressibility into tablet, tablet weight variation, granule flowability. Friability is determined carrying out tumbler test or using friability tester (Roche friabilator) and % loss is determined.

Moisture Content

It affects the granule flowability, compressibility as well as the stability of moisture sensitive drug and therefore, should be determined to evaluate the quality of granule.

DISINTEGRANT

Disintegrant are added to tablet to induce breakup of tablet when it comes in contact with aqueous fluid and this process of desegregation of constituent particles before the drug dissolution occurs, is known as disintegration process and excipients which causes this process are known as disintegrant (Fig. 3.1).

Mechanism of Tablet Disintegration

The tablet breaks to primary particles by one or more of the mechanisms listed below:
1. By capillary action
2. By swelling
3. Because of heat of wetting
4. Due to disintegrating particle/particle repulsive forces

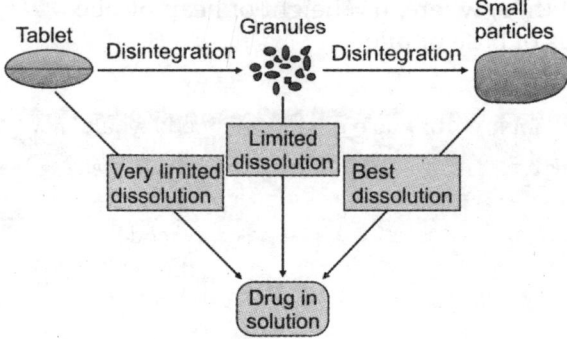

Fig. 3.1: Tablet disintegration and subsequent drug dissolution

5. Due to deformation
6. Due to release of gases
7. By enzymatic action

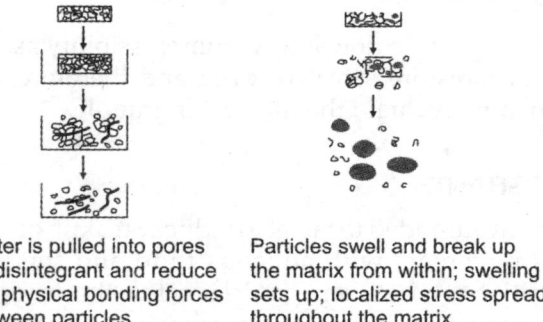

Wicking

Swelling

Water is pulled into pores by disintegrant and reduce the physical bonding forces between particles

Particles swell and break up the matrix from within; swelling sets up; localized stress spreads throughout the matrix

Fig. 3.2: Disintegration of tablet by wicking and swelling

Perhaps the most widely accepted general mechanism of action for tablet disintegration is swelling tablets with high porosity show poor disintegration due to lack of adequate swelling force. On the other hand, sufficient swelling force is exerted in the tablet with low porosity. It is worthwhile to note that if the packing fraction is very high, fluid is unable to penetrate in the tablet and disintegration is again slows down.

Methods of Addition of Disintegration

Disintegrating agent can be added either prior to granulation (intragranular) or prior to compression (after granulation, i.e. extragranular) or at the both processing steps. Extragranular fraction of disintegrant (usually, 50% of total disintegrant requires) facilitates break-up of tablets to granules and the intragranular addition of disintegrants produces further erosion of the granules to fine particles.

Table 3.11: List of disintegrants

Disintegrants	Concentration (w/w)	Special comments
Starch USP	5–20	Higher amount is required, poorly compressible
Explotab	2–8	Sodium starch glycolate, superdisintegrant.
Avicel (PH 101, PH 102)	10–20	Lubricant properties and directly compressible
AC-di-sol®	1–3	Direct compression
Alginic acid	1–5	Acts by swelling
Na alginate	2.5–10	Acts by swelling

Starch

Starch is widely used in tablet manufacturing. The mechanism of action of starch is wicking and restoration of deformed starch particles on contact with aqueous fluid and in doing so release of certain amount of stress which is responsible for disruption of hydrogen bonding formed during compression. The concentration of starch used is also very crucial part. If it is below the optimum concentration then there are insufficient channels for capillary action and if it is above optimum concentration then it will be difficult to compress the tablet.

Pregelatinized Starch

Pregelatinized starch is produced by the hydrolyzing and rupturing of the starch grain. It is a directly compressible disintegrants and its optimum concentration is 5–10%. The main mechanism of action of pregelatinized starch is through swelling.

Modified Starch

To have a high swelling properties and faster disintegration, starch is modified by carboxy methylation followed by cross-linking, which is available in market as cross-linked starch. One of them is SSG (Sodium starch glycolate). Even low and substituted carboxymethyl starches are also marketed as explotab and primojel. Mechanism of action of this modified starches are rapid and extensive swelling with minimum gelling. And concentration used is 4–6%.

Cellulose and its Derivatives

Sodium carboxymethyl cellulose (NaCMC) has highly hydrophilic structure and is soluble in water. But when it is modified by internally cross-linking we get modified cross-linked cellulose, i.e. crosscarmellose sodium which is nearly water insoluble due to cross-linking. It rapidly swells to 4–8 times its original volume when it comes in contact with water.

Microcrystalline Cellulose (MCC)

MCC exhibit very good disintegrating properties because MCC is insoluble and act by wicking action. The moisture breaks the hydrogen bonding between adjacent bundles of MCC. It also serves as an excellent binder and has a tendency to develop static charges in the presence of excessive moisture content. Hence, sometimes it causes separation in granulation.

Alginates

Alginates are hydrophilic colloidal substances which has high sorption capacity. Alginic acid is insoluble in water, slightly acidic in reaction. Hence, used in only acidic or neutral granulation. Unlike starch and MCC, alginates do not retard flow and can be successfully used with ascorbic acid, multivitamin formulations and acid salts of organic bases.

Superdisintegrants

Superdisintegrants which are effective at low concentration and have greater disintegrating efficiency and they are more effective. But have one drawback that it is hygroscopic therefore, not used with moisture sensitive drugs. Superdisintegrants act by swelling and due to swelling pressure exerted in the outer direction or radial direction, it causes tablet to burst or the accelerated absorption of water leading to an enormous increase in the volume of granules to promote disintegration. Example Ac-Di-Sol, Crosspovidone, Explotab, Primogel.

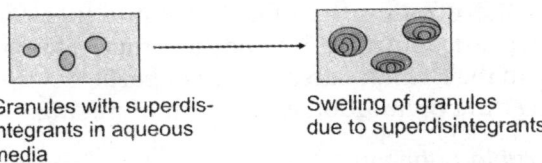

Granules with superdis-
integrants in aqueous
media

Swelling of granules
due to superdisintegrants

Fig. 3.3: Mechanism of superdisintegrants by swelling

Antifrictional Agents

Lubricants

Lubricants are the agents that act by reducing friction between the tablet constituents and the die wall during compression and ejection. Lubricants should be incorporated in the final mixing step, after granulation is complete. When hydrophobic lubricants are added to a granulation, they form a coat around the individual particles (granules), which may cause an increase in the disintegration time and a decrease in the drug dissolution rate. Surface area is important parameter for deciding lubricant efficiency. Lubricants with high surface area are more sensitive to changes in mixing time than lubricant with low surface area. Therefore, lubricant mixing time should be kept minimum. Tooling used to compress the tablet is important for deciding type and level of lubricant used. Additional lubricant is often added to the tablet formulations that are to be compressed with curved face punches. Further, the amount of lubricant increases as the particle size of the granulation decreases but its concentration should not exceed to 1% for producing maximum flow rate. Lack of adequate lubrication produces binding which can results in tablet machine strain and can lead to damage of lower punch heads, lower cam track, die seats and the tooling itself. And it may also yield tablets with scratched edges and are often fractured at the top edges. With excessive binding the tablet may be cracked and fragmented by ejection.

Classification of Lubricants

Lubricants are classified according to their water solubility, i.e. water insoluble and water soluble.

Water Insoluble Lubricants

Water insoluble lubricants are most effective and used at reduced concentration than water soluble lubricants. Since these lubricants function by coating, their effectiveness is related with their surface area, extent of particle size reduction, time, procedure of addition and length of mixing.

Water Soluble Lubricants

Water soluble lubricants are used when a tablet is completely soluble or when unique disintegration and dissolution characteristics are required. Tablet containing soluble lubricant shows higher dissolution rate than tablet with insoluble lubricants. Physical mixture of this lubricant, i.e. SLS or MLS with stearates can lead to the best compromise in terms of lubricity, tablet strength and disintegration.

Table 3.12: List of lubricants

S. no.	Lubricant	Concentration in table (wt%)	Comments
1.	Calcium stearate	0.5–2	Water insoluble
2.	Fumaric acid	5	Water soluble
3.	Glycery behenate	0.5–4	Water insoluble
4.	Glycery palmitostearate	0.5–5.0	Water insoluble
5.	Hydrogenated vegetable oil	1–6	Water insoluble
6.	Magnesium laury sulfate	1–2	Soluble in warm water
7.	Magnesium stearate	0.25–5	Water insoluble, excellent lubricant, reduce tablet strength, prolongs disintegration and dissolution times
8.	Polyethylene glycol 4000 or 6000	2–5	Soluble in water moderately effective, also known as macrogols

Contd.

Table 3.12: List of lubricants (Contd.)

S. no.	Lubricant	Concentration in table (wt%)	Comments
9.	Sodium lauryl sulfate	1–2	Water soluble moderate lubricant
10.	Starch	2–10	Moderate lubricant
11.	Stearic acid	1–3	Water insoluble
12.	Talc	1–10	Insoluble in water but not hydrophobic
13.	Zinc stearate	0.5–2	Water insoluble

Antiadherents

Some material have strong adhesive properties towards the metal of punches and dies or the tablet formulation containing excessive moisture which has tendency to result in picking and sticking problem. Therefore, antiadherents are added, which prevent sticking to punches and die walls. Talc, magnesium stearate and corn starch have excellent antiadherent properties.

Table 3.13: List of antiadherents

Antiadherent	Concentration (% W/W)	Comment
Talc	1–5	Lubricant with excellent antiadherents properties
Cornstarch	3–10	Lubricant with excellent antiadherents properties
Sodium lauryl sulfate	<1	Antiadherents with water soluble lubricant
Stearates	<1	Antiadherents with water insoluble lubricant

Glidants

Glidants are added to the formulation to improve the flow properties of the material which is to be fed into the die cavity. Starch is a popular glidant because it has additional value of disintegrant. Concentration of starch is common up to 10%, but beyond this it will worsen the flow of material. Talc is a glidant which is superior to starch; its concentration should be limited because it hinders dissolution and disintegration. Silaceous material like colloidal silica, i.e. syloid, pyrogenic silica (0.25%), hydrated sodium silioaluminate (0.75%) are also successfully used to induce flow.

Table 3.14: Glidant and there concentration used

S. no.	Glidant	Concentration in table (%)
1.	Calcium silicate	0.5–2
2.	Cellulose, powdered	1–2
3.	Magnesium carbonate	1–3
4.	Magnesium oxide	1–3
5.	Magnesium silicate	0.5–2
6.	Silicon dioxide, colloidal	0.05–0.5
7.	Starch	2–10
8.	Talc	1–10

MISCELLANEOUS EXCIPIENTS

Wetting Agents

Wetting agents in tablet formulation helps in water absorption and thereby helps in disintegration drug dissolution. Addition of Sodium Lauryl Sulphate (SLS) is known to enhance the dissolution. SLS improves permeation of drug through biological membrane by destroying the path through which drug has to pass and thus minimizing the path length for the drug to travel. Wetting agents are mainly added when hydrophobic drug is to be formulated.

Dissolution Retardants

Dissolution retardants are incorporated when controlled release of drug is required. Waxy materials like stearic acid and their esters can be used as dissolution retardants.

Dissolution Enhancers

They are the agents which decreases the molecular forces between ingredients to enhance the dissolution of solute in the solvent, e.g. fructose, povidone are used as dissolution enhancer.

Adsorbents

Adsorbents are the agents that can retain large quantities of liquids. Most commonly used adsorbents in pharmaceuticals are anhydrous calcium phosphate, starch, bentonite, kaolin, magnesium silicate, magnesium oxide and silicon dioxide. Generally the liquid to be adsorbed is first mixed with the adsorbent prior to incorporation into the formulation.

Buffers

Buffers are added to maintain a required pH since a change in pH because a small change in pH can cause great changes in the stability of drug. Examples are sodium bicarbonate, calcium carbonate, and sodium citrate.

Antioxidants

Antioxidants are added in tablet formulation to protect drug from undergoing oxidation. Antioxidants undergo oxidation in place of drug or they block the oxidation reaction. Most commonly used antioxidants include ascorbic acid and their esters, alpha-tocopherol, ethylene diamine tetra acetic acid, sodium metabisulfite, sodium bisulfite, Butylated Hydroxy Toluene (BHT), Butylated Hydroxy Anisole (BHA).

Preservatives

Preservatives prevent the growth of microorganisms in tablet formulation. They are generally used when the moisture content is bit high, i.e. beyound 4%. Parabens like methyl, propyl, benzyl, butyl p-hydroxy benzoate are used as preservatives.

Colouring Agent

They are used to overcome colours of active ingredient, for brand image in the market, to enhance the aesthetic appearance of the product to have better patient acceptance. Most widely used colourants are dyes and lakes which are FD and C and D and C approved. The list of 'permitted' colours is published under the authority of government. The following is the list of colours permitted under Drugs and Cosmetics Act 1940.

1. *Natural colours:* Annato, carotene, chlorophyll, cochineal, curcumin, red and yellow oxides of iron, titanium dioxide.
2. *Artificial colours:* Caramel
3. *Coaltar colours:*
   - Black   : Naphthol blue black 20470
   - Blue   : Brilliant blue FCS 42090
                Indigocarmine 73015
   - Brown : Resorcin brown 20170
   - Yellow : Tartrazine 19140
                Sunset yellow FCF 15185
                Quinoline yellow SS 4700
   - Green   : Fast green FCF 42053
                Quinazoline green 61565
                Green S 44090
                Alizarin cyanine green F 61570
   - Orange : Orange G 16230
   - Red   : Amaranth I. N. 16185
                Erythrosin 45430
                Ponceaux 4 R 16255
                Sudan III 26100
                Carminosine 14720
                Fast red E 16045
4. *Lakes:* These are those colours in which dyes are absorbed generally on aluminum hydroxide. The lakes consist of 15 to 40% of adsorbed dyes and are insoluble in water.

Flavoring Agents

Flavors are commonly used to improve the taste of chewable tablets as well as mouth dissolved tablets. Flavors are incorporated either as solids (spray dried flavors) or oils or aqueous (water soluble) flavors. The flavor of a pharmaceutical formulation is a very important characteristic so much that then very success or failure of a commercial product can be interlinked with the quality of its flavor. In the traditional context the term flavor was equated with odorific qualities of a product though in the modern concept a flavor includes initial impact, mouth feel and after impact of the preparations. The flavor should ultimately be in consonance with the taste as well as the colour of the product. They should also cater to specific liking of patient population. Some guidelines in this respect are given Table 3.15 and 3.16

Table 3.15: Matches between tastes and flavors

Taste	Flavor/flavors
Alkaline	Mint, chocolate, vanilla, custard
Acid (sour)	Lemon, orange, anise, liquorice, raspberry, cherry, strawberry
Bitter	Anise, mint, fennel, chocolate, spicy, cherry
Metallic	Grape, lemon, burgundy
Salty	Citrus flavors, maple, raspberry, fruity, melon
Sweet	Fruity, vanilla, maple, honey

Table 3.16: Matching flavors and colours

Flavors	Colours
Raspberry, cherry, strawberry, apple, rose	Pink to red
Chocolate, honey, molasses, walnut, caramel	Brown
Lemon, lime, orange, custard, cherry	Yellow to orange
Banana, mint, pistachio	Green
Mint, vanilla, spearmint, jasmine, banana	White to off white
Grape, liquorice, violet	Violet or purple
Blueberry, mixed fruit, plum, liquorice	Blue

Sweetening agents: Sweeteners are added primarily to chewable tablets.

Table 3.17: List of sweetening agents used in tablet formulations

Sweetening agent	Relative sweetness compared to sucrose
a. L-aspartyl-1-phenylalanine	250
b. Cyclamate	40
c. Dextrose	0.75
d. D-Fructose	1.73
e. Glycerrhizin	50
f. Lactose	0.16
g. Maltose	0.32

Contd.

Table 3.17: List of sweetening agents used in tablet formulations (Contd.)

Sweetening agent	Relative sweetness compared to sucrose
h. Mannitol	0.6
i. Neohesperidin dihydrochalone	2,000
j. Saccharin	450
k. Sorbitol	0.5
l. Sucrose	1
m. Xylitol	1

Amongst the other sweetening agents listed above saccharin and cyclamates have had an era of popularity chiefly because very small amounts of these substances can make formulations appreciably sweet. Saccharin has a structural formula as below and can be easily synthesized starting with toluene. Saccharin is also marketed as saccharin or saccharin sodium in which the hydrogen group in NH group is replaced by Na and which in crystalline form also has two molecules of water crystallization. Sodium saccharin can easily prepared by dissolving saccharin in equimolecular quantities of sodium hydroxide solution followed by crystallization. Sodium saccharin is nearly 200 times more soluble in water in comparison to saccharin. Saccharin is reputed to be nearly 450 times sweeter than sucrose in dilute solutions. Cyclamates are the sodium or potassium salts of cyclohexesulfonic acid.

Previously national formulary of USA included monographs on solutions and tablets containing sodium cyclamate·and sodium saccharin. The solution contained 60% of sodium cyclamate and 6% of sodium saccharin and sweetening power of 1 ml of this solution was reckoned to be equal to 4.8 gm of sucrose. Tablets used to contain 50 mg of sodium cyclamate and 5 mg of sodium saccharin and one tablet had a sweetening power equivalent to 4 gm of sucrose.

Both saccharin and the cyclamates have been very popular with the pharmaceutical and food manufacturers. At one time these compounds were considered to be absolutely safe but some recent reports have turned the tables against them. Some countries have banned the use of these compounds while some others in process of doing so because they are found to be carcinogenic. Hence, before including these sweeteners in a preparation the manufacturer should check up the law regarding their use.

TABLET MANUFACTURING

Tablets are made by compressing a formulation containing a drug or drugs with excipients on stamping machine called presses. Solid, in the form of relatively small particles, is contained in a die and a compressing force of several tonnes is applied to it by means of punches. The shape of the die governs the cross-sectional shape of the tablet, and the distance between the punch tips at the point of maximum compression governs its thickness. The conformation of the tablet faces, usually flat or convex, is a refection of those of the punches. The tip of the lower punch moves within the die, but never actually leaves it. The upper punch descends to penetrate the die and apply the compressive force. It is then withdrawn to permit ejection of the tablet, brought about by an upward movement of the lower punch. There are two types of tablet press. The excentric press has one die and one pair of punches. The rotary press has a larger number of dies which are fitted, with their corresponding punches, into a rotating turret. Traditionally, tablets have been made by granulation, a process that imparts two primary requisites to formulate: compactibility and fluidity. Both wet granulation and dry granulation (slugging and roll compaction) are used. Regardless of weather tablets are made by direct compression or granulation, the first step, milling and mixing, is the same; subsequent step differ. Numerous unit processes are involved in making tablets, including particle size reduction and sizing, blending, granulation, drying, compaction, and (frequently) coating. Various factors associated with these processes can seriously affect content uniformity, bioavailability, or stability (Fig. 3.4).

Dispensing

Dispensing is the first step in tablet manufacturing process. Dispensing may be done by purely manual by hand scooping

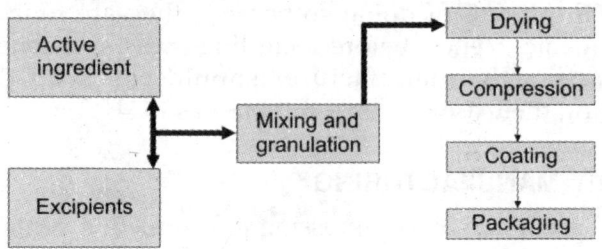

Fig. 3.4: Various steps in tablet manufacturing

from primary containers and weighing each ingredient by hand on a weigh scale, manual weighing with material lifting assistance like vacuum transfer and bag lifters, manual or assisted transfer with automated weighing on weigh table, manual or assisted filling of loss-in weight dispensing system, automated dispensaries with mechanical devices such as vacuum loading system and screw feed system. Issues like weighing accuracy, dust control (laminar air flow booths, glove boxes), during manual handling, lot control of each ingredient, material movement into and out of dispensary should be considered during dispensing.

Size Reduction

The size reduction is an important step in the tablet manufacturing. In manufacturing of tablet, the mixing or blending of several solid ingredients of pharmaceuticals is easier and more uniform when the ingredients are approximately of same size. This provides a greater uniformity of dose. A fine particle size is essential in case of lubricant mixing with granules for its proper function.

Advantages of size reduction in tablet manufacture are as follows:

i. It increases surface area, which increases dissolution rate and bioavailability.

ii. Increases tablet content uniformity.

iii. Better particle size distribution of dry granulation and mixing.

iv. Better flow properties of powders and granules.

Mixing or Blending

The powder/granules blending are involved at stage of pre-granulation and/or post-granulation stage of tablet manufacturing. Each process of mixing has optimum mixing time and so prolonged mixing may result in an undesired product. So, the optimum mixing time and mixing speed are to be evaluated. The various blenders used include blender, oblicone blender, container blender, tumbling blender, agitated powder blender, etc.

Granulation

After particle size reduction and blending, the active ingredient along with the excipients are granulated to form granules with the help of a binder, which provides homogeneity of drug distribution in blend.

Drying

Drying is a one of the important step in the formulation. It is important to keep the residual moisture low enough to prevent product deterioration and ensure free flowing properties. The commonly used dryer includes fluidized bed dryer, vacuum tray dryer, microwave dryer, spray dryer, freeze dryer, turbo - tray dryer, pan dryer.

Compression

After the preparation of granules (in case of wet granulation) or sized slugs (in case of dry granulation) or mixing of ingredients (in case of direct compression), they are compressed to get final product. The compression is done either by single punch machine (stamping press) or by multi-station machine (rotary press).

The tablet press is a high-speed mechanical device. It 'squeezes' the ingredients into the required tablet shape with extreme precision. It can make the tablet in many shapes, although they are usually round or oval. Also, it can press the name of the manufacturer or the product into the top of the tablet. Each tablet is made by pressing the granules inside a die, made-up of hardened steel. The die is a disc shape with a hole cut through its centre. The powder is compressed in the centre of the die by two hardened steel punches that fit into the top and bottom of the die. Tablet presses are designed with following basic components:

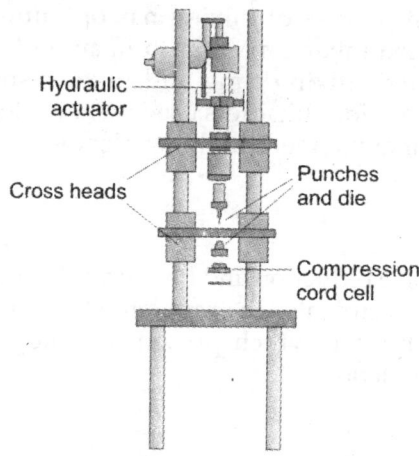

Fig. 3.5: Schematic diagram of a compression machine

1. Hopper for holding and feeding granulation.
2. Dies that define the size and shape of the tablet.
3. Punches for compressing the granulation within the dies.
4. Cam tracks for guiding the movement of the punches.
5. A feeding mechanism for moving granulation from hopper into the dies. The compression is divided into mainly three steps.

Step 1: Filling

The lower punch falls within the die, leaving a cavity into which particulate matter flows under the influence of gravity from a hopper. Though tablets are usually described in terms of weight, the die is filled by a volumetric process. The volume is determined by the depth to which the lower punch descends in the die. Unless this volume is fillled reproducibly on each occasion, then the mass of the tablet will vary, and with it the drug content of each tablet.

Therefore, uniform filling is essential. However, it must be borne in mind that the die cavity has a cross-section of only a few millimetres, and only a fraction of a second is available for filling each die. It therefore follows that the particles must flow easily and reproducibly.

Step 2: Compression

The upper punch descends, and its tip enters the die, confining the particles. The distance separating the punch faces decreases, either by movement of the upper punch alone or by movement of both punches as in rotary presses. The porosity of the contents of the die is progressively reduced, and the particles are forced into ever-closer proximity to each other. This process is facilitated by the particles fragmenting and/or deforming. Once the particles are close enough together, interparticulate forces then cause the individual particles to aggregate, forming a tablet. The magnitude of the force is governed by the minimum distance separating the punch faces. Hence a second essential property of the particles is that they cohere under the influence of a compressive force.

Step 3: Ejection

The upper punch is withdrawn from the die, and so the force being applied to the tablet is removed. As the upper punch leaves the die, the lower punch moves upwards, pushing the tablet before it.

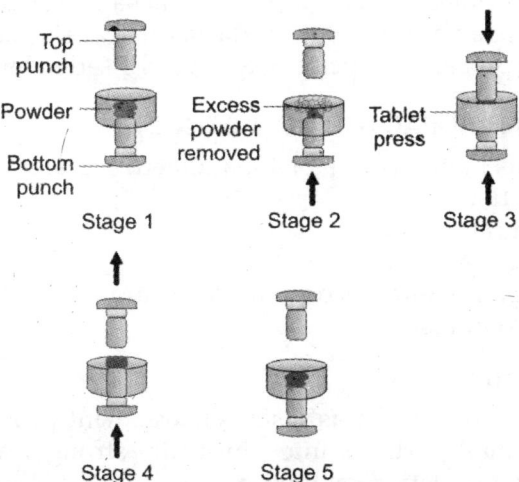

Fig. 3.6: Various stages during compression

Common Stages Occurring during Compression

Stage 1: Top punch is withdrawn from the die by the upper cam. Bottom punch is low in the die so powder falls in through the hole and fills the die.

Stage 2: Bottom punch moves up to adjust the powder weight-it raises and expels some powder.

Stage 3: Top punch is driven into the die by upper cam, bottom punch is raised by lower cam. Both punch heads pass between heavy rollers to compress the powder.

Stage 4: Top punch is withdraw by the upper cam. Lower punch is pushed up and expels the tablet. Tablet is removed from the die surface by surface plate.

Stage 5: Return to stage 1.

Packaging

'Blister packs' are a common form of packaging used for a wide variety of products. They are safe and easy to use and they allow the consumer to see the contents without opening the pack. This saves the cost of different tools and to change the production machinery between products. Sometimes the pack may be perforated so that individual tablets can be detached. This means that the expiry date and the name of the product have to be printed on each part of the package. The blister pack itself-must remain absolutely flat as it travels through the packaging processes, especially when it is inserted into a carton.

TABLET MANUFACTURING METHODS

The various methods of tablet manufacturing are:
1. Granulation
   a. Wet granulation
   b. Dry granulation
   c. Dry granulation incorporating bound moisture
2. Direct compression.

Granulation

Granulation is defined as a size enlargement process which converts small particles into physically stronger and larger particles. Granulation method can be broadly classified into three types: Wet granulation, dry granulation, and dry granulation incorporating bound moisture. The process of granulation is essentially one of size enlargement, and it serves several purposes in the tablet manufacturing process:

1. It improves flow by increasing particle size, since large particles flow more readily than small ones.
2. It improves compression characteristics, adding to the cohesive strength of the tablet.
3. Once a homogeneous mixture has been achieved, segregation is prevented, since particles that are stuck together cannot separate.
4. It reduces dust.

Ideal Characteristics of Granules

The ideal characteristics of granules include uniformity, good flow, and compatibility. Spherical shape, narrow particle size distribution with sufficient fines to fill void spaces between granules, adequate moisture (between 1 and 2%), and addition of binder.

The effectiveness of granulation depends on the following properties:

i. Particle size of the drug and excipients
ii. Type of binder
iii. Volume of binder
iv. Wet massing time
v. Amount of force applied to distribute drug, binder and moisture
vi. Drying rate.

Wet Granulation

The most widely used process in pharmaceutical industry is wet granulation. This is the traditional method of pretreatment of solids prior to tabletting. Despite its complexity and inherent disadvantages, even now about half the tablets produced worldwide are manufactured by this process. Its essence is that particles of active ingredient, with a diluent if necessary, are stuck together using an adhesive, the latter usually being water-based. The result is a granular product which flows more readily and has an improved ability to cohere during compression. Wet granulation process simply involves mixing of wet powder mass with a granulating liquid, wet sizing and drying.

Important steps involved in the wet granulation:
i. Mixing of the drug (s) and excipients.
ii. Preparation of binder solution.
iii. Mixing of binder solution with powder mixture to form wet mass.
iv. Coarse screening of wet mass using a suitable sieve (6–12 screens).
v. Drying of moist granules.
vi. Screening of dry granules through a suitable sieve (14–20 screen).
vii. Mixing of screened granules with disintegrant, glidant, and lubricant (Fig. 3.7).

Disadvantage

The various disadvantage of wet granulation are:
- It is an expensive process because of labor, time, equipment, energy and space requirements.
- Loss of material during various stages of processing.
- Not suitable for moisture sensitive and thermo labile drugs.
- Multiple processing steps add complexity and make validation and control difficult.

Special wet granulation techniques:
i. High shear mixture granulation
ii. Fluid bed granulation
iii. Extrusion-spheronization
iv. Spray drying

High Shear Mixture Granulation

High shear mixture has been widely used in pharmaceutical industries for blending and granulation. Blending and wet granulation is accompanied by high mechanical agitation. Mixing, densification and agglomeration are achieved through shear and compaction force exerted by the impeller.

Advantages

i. Short processing time.
ii. Less amount of liquid binders required compared with fluid bed.
iii. Highly cohesive material can be granulated.

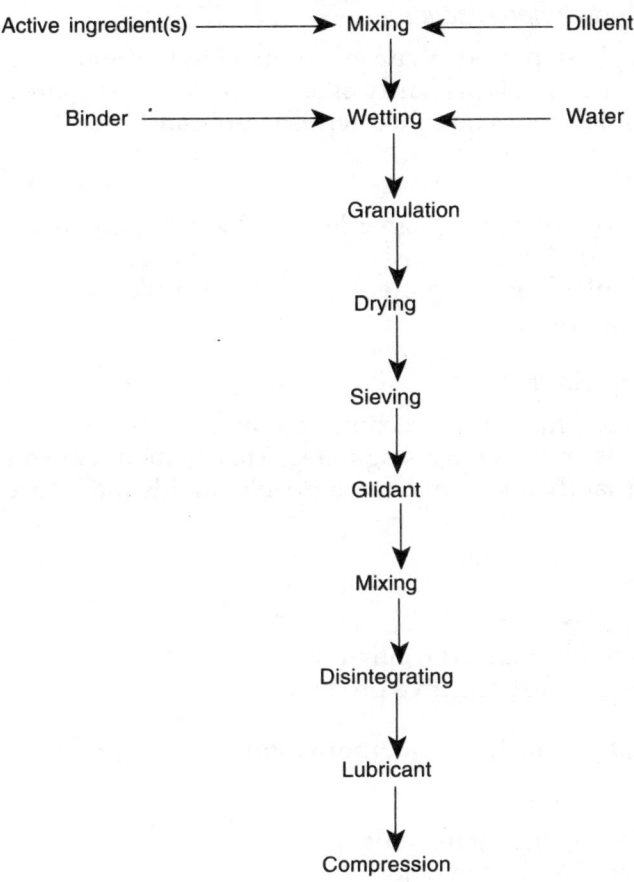

Fig. 3.7: Tablet manufacture (wet granulation process)

Fluid Bed Granulation

Fluidization is the operation by which fine solids are transformed into a fluid like state through contact with a gas. At certain gas velocity the fluid will support the particles giving them free mobility without entrapment. Fluid bed granulation is a process by which granules are produced in a single equipment by spraying a binder solution onto a fluidized powder bed. The material processed by fluid bed granulation are finer, free flowing and homogeneous.

Extrusion and Spheronization

It is a multiple step process capable of making uniform sized spherical particles. It is primarily used as a method to produce multi-particulates for controlled release application.

Advantages

i. Ability to incorporate higher levels of active components without producing excessively larger particles.
ii. Applicable to both immediate and controlled release dosage form.

Spray Drying Granulation

It is a unique granulation technique that directly converts liquids into dry powder in a single step. This method removes moisture instantly and converts pumpable liquids into a dry powder.

Advantages

i. Rapid process
ii. Ability to be operated continuously
iii. Suitable for heat sensitive product.

Lists of Equipment for Wet Granulation

High Shear Granulation

i. Little ford lodgie granulator
ii. Little ford MGT granulator
iii. Diosna granulator
iv. Gral mixer

Granulator with Drying Facility

i. Fluidized bed granulator
ii. Day nauta mixer processor
iii. Double cone or twin shell processor
iv. Topo granulator

Special Granulator

i. Roto granulator
ii. Marumerizer

Dry Granulation

In dry granulation process the powder mixture is compressed without the use of heat and solvent. It is less frequently used methods of granulation. The two basic procedures are to form a compact of material by compression and then to mill the compact to obtain a granules. Two methods are used for dry granulation.

1. Slugging, where the powder is precompressed and the resulting tablet or slug are milled to yield the granules.
2. To precompress the powder with pressure rolls using a machine such as chilosonator.

Advantages

The main advantages of dry granulation or slugging are that it uses less equipment and space. It eliminates the need for binder solution, heavy mixing equipment and the costly and time consuming drying step required for wet granulation. Slugging can be used for advantages in the following situations:

   i. For moisture sensitive material
   ii. For heat sensitive material
   iii. For improved disintegration since powder particles are not bonded together by a binder.

Disadvantages

   i. It requires a specialized heavy duty tablet press to form slug.
   ii. It does not permit uniform colour distribution.
   iii. More dust is formed than wet granulation, increasing the chances of contamination.

Steps in Dry Granulation

   i. Milling of drugs and excipients
   ii. Mixing of milled powders
   iii. Compression into large, hard tablets to make slug
   iv. Screening of slugs
   v. Mixing with lubricant and disintegrating agent
   vi. Tablet compression

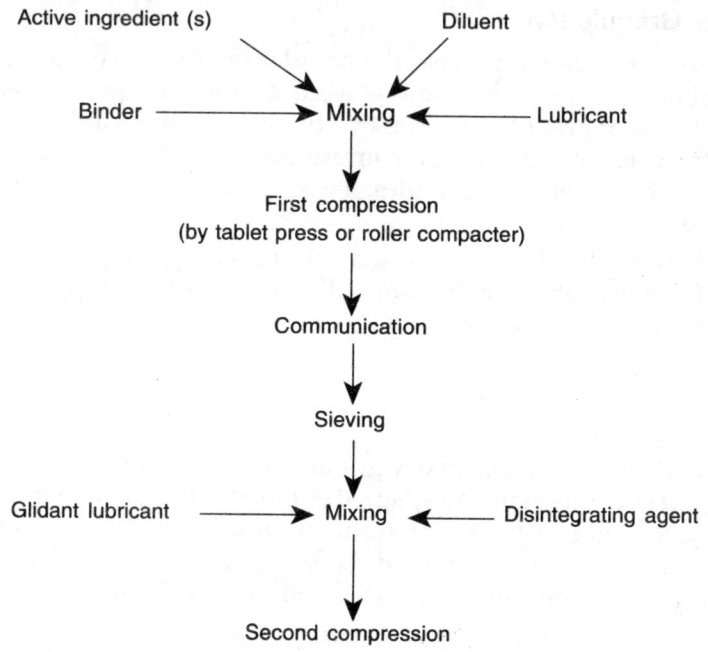

Fig. 3.8: Tablet manufacture (dry granulation process)

Two Main Dry Granulation Processes

Slugging Process

Granulation by slugging is the process of compressing dry powder of tablet formulation with tablet press having die cavity large enough in diameter to fill quickly. The accuracy or condition of slug is not too important. Only sufficient pressure to compact the powder into uniform slugs should be used. Once slugs are produced they are reduced to appropriate granule size for final compression by screening and milling.

Factors Affecting Slugging

   i. Compressibility or cohesiveness of the mater
  ii. Compression ratio of powder
 iii. Density of the powder
 iv. Machine type

v. Punch and die size
vi. Slug thickness
vii. Speed of compression
viii. Pressure used to produce slug.

Roller Compaction

The compaction of powder by means of pressure roll can also be accomplished by a machine called chilsonator. Unlike tablet machine, the chilsonator turns out a compacted mass in a steady continuous flow. The powder is fed down between the rollers from the hopper which contains a spiral auger to feed the powder into the compaction zone. Like slugs, the aggregates are screened or milled for production into granules.

Formulation for Dry Granulation

The excipients used for dry granulation are basically same as that of wet granulation or that of direct compression. With dry granulation it is often possible to compact the active ingredient with a minor addition of lubricant and disintegrating agent. Fillers that are used in dry granulation include the following examples: Lactose, dextrose, sucrose, MCC, calcium sulphate, etc.

Direct Compression

The term "direct compression" is defined as the process by which tablets are compressed directly from powder mixture of API and suitable excipients. No pretreatment of the powder blend by wet or dry granulation procedure is required. Amongst the techniques used to prepare tablets, direct compression is the most advanced technology. It involves only blending and compression. Thus offering advantage particularly in terms of speedy production. Because it requires fewer unit operations, less machinery, reduced number of personnel and considerably less processing time along with increased product stability.

Advantages over Wet Granulation Process

The variables faced in the processing of the granules can lead to significant tableting problems. Properties of granules formed can be affected by viscosity of granulating solution, the rate of addition of granulating solution, type of mixer used and duration of mixing, method and rate of dry and wet blending. The above variables can change the density and the particle size of the resulting granules and may have a major influence on fill weight and compaction qualities. Drying can lead to unblending as soluble API migrates to the surface of the drying granules.

   i. Direct compression is more efficient and economical process as compared to other processes, because it involves only dry blending and compaction of API and necessary excipients.

   ii. Decreases processing time, reduced labor costs, fewer manufacturing steps, and less number of equipment are required, less process validation, reduced consumption of power.

   iii. Elimination of heat and moisture, thus increasing not only the stability but also the suitability of the process for thermolabile and moisture sensitive APIs.

   iv. Particle size uniformity.

   v. Provides stability against the effect of aging.

   vi. The chances of batch-to-batch variation are negligible.

   vii. Chemical stability problems for API and excipient would be avoided.

Disadvantages

   i. Problems in the uniform distribution of low dose drugs.

   ii. High dose drugs having high bulk volume, poor compressibility and poor flowability are not suitable for direct compression. For example, aluminium hydroxide, magnesium hydroxide.

   iii. The choice of excipients for direct compression is extremely critical. Direct compression diluents and binders must possess both good compressibility and good flowability.

   iv. Many active ingredients are not compressible either in crystalline or in amorphous forms.

   v. Direct compression blends may lead to unblending because of difference in particle size or density of drug and excipients. Similarly the lack of moisture may give rise to static charges, which may lead to unblending.

   vi. Non-uniform distribution of colour, especially in tablets of deep colours.

Manufacturing Steps for Direct Compression

Direct compression involves comparatively few steps:
  i. Sizing of drug and excipients.
 ii. Mixing of drug and excipients.
iii. Tablet compression.

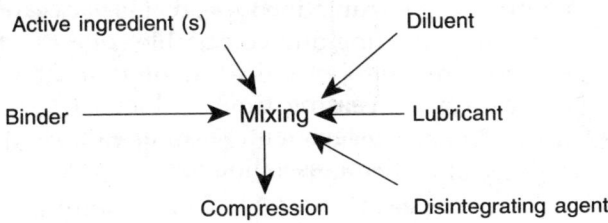

Fig. 3.9: Tablet manufacture (direct compression process)

Direct Compression Excipients

Direct compression excipients mainly include diluents, binders and disintegrants. Generally these are common materials that have been modified during the chemical manufacturing process, in such a way to improve compressibility and flowability of the material. The physico-chemical properties of the ingredients such as particle size, flowability and moisture are critical in direct compression tableting. The success of direct compression formulation is highly dependent on functional behavior of excipients.

An Ideal Direct Compression Excipient Should Possess the Following Attributes

  i. It should have good compressibility.
 ii. It should possess good hardness after compression, that is material should not possess any deformational properties; otherwise this may lead to capping and lamination of tablets.
iii. It should have good flowability.
 iv. It should be physiologically inert.
  v. It should be compatible with wide range of API.
 vi. It should be stable to various environmental conditions (air, moisture, heat, etc.).

vii. It should not show any physical or chemical change in its properties on aging.
viii. It should have high dilution potential, i.e. able to incorporate high amount of API.
ix. It should be colourless, odorless and tasteless.
x. It should accept colourants uniformity.
xi. It should possess suitable organoleptic properties according to formulation type, that is in case of chewable tablet diluent should have suitable taste and flavor. For example, mannitol produces cooling sensation in mouth and also sweet test.
xii. It should not interfere with bioavailability and biological activity of active ingredients.
xiii. It should be easily available and economical in cost.

Major Excipients Required in Direct Compression

I. Diluents
II. Binders
III. Disintegrants

Diluents

Selection of direct compression diluent is extremely critical, because the success or failure of direct compression formulation completely depends on characteristics of diluents. There are number of factors playing key role in selection of optimum diluent. Factors like-primary properties of API (particle size and shape, bulk density, solubility), the characteristics needed for processing (flowability, compressibility), and factors affecting stability (moisture, light, and other environmental factors), economical approach and availability of material. After all, one can say that raw material specifications should be framed in such a way that they provide an ease in manufacturing procedures and reduce chances of batch to batch variation.

Binders

Binders are the agents used to impart cohesive qualities to the powdered material. The quality of binder used has considerable influence on the characteristic of the direct compression tablets. The direct compression method for preparing tablets requires materials which are not only free flowing but also sufficiently cohesive to act as binder.

Disintegrants

Tablet formulations often include a disintegrating agent, which when it comes into contact with water, disrupts the tablet structure and leads to fragmentation. A larger surface area is thus exposed to the dissolving fluid and dissolution is facilitated. Tablets which contain a large proportion of solids that are freely soluble in water have less need of a disintegrating agent, since such tablets tend to erode from their exterior surfaces rather than disintegrate.

Table 3.18: Comparison among wet granulation, dry granulation and direct compression

Wet granulation	Dry granulation	Direct compression
1. Milling and mixing of drugs and excipients	1. Milling and mixing of drugs and excipients	1. Milling and mixing of drugs and excipients
2. Preparation of binder	2. Compression into slugs	2. Compression of tablet
3. Wet massing by addition of binder solution	3. Milling and screening of slugs and compacted powder	–
4. Screening of wet mass	4. Mixing with lubricant and disintegrant	–
5. Drying of the wet granules	5. Compression of tablet	–
6. Screening of dry granules	–	–
7. Blending with lubricant and disintegrant to produced	–	–
8. Compression of tablet	–	–

ADVANCEMENT IN GRANULATIONS

Steam Granulation

It is modification of wet granulation. Here, steam is used as a binder instead of water. Its various benefits includes higher distribution uniformity, higher diffusion rate into powders, more favourable thermal balance during drying step, steam granules are more spherical, have large surface area hence increased dissolution rate of the drug from granules, processing time is shorter therefore more number of tablets are produced per batch, compared to the use of organic solvent water vapour is environmentally friendly, no health hazards to operators, freshly distilled steam is sterile and therefore the total count can be kept under control, lowers dissolution rate so can be used for preparation of taste masked granules without modifying availability of the drug. But it is unsuitable for thermolabile drugs. Moreover special equipment are required and are unsuitable for binders that cannot be later activated by contact with water vapour.

Melt Granulation (Thermoplastic Granulation)

Here granulation is achieved by the addition of meltable binder. That is binder is in solid state at room temperature but melts in the temperature range of 50–80°C. Melted binder then acts like a binding liquid. There is no need of drying phase since dried granules are obtained by cooling it to room temperature. It is useful for granulating water sensitive material and producing SR granulation or solid dispersion. But this method is not suitable for thermolabile substances. When water soluble binders are needed, Polyethylene Glycol (PEG) is used as melting binders. When water insoluble binders are needed, Stearic acid, cetyl or stearyl alcohol are used as melting binders.

Moisture Activated Dry Granulation (MADG)

It involves minimum moisture addition, distribution and agglomeration. No drying step is required. Water distribution is via high shear mixer, or low-shear mixer with highly atomized water spray. Tablets prepared using MADG method have better content uniformity than direct compression. This method utilizes very little granulating fluid and requires no drying, since any excess moisture is absorbed by hydrophilic polymers such as cellulose or silica added to the moist pre-blend. It produces granules with excellent flowability and uniformity, and is applicable to controlled release.

Thermal Adhesion Granulation Process (TAGP)

It is applicable for preparing direct tableting formulations. TAGP is performed under low moisture content or low content of pharmaceutically acceptable solvent by subjecting a mixture containing excipients to heating at a temperature in the range from about 30°C to 130°C in a closed system under mixing by tumble rotation until the formation of granules. This method utilizes less water or solvent than traditional wet granulation method. It provides granules with good flow properties and binding capacity to form tablets of low friability, adequate hardness and have a high uptake capacity for active substances whose tableting is poor.

Foam Granulation

Here liquid binders are added as aqueous foam. It has several benefits over spray (wet) granulation such as it requires less binder than spray granulation, requires less water to wet granulate, rate of addition of foam is greater than rate of addition of sprayed liquids, no detrimental effects on granulate, tablet, or in vitro drug dissolution properties, no plugging problems since use of spray nozzles is eliminated, no overwetting, useful for granulating water sensitive formulations, reduces drying time, uniform distribution of binder throughout the powder bed, reduce manufacturing time, less binder required for Immediate Release (IR) and Controlled Release (CR) formulations.

PROBLEMS IN TABLET MANUFACTURING

A manufacturing chemist faces number of problems during tablet manufacture. Majority of defects are due to inadequate fines or inadequate moisture in the granules ready for compression or due to faulty machine setting. These manufacturing problems requires an in-depth knowledge of granulation processing and tablet presses, and is acquired only through an in depth study and a vast experience.

The manufacturing problems found in tablets alongwith their causes and related remedies are discussed below. These manufacturing problems are due to:

I. Tableting process

II. Excipient

III. Machine

Tableting Process Problems are:

- Capping
- Lamination:
- Cracking

Excipients Related Problems are:

- Chipping.
- Sticking
- Picking
- Binding
- Mottling

Defect Related to Machine is:

- Double impression

Capping

'Capping' is defined as, when the upper or lower segment of the tablet separates horizontally, either partially or completely from the main body of a tablet and comes off as a cap, during ejection from the tablet press, or during subsequent handling.

Cause: Capping is usually due to the air-entrapment in a compact during compression, and subsequent expansion of tablet on ejection of a tablet from a die.

Table 3.19: Causes and remedies of capping related to granulation

S. no.	Causes	Remedies
1.	Large amount of fines in the granulation.	Remove fines through 100 to 200 mesh screen.
2.	Too dry or very low moisture content.	Moisten the granules. Add hygroscopic substance, e.g. sorbitol, methyl-cellulose or PEG-4000.
3.	Not properly dried granules.	Dry the granules properly.
4.	Less amount of binder.	Increasing the mount of binder or by adding dry binder like gum acacia, powdered sorbitol, PVP, hydrophilic silica or powdered sugar.
5.	Less or improper lubricant.	Increase the amount of lubricant or by changing the lubricant.

Table 3.20: Causes and remedies of capping related to dies, punches and tablet press

S. no.	Causes	Remedies
1.	Improper finished dies.	Polish dies properly.
2.	Deep concave punches or beveled-edge faces of punches.	By using flat punches.
3.	Lower punch remains below the face of die during ejection.	By proper setting of lower punch during ejection.
4.	Sweep off blade is not adjusted properly.	By adjusting sweep-off blade properly.
5.	High speed of turret.	Reduce speed of turret .

Lamination

'Lamination' is the separation of a tablet into two or more distinct horizontal layers.

Cause: Air-entrapment during compression and subsequent release on ejection,which worsen by high speed of turret.

Table 3.21: Causes and remedies of lamination related to granulation

S. no.	Causes	Remedies
1.	Oily or waxy materials in granules.	By Adding adsorbent or absorbent.
2.	High amount of hydrophobic lubricant, e.g. magnesium-stearate.	By using less amount of lubricant or changing the lubricant.

Table 3.22: Causes and remedies of lamination related to dies, punches and tablet press

S. no.	Causes	Remedies
1.	Rapid relaxation of the peripheral regions of a tablet during ejection from die wall cavity.	• By using tapered dies, i.e. upper part of the die bore having an outward taper of 3°–5°.

Chipping

'Chipping' is defined as the breaking of tablet edges during ejection of tablet from the press or handling and coating process.

Cause: Incorrect machine settings, specially improper ejection.

Table 3.23: Causes and remedies of chipping related to granulation

S. no.	Causes	Remedies
1.	Sticking on punch faces.	Drying the granules properly or increasing the amount of lubricant.
2.	Too dry granules.	Moisten the granules and by adding hygroscopic substances.

Table 3.24: Causes and remedies of chipping related to dies, punches and tablet press

S. no.	Causes	Remedies
1.	Groove of die damaged at compression point.	Polish to open end and replacing the die.
2.	Center of the die wider than ends.	Polish the die to make it cylindrical.

Contd.

Table 3.24: Causes and remedies of chipping related to dies, punches and tablet press (Contd.)

S. no.	Causes	Remedies
3.	Edge of punch face turned inside/inward.	Polish the punch edges
4.	Concavity is high to compress properly.	Reducing concavity of punch faces and using flat punches.

Cracking

Small, fine cracks observed on the upper and lower central surface of tablets, or very rarely on the sidewall are referred to as 'Cracks'.

Cause: It is due to rapid expansion of tablets, especially when deep concave punches are used.

Table 3.25: Causes and remedies of cracking related to granulation

S. no.	Causes	Remedies
1.	Large size of granules.	Reducing granule size and by adding fines.
2.	Granules are very dry.	Moisten the granules properly and add proper amount of binder.
3.	Granulation too cold.	Compress at room temperature.

Table. 3.26: Causes and remedies of cracking related to dies, punches and tablet press

S. no.	Causes	Remedies
1.	Tablet expands on ejection due to air entrapment.	Using tapered die.
2.	Deep concavities during ejection.	Using special takeoff.

Sticking and Filming

'Sticking' refers to the tablet material adhering to the die wall. Filming is a slow form of sticking and is largely due to excess moisture in the granulation.

Cause: Improperly dried or improperly lubricated granules.

Table 3.27: Causes and remedies of sticking related to granulation

S. no.	Causes	Remedies
1.	Granules not dried properly.	Drying the granules properly.
2.	Less or improper lubrication.	Increasiing or changing the lubricant.
3.	Too much binder.	Reduce the amount of binder.
4.	Soft or weak granules.	Optimize the amount of binder and granulation technique.
5.	Oily or way materials.	Modify mixing process. Add an absorbent.

Table 3.28: Causes and remedies of sticking related to dies, punches and tablet press

S. no.	Causes	Remedies
1.	Concavity too deep for granulation.	Reducing concavity.
2.	Too little pressure.	Increase pressure.
3.	Compressing too fast.	Reducing the speed of compression.

Picking

'Picking' is the term used when a small amount of material from a tablet is sticking to and being removed off from the tablet-surface by a punch face. The problem is more frequent on the upper punch faces than on the lower ones. The problem becomes more severe when tablets are repeatedly manufactured in same station because of the more and more material getting added to the already stuck material on the punch face.

Cause: When punch tips have engraving or embossing letters, as well as the granular material is improperly dried (Tables 3.29 and 3.30).

Binding

'Binding' in the die, is the term used when the tablets sticks, seize or tear in the die. A film is formed in the die and ejection of tablet is hindered. With excessive binding, the tablet sides are cracked and it may crumble apart.

Cause: Binding is usually due to excessive amount of moisture in granules, lack of lubrication and use of worn dies (Tables 3.31 and 3.32).

Table 3.29: Causes and remedies of picking related to granulation

S. no.	Causes	Remedies
1.	Excessive moisture in granules.	Dry properly the granules.
2.	Less or improper lubrication.	Increase lubrication; use colloidal silica as a 'polishing agent', so that material does not cling to punch faces.
3.	Low melting point substances, may soften from the heat of compression and lead to picking.	Add high melting point materials. Use high meting point lubricants.
4.	High amount of binder.	Reduce the amount of binder or by changing the type of binders.
5.	Too warm granules when compressing.	Compress at room temperature. Cool sufficiently before compression.

Table 3.30: Causes and remedies of picking related to dies, punches and tablet press

S. no.	Causes	Remedies
1.	Rough or scratched punch faces.	Polish faces to high luster.
2.	Embossing or engraving letters on punch faces such as B, A, O, R, P, Q, G.	Designing letter as large as possible and coating the punch faces with chromium to produce a smooth and non-adherent face.
3.	Pressure applied is not enough.	Increase pressure to optimum.

Mottling

'Mottling' is define as the unequal distribution of colour on a tablet, with light or dark spots standing out in an otherwise uniform surface.

Cause: Major cause of mottling is coloured drug, whose colour differs from the colour of excipients used for granulation (Table 3.33).

Table 3.31: Causes and remedies of binding related to granulation

S. no.	Causes	Remedies
1.	High moisture content in granules.	Dry the granules properly.
2.	Insufficient or improper lubricant.	Increase the amount of lubricant.
3.	Too coarse granules.	Reduce granular size, add more fines, and increase the quantity of lubricant.
4.	Granular material too warm, sticks to the die.	Reduce temperature.
5.	Granular material very abrasive and cutting into dies.	Using wear-resistant dies.

Table 3.32: Causes and remedies of binding related to dies, punches and tablet press

S. no.	Causes	Remedies
1.	Poorly finished dies.	Polish the dies properly.
2.	Rough dies due to abrasion, corrosion.	Changing the granulation.
3.	Too much pressure in the tablet press.	Reduce pressure.

Table 3.33: Causes and remedies of mottling

S. no.	Causes	Remedies
1.	A coloured drug used along with colourless or white-coloured excipients.	Using appropriate colourants.
2.	A dye migrates to the surface of granulation.	Changing the solvent system, while drying. and binder reducing drying temperature and using a smaller particle size.
3.	Improperly mixed dye.	Mixing properly and reducing size to prevent segregation.

Double Impression

'Double impression' involves only those punches, which have a monogram or other engraving on them.

Cause: During compression, the tablet receives the imprint of the punch. Also when the lower punch freely drops and travels uncontrolled for a short distance before riding up the ejection cam to push the tablet out of the die, now during this free travel, the punch rotates and at this point, the punch may make a new impression on the bottom of the tablet, resulting in 'Double Impression'. If the upper punch is uncontrolled, it can rotate during the short travel to the final compression stage and create a double impression.

Table 3.34: Causes and remedies of double impression

Cause	Remedy
Free rotation of either upper punch or lower punch during ejection of a tablet.	Preventing punch rotation.

TABLET TESTING

For establishing the quality of a tablet product, the fundamentals remain the same, i.e. to ascertain that the product delivers the intended active ingredient in an accurate and reproducible manner. Therefore, tablet testing are broadly divided into three aspects.

1. Confirmation of the nature of the active ingredient and the product (identity, quantity, impurities, integrity, etc.).
2. Establishing pharmaceutical availability of the active moiety both in vitro and in vivo in humans and, if required, also in animals
3. Establishing stability profiles to achieve shelf life.

In this category, one seeks to establish whether the tablets are within specifications, for example, the nature of the active ingredient (identification), expected amount (assay), purity (related compounds), and uniformity of the amount of drug from tablet-to-tablet (uniformity of dosage units). Commonly these testing procedures are described in pharmacopoeias under a specific name, for example, the names given in parentheses are referred to as the USP (US Pharmacopoeia). In addition to these tests, some other tests such as friability, hardness, disintegration, etc. are also conducted and are described below. Although a number of procedures could be described for individual tests, most emphasis will be given to procedures described in the pharmacopoeias because these are usually relatively simpler to conduct and are generally recognized around the world. The various quality control test prescribed in pharmacopoeias regarding the quality of pharmaceutical tablets are diameter, size, shape, thickness, weight, hardness, disintegration and dissolution characteristics of tablets.

General Appearance

The general appearance of tablets, its visual identity and overall 'elegance' effects the consumer acceptance. The general appearance test involves characteristics like tablet's size, shape, color, taste, surface textures and consistency.

Size and Shape

The shape and dimensions of compressed tablets are determined by the type of tooling during the compression process. Tablet thickness is consistent from batch to batch or within a batch only when tablet granulation is consistent in particle size and particle size distribution, if the punch tooling is of consistent length, and if the tablet press is clean and in good working condition. The thickness of individual tablets may be measured with a micrometer, which permits accurate measurements and provides information of the variation between tablets. Tablet thickness should be controlled within ± 5% variation of a standard value. The size and shape of the tablet can also influence the choice of tablet machine to use, the best particle size for granulation, production lot size that can be made, the best type of tableting processing that can be used, packaging operations, and the cost of production. The USP has provided limits for the average weight of uncoated compressed tablets. These are applicable when the tablet contains 50 mg or more of the drug substance or when the latter comprises 50% or more, by weight of the dosage form. Twenty tablets are weighed individually and the average weight is calculated. The individual tablet weights are then compared to the average weight. Not more than two of the tablets must differ from the average weight by not more than the percentages stated in table. No tablet should differ by more than double the relevant percentage.

Table 3.35: Weight variation parameters

Average weight	Percentage difference
130 mg or less	10
More than 130 mg through 324 mg	7.5
More than 324 mg	5

Organoleptic Properties

The color of the product should be uniform in a single tablet, tablet to tablet and from batch to batch. Non-uniformity of coloring not only lack esthetic appeal but could be associated by the consumer with non-uniformity of content and general poor product quality. The eye cannot differentiate small differences in color hence eflectance spectrophotometry, and micro reflectance photometer have been used to measure color uniformity. Taste is also important especially chewable tablets for this companies utilize taste panels to judge the preference of different flavors and flavor levels in the development of a product. Taste preference is however subjective and the control of taste in the production of chewable tablets is usually based on the presence or absence of a specified taste.

Assay

Quantitative test, in this 10–20 tablets are ground and the active ingredient is dissolved or extracted in a suitable solvent using the described procedure. The concentration of the extracted solution is determined using a specific and validated spectroscopic or chromatographic method against a solution of reference standard. These results are reported as percent of expected/labeled value. Although the specifications for assay results differ from product-to-product, generally the expected range for individual active ingredient is to be within 90–110% of the labeled amount.

Content Uniformity Test

This test is done to make sure that every tablet should contains the same amount of Active ingredient with little or no variation within a batch. Due to increased awareness of physiological availability, the content uniformity test has been included in the monographs of all coated and uncoated tablets where the range of size of the dosage form available include 50 mg or smaller sizes. For content uniformity test, 30 tablets are selected and 10 are assayed individually. At least 9 must assay within ±15% of the declared potency and none may exceed ± 25%. According to United States Pharmacopoeia(USP), the procedure for content uniformity test is:

- *Step1:* Take 10 tablets randomly and perform the assay. It passes the test if the relative standard deviation (RSD) is less than 6% and no value is outside 85–115%. Fails the test if one or more values are outside 75–125%.
- *Step2:* Take 20 more units and perform the assay procedure. Passes the test if RSD of all the 30 tablets is less than 7.8%, not more than one value is outside 85–115%, and no value is outside 75–125%. Or else the batch fails the test. Procedure for content uniformity tests according to British pharmacopoeia (BP) is as follows:

Test A: Applicable for tablets, powders for parenteral use and suspensions for injection.

Take 10 tablets randomly. Passes the test if each individual unit is between 85% and 115% of the average content. Fails the test if more than one individual unit is outside these limits or if even one is outside the limits of 75 to 125% of the average content. But if one unit is outside the limits of 85 to 115% and within 75 to 125%, then take another 10 units at random and perform the assay. The lot passes the test if not more than one unit of the thirty units is outside 85 to 115%, and not even one unit is outside the limits of 75 to 125% of the average content.

Test B: Applicable for capsules, powders other than for parenteral use, granules, suppositories and pessaries.

The batch passes the test if not more than one individual tablet (out of 10 tablets selected randomly) is outside the limits of 85 to 115% and none is outside the limits of 75 to 125% of the labelled content. The batch fails the test if more than three units are outside the limits of 85 to 115% or if one or more units are outside the limits of 75 to 125% of the labelled content.

If two or three tablets are outside the limits of 85 to 115%, but within the limits of 75 to 125%, then select another 20 units at random. The batch complies the test when not more than three units out of these thirty units are outside the limits of 85 to 115%, and not even one unit is outside the limits of 75 to 125% of the labelled content.

Test C: Applicable only for transdermal patches.

The preparation passes test only if the average content of the 10 units is between 90% and 110%, and if the content of each unit is between 75% and 125% of the average content.

Hardness or Crushing Strength

The resistance of tablets to capping, abrasion or breakage under conditions of storage, transportation and handling before usage depends on its hardness. The instrument measures the force required to break the tablet when the force generated by a coil spring is applied diametrally to the tablet. Hardness, which is now more appropriately called crushing strength determinations are made during tablet production and are used to determine the need for pressure adjustment on tablet machine. If the tablet is too hard, it may not disintegrate in the required period of time to meet the dissolution specifications; if it is too soft, it may not be able to withstand the handling during subsequent processing such as coating or packaging and shipping operations. The force required to break the tablet is measured in kilograms and a crushing strength of 4 kg is usually considered to be the minimum for satisfactory tablets . Oral tablets normally have a hardness of 4 to 10 kg; however, hypodermic and chewable tablets are usually much softer (3 kg) and some sustained release tablets are much harder (10–20 kg). Tablet hardness have been associated with other tablet properties such as density and porosity. Hardness generally increase with normal storage of tablets and depends on the shape, chemical properties, binding agent and pressure applied during compression (Fig. 3.10).

Tablet Disintegration

For a drug to be absorbed from a solid dosage form after oral administration, it must first be in solution, and the first important step toward this condition is usually the break-up of the tablet; a process known as disintegration. The disintegration test is a measure of the time required under a

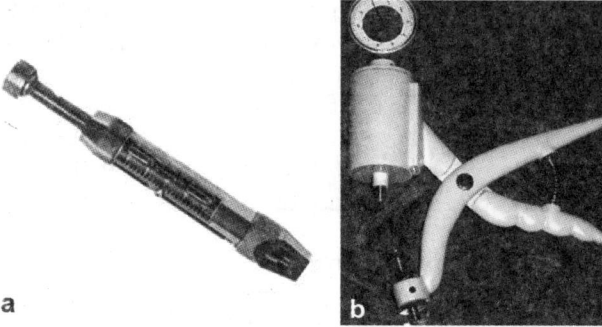

a   b

Figs 3.10a and b: Tablet hardness tester: (a) Monsanto type, (b) Pfizer type

given set of conditions for a group of tablets to disintegrate into particles which will pass through a 10 mesh screen. The disintegration test is carried out using the disintegration tester which consists of a basket rack holding 6 plastic tubes, open at the top and bottom, the bottom of the tube is covered by a 10 mesh screen. The basket is immersed in a bath of suitable liquid held at 37°C, preferably in a 1 L beaker. For compressed uncoated tablets, the testing fluid is usually water at 37°C but some monographs direct that simulated gastric fluid be used. If one or two tablets fail to disintegrate, the test is repeated using 12 tablets. For most uncoated tablets, the BP requires that the tablets disintegrate in 15 minutes (although it varies for some uncoated tablets) while for coated tablets, up to 2 hours may be required. The individual drug monographs specify the time disintegration must occur to meet the Pharmacopoeial standards. Each of the pharmacopoeia like the USP, BP, IP, etc. each have their own set of standards and specify disintegration tests of their own. USP, European pharmacopoeia and Japanese pharmacopoeia have been harmonised by the International Conference on Harmonisation (ICH) and are interchangeable. The disintegration test is performed to find out the time it takes for a solid oral dosage form like a tablet or capsule to completely disintegrate. The time of disintegration is a measure of the quality. This is because, for example, if the disintegration time is too high; it means that the tablet is too highly compressed or the capsule shell gelatin is not of pharmacopoeial quality or it may imply several other reasons. And also if the disintegration time is not uniform in a set of samples being analysed, it indicates batch inconsistency and lack of batch uniformity.

Disintegration Test Apparatus

The disintegration test is conducted using the disintegration apparatus. Although there are slight variations in the different pharmacopoeias, the basic construction and the working of the apparatus remains the same. The apparatus consists of a basket made of transparent polyvinyl or other plastic material. It has 6 tubes set into the same basket with equal diameter and a wire mesh made of stainless steel with uniform mesh size is fixed to each of these six tubes. Small metal discs may be used to enable immersion of the dosage form completely. The entire basket-rack assembly is movable by reciprocating motor which is fixed to the apex of the basket-rack assembly. The entire assembly is immersed in a vessel containing the medium in which the disintegration test is to be carried out. The vessel is provided with a thermostat to regulate the temperature of the fluid medium to the desired temperature (Fig. 3.11).

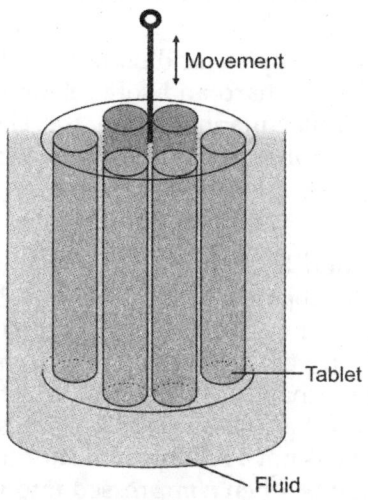

Fig. 3.11: Schematic representation of disintegration test apparatus

Disintegration Test Method

The disintegration test for each dosage form is given in the pharmacopoeia. There are some general tests for typical types of dosage forms. However, the disintegration test prescribed in the individual monograph of a product is to be followed. If the monograph does not specify any specific test, the general test for the specific dosage form may be employed. Some of the types of dosage forms and their disintegration tests are:

1. *Uncoated tablets:* Tested using distilled water as medium at 37 + /–2C at 29–32 cycles per minute; test is completed after 15 minutes. It is acceptable when there is no palpable core at the end of the cycle (for at least 5 tablets or capsules) and if the mass does not stick to the immersion disc.

2. *Coated tablets:* The same test procedure is adapted but the time of operation is 30 minutes.

3. *Enteric coated/gastric resistant tablets:* The test is carried out first in distilled water (at room temperature for 5 min. USP and no distilled water per BP and IP), then it is tested in 0.1 M HCL (up to 2 hours; BP) or Stimulated gastric fluid (1 hour; USP) followed by phosphate buffer, pH 6.8 (1 hour; BP) or stimulated intestinal fluid without enzymes (1 hour; USP).

4. *Chewable tablets:* Exempted from disintegration test (BP and IP), 4 hours (USP).

These are a few examples for illustration. The disintegration tests for capsules, both hard and soft gelatin capsules are also performed in a similar manner. Also, the USP also provides disintegration tests for suppositories, pessaries, etc.

Friability Test

This test is intended to determine the friability of uncoated tablets, tablets are subjected to abrasion and shock by utilizing a plastic chamber by mechanical shock or attrition the strength of a tablet plays an very important role in its marketing and dissolution. The mechanical strength of tablet or granules can be determined by its hardness and friability test. Measuring the hardness of a tablet is not a reliable indicator for tablet strength as some formulations when compressed into very hard tablets tend to 'cap' or lose their crown portions on attrition. Such tablets tend to powder, chip and fragment. The commonly used friabilator in laboratories is the roche friabilator. This instrument consists of a plastic chamber for placing the tablets which is attached to a horizontal axis. The drum has an inside diameter of 287 mm and is about 38 mm in depth, made of a transparent synthetic polymer with polished internal surface. A set of pre weighed tablets (if one tablet weigh 650 mg or less than approx 6.5 g of total weight should be taken and for more than 650 mg/tablet weight, 10 tablets should be taken) are placed in the plastic chamber revolving at 24–25 rpm for 4 min. The tablets are subjected to combined effects of abrasion and shock. The tablets are dropped at a dista nce of six inches on each revolution.

If the tablet size or shape becomes irregular adjust the drum so that base forms an angle of about 10 degrees with bench top and the tablets fall freely when drum is rotated. The instrument is operated for 100 revolutions after which the tablets are dusted and reweighed.

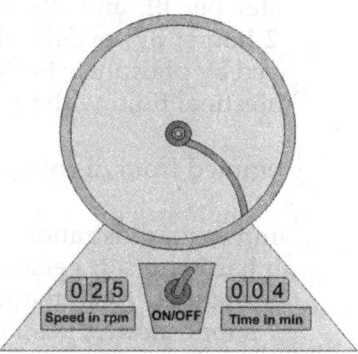

Fig. 3.12: Schematic representation of roche friabilator

Conventional compressed tablets that lose less than 0.5 to 1% of weight are considered acceptable. Most effervescent tablets and some chewable tablets undergo high friability weight loss which is an indication for the special stack packing that is required for these types of tablets. In case of hygroscopic tablets a humidity-controlled environment (relative humidity less than 40%) is required for testing. Normally compressed tablet which lose less than 0.5 to 1.0%

acceptable. The tablets roll or slide and fall onto the drum wall or onto each other. Usually, a sample of 10 tablets are tested at a time, unless tablet weight is 0.65 g or less, where 20 tablets are tested. After 100 turns, the tablet samples are evaluated by weighing. If the reduction in the total mass of the tablets is more than 1%, the tablets fail the friability test. Generally, the tests done once. If cracked, cleaved, or broken tablets are obvious, then the sample also fails the test.

Friability is affected by various external and internal factors like:

1. Punches that are in poor condition or worn at their surface edges, resulting in 'whiskering' at the tablet edge.
2. Friability test is influenced by internal factors like the moisture content of tablet granules and finished tablets.

DISSOLUTION

Dissolution is pharmaceutically defined as the rate of mass transfer from a solid surface into the dissolution medium or solvent under standardized conditions of liquid/solid interface, temperature and solvent composition. It is a dynamic property that changes with time and explains the process by which a homogenus mixture of a solid or a liquid can be obtained in a solvent. Dissolution is considered one of the most important quality control tests performed on tablet and is used for predicting bioavailability, and in some cases, replacing clinical studies to determine bioequivalence the dissolution test measures the amount of time required for certain percentage of the drug substance in a tablet to go into solution under a specified set of conditions. It describes a step towards physiological availability of the drug substance, but it is not designed to measure the safety or efficacy of the tablet being tested. It provides in vitro control procedure to eliminate variation among production batches. The dissolution medium must be aqueous and the pH of the medium should be controlled and should simulate in vivo conditions (Fig. 3.13).

• Dissolution testing is widely used in the pharmaceutical industry for optimization of formulation and quality control.
• To identify the critical manufacturing variable, like the binding agent effect, mixing effects, granulation procedure, coating parameters and comparative profile studies.

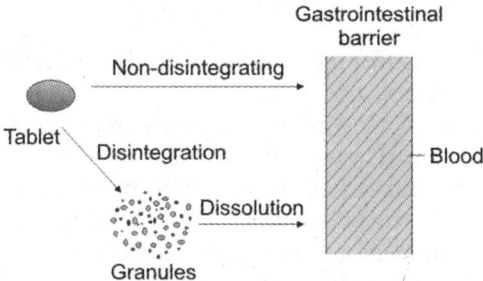

Fig. 3.13: Schematic diagram of the dissolution process

- To comply with guidelines set in the scale up and post approval changes (SUPAC) and ICH.
- Routine assessment of production quality to ensure uniformity between production lots.
- Assessment of 'bioequivalence', that is to say, production of the same biological availability from discrete batches of products from one or different manufacturers.
- Prediction of 'in vivo' availability, i.e. bioavailability (where applicable) (Fig. 3.14).

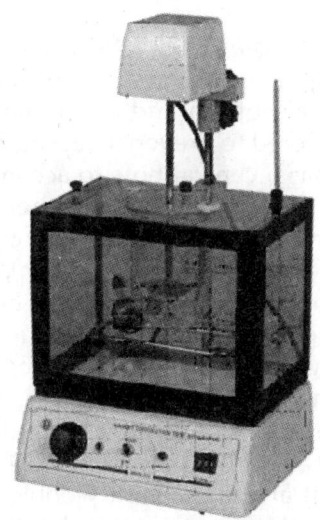

Fig. 3.14: Dissolution test apparatus

Procedure

Ensure that the equipment has been calibrated within the past 6–12 months. Place the volume of dissolution medium, as stipulated in the individual monograph, in the vessel; assemble the apparatus and place it in the water-bath; allow the temperature of the dissolution medium to reach 37 ± 0.5°C and remove the thermometer. When apparatus "Paddle" is used, allow either one tablet or one capsule of the preparation to be tested to sink to the bottom of the vessel before starting the rotation of the blade, taking care that no air bubbles are present on the surface of the dosage form. In order to stop the dosage form from floating, anchor it to the bottom of the vessel using a suitable device such as a wire or glass helix. When apparatus "Basket" is used, place either one tablet or one capsule of the preparation to be tested in a dry basket at the beginning of each test. Lower the basket into position before rotation. Immediately start rotation of the blade or basket at the rate specified in the individual monograph. Withdraw a sample from a zone midway between the surface of the dissolution medium and the top of the rotating blade or basket, not less than 10 mm below the surface and at least 10 mm from the vessel wall, at the time or time intervals specified.

The apparatus "Paddle" (Fig. 3.14) consists of a cylindrical vessel of suitable glass or other suitable transparent material with a hemispherical bottom and a nominal capacity of 1000 ml. The vessel is covered to prevent evaporation of the medium with a cover that has a central hole to accommodate the shaft of the stirrer and other holes for the thermometer and for devices for withdrawal of liquid. The stirrer consists of a vertical shaft with a blade at the lower end. The blade is constructed around the shaft so that it is flush with the bottom of the shaft. When placed inside the vessel, the shaft's axis is within 2 mm of the axis of the vessel and the bottom of the blade is 25 ± 2 mm from the inner bottom of the vessel. The upper part of the shaft is connected to a motor provided with a speed regulator so that smooth rotation of the stirrer can be maintained without any significant wobble. The apparatus is placed in a water-bath that maintains the dissolution medium in the vessel at 37 ± 0.5°C.

The apparatus "Basket" (Fig. 3.15) consists of the same apparatus as described for "Paddle", except that the paddle stirrer is replaced by a basket stirrer. The basket consists of two parts. The top part, with a vent, is attached to the shaft. It is fitted with three spring clips, or other suitable attachments, that allow removal of the lower part so that the preparation being examined can be placed in the basket. These three spring clips firmly hold the lower part of the basket concentric with the axis of the vessel during rotation. The lower detachable part of the basket is made of welded-seam cloth, with a wire thickness of 0.254 mm diameter and with 0.381 mm square openings, formed into a cylinder with a narrow rim of sheet metal around the top and the bottom. If the basket is to be used with acidic media, it may be plated with a 2.5 μm layer of gold. When placed inside the vessel, the distance between the inner bottom of the vessel and the basket is 25 ± 2 mm.

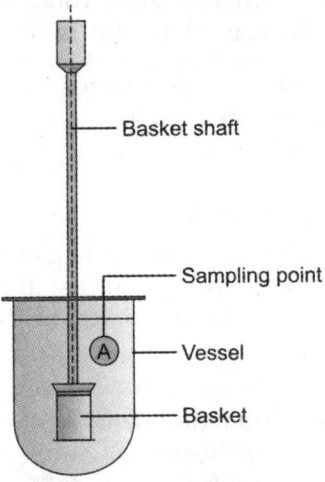

Basket shaft

Sampling point

Vessel

Basket

Fig. 3.15: Apparatus basket

Basket Type Dissolution Test Apparatus

Test conditions: The following specifications are given in the individual monographs:

• The apparatus to be used
• The composition and volume of the dissolution medium

- The rotation speed of the paddle or basket
- The preparation of the sample and reference solutions
- The time, the method, and the amount for sampling of the test solution.
- The method of analysis and
- The limits of the quantity or quantities of active ingredient (s) required to dissolve within a prescribed time.

Dissolution media: If a buffer is added to the dissolution medium, adjust its pH to within ± 0.05 units of the prescribed value. Prior to testing, if necessary, remove any dissolved gases that could cause the formation of bubbles.

Dissolution Buffer pH 1.3

Dissolve 2 g of sodium chloride R in 800 ml of deionized water, adjust the pH to 1.3 with hydrochloric acid (~70 g/l), and dilute to 1000 ml with water.

Dissolution Buffer pH 2.5

Dissolve 2 g of sodium chloride R in 800 ml of deionized water, adjust the pH to 2.5 with hydrochloric acid (~70 g/l), and dilute to 1000 ml with water.

Dissolution Buffer pH 3.5

Dissolve 7.507 g of glycine R and 5.844 g of sodium chloride R in 800 ml of deionized water, adjust the pH to 3.5 with hydrochloric acid (~70 g/l), and dilute to 1000 ml with water.

Dissolution Buffer pH 4.5

Dissolve 6.8 g of potassium dihydrogen phosphate R in 900 ml of deionized water, adjust the pH to 4.5 either with hydrochloric acid (~70 g/l) or sodium hydroxide (~80 g/l), and dilute to 1000 ml with water.

Dissolution Buffer pH 6.8

Dissolve 6.9 g of sodium dihydrogen phosphate R and 0.9 g of sodium hydroxide R in 800 ml of water R, adjust the pH to 6.8 with sodium hydroxide (~80 g/l) and dilute to 1000 ml with water R.

Dissolution Buffer pH 6.8, 0.25% SDS

Dissolve 6.9 g of sodium dihydrogen phosphate R, 0.9 g of sodium hydroxide R and 2.5 g of sodium dodecyl sulfate R in 800 ml of water R, adjust the pH to 6.8 with sodium hydroxide (~80 g/l) and dilute to 1000 ml with water R.

Dissolution Buffer pH 7.2

Dissolve 9.075 g of potassium dihydrogen phosphate R in deionized water to produce 1000 ml (solution A). Dissolve 11.87 g of disodium hydrogen phosphate R in sufficient water to produce 1000 ml (solution B). Mix 300 ml of solution A with 700 ml of solution B.

Gastric Fluid, Simulated

Dissolve 2.0 g of sodium chloride R and 3.2 g of pepsin R in 7.0 ml of hydrochloric acid (~420 g/l) TS and sufficient water to produce 1000 ml. This test solution has a pH of about 1.2.

Intestinal Fluid, Simulated

Dissolve 6.8 g of potassium dihydrogen phosphate R in 250 ml of water, mix, and add 190 ml of sodium hydroxide (0.2 mol/l) and 400 ml of water. Add 10.0 g of pancreatin R, mix, and adjust the resulting solution with sodium hydroxide (0.2 mol/l) to a pH of 7.5 ± 0.1. Dilute with sufficient water to produce 1000 ml.

The requirements are met if the quantities of active ingredient (s) dissolved from the dosage forms tested conform to the following table, unless otherwise specified in the individual monograph.

Stage	Samples tested	Acceptance criteria
S_1	6	Each unit is not less than Q + 5%
S_2	6	Average of 12 units (S_1 + S_2) is equal to or greater than Q, and no unit is less than Q–15%
S_3	12	Average of 24 units (S_1 + S_2 + S_3) is equal to or greater than Q; not more than 2 units are less than Q–15%; no unit is less than Q–25%

Continue testing through the three stages unless the results conform at either S_1 or S_2. The quantity, Q, is the released labelled content of active ingredient as a percentage as specified in the individual monograph; both the 5% and 15% values in the acceptance table are percentages of the labelled content so that these values and Q are in the same terms.

Isolated Key Points

- Sublingual tablet is designed to dissolve in small quantity of saliva and used when immediate action within few minutes is desired.
- Implants are inserted into subcutaneous tissue by surgical procedures where they are very slowly absorbed over a period of a month or a year.
- Excipients are any component other than active pharmaceutical ingredient (s) intentionally added to the formulation of a dosage form.
- Excipients play a crucial role in determining the final suitable dosage form and determining the bioavailability.
- Various excipients used in tablet formulation are diluents, binders, disintegrants, lubricants, antiadherents, glidants, wetting agents, dissolution retardants, dissolution enhancers, absorbents, buffers, antioxidants, chelating agents, preservatives, colours, flavours, sweeteners, etc.
- Diluents make the required bulk of the tablet when the drug dosage itself is inadequate to produce tablets of adequate weight and size.
- Microcrystalline cellulose (MCC) is perhaps the most widely used direct-compression at binders are added in tablet formulation to have required flow property and compressibility of powders.
- Wet granulation, dry granulation/slugging, direct compression are major granule manufacturing methods.
- Disintegrants are added to tablet to induce break-up when it comes in contact with aqueous fluid.
- Disintegration by capillary action or by swelling is the major mechanism for disintegrants.
- Lubricants are added to reduce the friction during compression.
- Glidants improve the flow property of material/granules.
- Only FD and C or D and C approved colourants can be incorporated into tablet formulation.

- Direct compression is one of the most advanced technologies to prepare tablets.
- Wet granulation has been and continues to be the most widely used agglomeration process.
- In the dry granulation process granulation takes place without utilizing liquid.

Tablets Problems

- Capping and lamination are the defects arising as a result of air-entrapment in the granular material
- Cracking is due to rapid expansion of tablets, when deep concave punches are used
- Sticking, Picking and Binding are the imperfections related to more amount of binder in granules
- Mottling is an imperfection arising due to more than one factor: a coloured drug, dirt in granules or the use of an oily lubricant
- Double-impression is related to a machine defect: It is caused by the free rotation of punches that have some engraving on the punch-faces.

PRACTISE QUESTIONS

1. Define the term "Tablets"? Name the different categories of excipients used in the preparation of compressed tablets.
2. Define the term "Excipient". Enlist the various excipients used in the formulation of tablet.
3. Name of the various diluents commonly used in the formulation of a tablet.
4. Why is a binding agent required in certain types of tablets?
5. Give a list of the granulating agents which are commonly used in the moist granulation method.
6. What are the various tests usually employed for the purpose of evaluation of tablets?
7. What materials, are commonly used in the enteric coating of tablets?
8. Name the materials commonly used in film coating of tablets.
9. What are the various type of lubricants used as excipients in compressed tablets?
10. What are advantages and disadvantages of tablets?

11. Give the advantages of film coating of tablets.
12. How does a disintegrating agent help to disintegrate a tablet in the stomach?
13. Mention the properties of an ideal enteric coating material.
14. Why are tablets still considered to be a formulation of choice among oral preparations?
15. Give in brief the various steps involved in the manufacturing of compressed tablets.
16. Describe the various stages, construction and working of a "single-punch tablet making machine".
17. Discuss in brief the various tests which are generally done to maintain the quality control of tablets.
18. Discuss in brief the common defects which can occur in compressed tablets. How can such defects be removed.
19. Write short notes on the following:
    i. Effervescent tablets
    ii. Enteric coated tablets
    iii. Multiple compressed tablets
    iv. Hypodermic tablets
    v. Lozenges
    vi. Sustained action tablets
    vii. Sublingual tablets
20. Write short notes on:
    a. Disintegration test
    b. Dissolution test
    c. Excipients used in tablet formulation
    d. Common defects which occurs in compressed tablets.

OBJECTIVE TYPE QUESTIONS

1. Precompression can be used to solve the problem:
   i. Capping and lamination
   ii. Mottling
   iii. Picking and sticking
   iv. Double impression
2. Picking and sticking problems may be observed due to:
   i. Excess glidant
   ii. Excess diluent
   iii. Insufficient lubrication
   iv. Insufficient compression

3. Engraving or embossing or debossing on the upper punch tip like small enclosed areas in the letters like "D", "O" or "Q" may result in:
   i. Sticking
   ii. Picking
   iii. Mottling
   iv. Tablet breaking

4. Unequal distribution of colour on tablet surface is called as:
   i. Mottling
   ii. Sticking
   iii. Picking
   iv. Chipping

5. Using bright coloring agent that will mask all the color variations of the ingredients in the formula helps in avoiding:
   i. Picking
   ii. Capping
   iii. Mottling
   iv. Sticking

6. The reason for mottling may be:
   i. Double impression
   ii. Migration of dye to the surface of granulation during drying
   iii. Improper mixing
   iv. Excess lubrication

7. Bridging/arching and rat-holing of granules at the bottom of the hopper results in:
   i. Poor mixing
   ii. Poor flow
   iii. Mottling
   iv. Capping

8. The processing problem of tablets that can be revealed by friability test is:
   i. Picking
   ii. Capping and lamination
   iii. Mottling
   iv. Sticking
   v. None of the above

9. In general the disintegration time of uncoated compressed tablet is _____.

10. According to IP the shape of a tablet is defined as _____.

11. The film coating of tablets protects their medicaments from _____.

12. The vaginal tablets are _____or _____ shaped to facilitate _____ in the vagina.

13. The dry cota tablet machine is used for the manufacturing of _____, _____ and _____ tablets .

14. The film coating of tablets is done to make them _____before sugar coating.

15. In capping, there is _____ or _____ removal of _____ or _____ portion of the tablet.

16. In picking the material is _____ or _____ by the upper punch form the _____ surface of the tablet.

17. The enteric coated tablets are made to get disintegrated in the _____.

18. The tablets are tested for their mechanical strength in order to ensure that they can withstand _____ handling and _____.

19. Lozenges are so designed as the exert a local effect in the _____ or _____.

20. Buccal tablets are placed between the _____ and _____ or check so that they are dissolved and _____ directly.

21. Match the following.

Column I	Column II
a. Sugar coating of tablet	i. Is done to disintegrate it in the intestine.
b. The disintegration technique in not required	ii. For sugar coating, film coating and enteric coating.
c. Pan coating technique is used	iii. In lozenge tablets and chewable tablets.
d. The enteric coating of tablet	iv. Is done to mask the unpleasant odour and taste of the medicament.

ANSWERS

1. i
2. iii
3. ii
4. i
5. iii
6. ii
7. ii
8. ii
9. 15 mts
10. Circular with flat or convex faces
11. Atmospheric effect
12. Ovoid, pear, retention
13. Multiple compressed, multicoloured press coated
14. Water proof
15. Partial, complete, top, bottom
16. Removed, picked up, upper
17. Intestine
18. Normal risk, transportation
19. Mouth, throat
20. Gum, lips, absorbed
21. A (iv) B (iii) C (ii) D (i)

4

Tablet Coating

Coating is defined as "tablets covered with one or more layers of mixture of various substances such as natural or synthetic resins, gums, inactive and insoluble filler, sugar, plasticizer, polyhydric alcohol, waxes, authorized colouring material and sometimes flavoring material. Coating may also contain active ingredient. Substances used for coating are usually applied as solution or suspension under conditions where vehicle evaporates.

Advantages of Tablet Coating

    i. Prevent irritation of oesophagus and stomach

    ii. Prevent bad taste

    iii. Prevent inactivation of drug in the stomach

    iv. Improve drug effectiveness

    v. Prolong dosing interval in the form of sustain release or prolong release dosage form.

    vi. Improve dosing interval

    vii. Better patient compliance

    viii. Prevent the active drug from moisture

    ix. Prevent dust formation

    x. Reduce influence of atmosphere

    xi. Improve drug stability

    xii. Prolong shelf life

    xiii. Overcome bad taste

    xiv. Improve product identity

    xv. Improve appearance and acceptability.

Tablet coating is the application of coating composition to moving bed of tablets with concurrent use of heated air to facilitate evaporation of solvent.

Type of Tablet Coating Process

- Sugar coating
- Film coating
- Enteric coating
- Specialized coating

1. Sugar Coating

The sugar coating protects the drug from the atmosphere and provides a barrier to objectionable taste. The coating is water soluble and quickly dissolves after swallowing sugar coating helps in taste masking, smoothing the tablet core, colouring and modified release. The disadvantages of sugar coating are that it requires more time and expertise also it increases size, weight and shipping costs.

Sugar coating process involves following steps:

i. *Sealing/water proofing:* Provides a moisture barrier and harden the tablet surface.

ii. *Subcoating:* Increases the bulk and round off the tablet edges.

iii. *Grossing/smoothing:* Smoothes out the subcoated surface and increases the tablet size.

iv. *Colouring:* Gives colour to the tablet.

v. *Polishing:* Give characteristics gloss.

Sealing

It is also called as water proofing, it provides a moisture barrier and hardness the surface of the tablet in order to minimize attritional effects. The sealants are generally water-insoluble polymers/film formers applied from an organic solvent solution. The quantities of material applied as a sealing coat will depend primarily on the tablet porosity, since highly porous tablets will tend to soak up the first application of solution, thus preventing it from spreading uniformly across the surface of every tablet in the batch. Therefore, one or more further application of resin solution may be required to ensure that the tablet cores are sealed effectively.

Common materials used as a sealant include shellac, cellulose acetate phthalate (CAP), polyvinylacetate phthalate (PVAP), hyroxypropyl cellulose, hydroxypropyl methylcellulose (HPMC), etc.

Subcoating

It is the actual sugar coating process and provides the rapid buildup necessary to round up the tablet edge. It also acts as the foundation for the smoothing and colour coats. The methods used for subcoating are:

- The application of gum based solution followed by dusting with powder and then drying.
- The application of a suspension of dry powder in gum/ sucrose solution followed by drying.

Thus subcoating is a sandwich of alternate layer of gum and powder. It is necessary to remove the bulk of the water after each application of coating syrup.

Table 4.1: Binder solution used for subcoating

Ingredient	% w/w	
Gelatin	6	3.3
Gum acacia (powdered)	8	8.7
Sucrose (powdered)	45	55.3
Distilled water	upto 100	upto 100

Table 4.2: Dusting powder used for subcoating

Ingredient	% w/w	
Calcium carbonate	40.0	–
Titanium dioxide	5.0	1.0
Talc, asbestos free	25.0	61.0
Sucrose (powdered)	28.0	38.6
Gum acacia (powdered)	2.0	–

Smoothing

It is also called as grossing, in this process smoothing and filling of the irregularity on the surface generated during subcoating is done. If the subcoating is rough with high amount of

Table 4.3: Suspension used for subcoating

Ingredient	% w/w
Sucrose	40.0
Calcium carbonate	20.0
Talc, asbestos free	12.0
Gum acacia (powdered)	2.0
Titanium dioxide	1.0
Distilled water	25.0

irregularities then the use of grossing syrup containing suspended solids will provide better texture it also help in increasing the bulk of tablet. Smoothing is generally done by application of a simple syrup solution (approximately 60–70% sugar solid). This syrup generally contains pigments, starch, gelatin, acacia and opacifier.

Colour Coating

This stage is very important in the successful completion of a sugar coating process and involves the multiple application of syrup solution (60–70% sugar) containing the desired colouring matter. Mainly soluble dyes were used in the sugar coating to achieve the desired colour, since the soluble dye will migrate to the surface during drying. But nowadays the insoluble certified lakes are more frequently used.

Polishing

Polishing is achieved by applying the mixture of waxes like beeswax, carnubawax, candelila wax or hard paraffin wax to tablets in polishing pan.

2. Film Coating

Film coating is deposition of a thin film of polymer over the tablet core. Conventional pan equipment may be used but nowaday's more sophisticated equipment are employed to have a high degree of automation and coating time. Firstly the polymer is dissolved in the solvent. Other additives like plasticizers and pigments are added. Resulting solution is sprayed onto a rotated tablet bed. Continuous drying is done which cause removal of the solvent, giving thin deposition of coating material over the tablet.

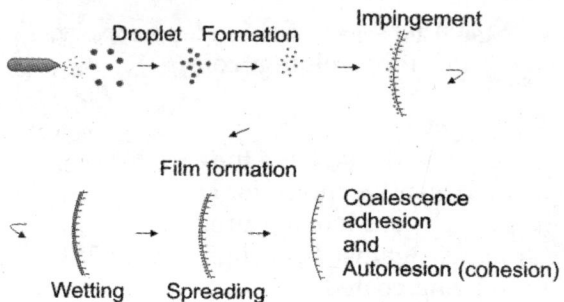

Fig. 4.1: Showing film coating process

Generally spray process is used in preparation of film coated tablets. Accela-cota is the prototype of perforated cylindrical drum providing high drying air capacity. Fluidized bed equipment has made considerable impact where tablets are moving in a stream of air passing through the perforated bottom of a cylindrical column. For fluidized bed coating, very hard tablets (hardness >20 N) have to be used. Film coating is more favored over sugar coating.

Table 4.4: Difference between film coating and sugar coating

Features	Film coating	Sugar coating
Tablet appearance	Usually not as shiny as sugar coat type.	Rounded with high degree of polish
Tablet weight increase	2–3%	30–50%
Tablet logo or 'break lines'	Possible	Not possible
Process stages	Usually single stage	Multistage process
Operator training required	Easy training of operator	Moderate

Materials Used in Film Coating

- Film formers, which may be enteric or nonenteric
- Solvents
- Plasticizers
- Colourants

- Opaquant-extenders
- Miscellaneous coating solution components.

Film Formers

An ideal film former should have the following characteristics:
i. Soluble in solvent of choice for coating preparation
ii. Should give elegant looking product
iii. High stability against heat, light, moisture, air and the substance being coated
iv. No inherent colour, taste or odor
v. Nontoxic and should have no pharmacological activity
vi. High resistance to cracking
vii. Compatible to printing procedure.

Table 4.5: Some commonly used film former polymers

Nonenteric polymers	Enteric polymers
Hypromellose	Hypromellose phthalate
Hydroxyethyl cellulose	Polyvinyl acetate phthalate
Hydroxyethylmethyl cellulose	Cellulose acetate phthalate
Carboxymethyl cellulose sodium	Polymethacrylates
Hydroxypropyl cellulose	Shellac
Ethyl cellulose	
Polyethylene glycol	

Hydroxypropyl Methylcellulose (HPMC)

It is a polymer of choice for air suspension and pan spray coating systems because of solubility characteristic in gastric fluid, organic and aqueous solvent system. Advantages are: it does not affect tablet disintegration and drug availability, it is cheap, flexible, highly resistant to heat, light and moisture, it has no taste and odor, colour and other additives can be easily incorporated.

Disadvantage: When it is used alone, the polymer has tendency to bridge or fill the debossed tablet surfaces. Hence, mixture of HPMC and other polymers is used.

Ethyl Cellulose (EC)

It is completely insoluble in water and gastric fluids. Hence, it is used in combination with water-soluble additives like HPMC and not alone. Unplasticized ethyl cellulose films are brittle and require film modifiers to obtain an acceptable film formulation. Aqua coat is aqueous polymeric dispersion utilizing ethyl cellulose. These pseudolatex systems contain high solids, low viscosity compositions that have coating properties quite different from regular ethyl cellulose solution.

Hydroxypropyl Cellulose (HPC)

It is soluble in water below 40°C (insoluble above 45°C), gastric fluid and many polar organic solvents. HPC is extremely tacky as it dries from solution system. It is used for sub-coat and not for colour or glass coat. It gives very flexible film.

Sodium Carboxymethyl Cellulose

It is available in medium, high and extra high viscosity grades. It is easily dispersed in water to form colloidal solutions but it is insoluble in most organic solvents and hence not a material of choice for coating solution based on organic solvents. Films prepared by it are brittle but adhere well to tablets. Partially dried films of are tacky. So coating compositions must be modified with additives.

Polyethylene Glycols (PEG)

Lower molecular weights PEG (200–600) are liquid at room temperature and are used as plasticizers. High molecular weights PEG (900–8000 series) are white, waxy solids at room temperature. Combination of PEG waxes with CAP gives films that are soluble in gastric fluids.

Acrylate Polymers

It is marketed under the name of Eudragit® E is freely soluble in gastric fluid up to pH 5 and co-polymer. Only eudragit expandable and permeable above pH 5. This material is available as organic solution (12.5% in isopropanol/acetone), solid material or 30% aqueous RL dispersion. Eudragit® and RS are co-polymers with low content of quaternary ammonium groups. These are available only as organic solutions and solid materials. They produce films for delayed action (pH dependent).

Solvents

Solvents are used to dissolve or disperse the polymers and other additives and convey them to substrate surface. Ideal solvent should have the following characteristics:

i. Should be either dissolve/disperse polymer system.
ii. Should easily disperse other additives.
iii. Only small concentration of polymers (2–10%) is required.
iv. Should be colourless, tasteless, odorless, inexpensive, inert and nontoxic.
v. Rapid drying rate.
vi. Should not cause environmental pollution.

Mostly solvents are used either alone or in combination with water, ethanol, methanol, isopropanol, chloroform, acetone, methylene chloride, etc. water is most frequently used it is economic and easily available. For drugs sensitive to water, non-aqueous solvents are used.

Plasticizers

Plasticizers are simply relatively low molecular weight materials which have the capacity to alter the physical properties of the polymer to render it more useful in performing its function as a film-coating material. They are generally used in concentration (0.5–2.0%).

When solvent is removed, most polymeric materials tend to pack together in 3-D honey comb arrangement. "Internal" or "External" plasticizing technique is used to modify quality of film. Combination of plasticizer may be used to get desired effect.

Commonly used plasticizers are castor oil, PG, glycerin, lower molecular weight (200–400 series), PEG, surfactants, etc. For aqueous coating PEG and PG are more used while castor oil and spans are primarily used for organic-solvent based

Table 4.6: Some common plasticizers

Polyols	Organic esters	Oils/glycerides
Glycerol	Phthalate esters	Castor oil
Propylene glycol	Citrate esters	Fractionated coconut oil
Polyethylene glycol (PEG)	Triacetin	Acetylated Monoglycerides

coating solution. External plasticizer should be soluble in the solvent system used for dissolving the film former and plasticizer. The plasticizer and the film former must be at least partially soluble or miscible in each other.

Colourants

These materials are generally used as ingredients in film coating formulae to contribute to the visual appeal of the product, but they also improve the product in other ways they are used in concentration (2.5–8%).

Table 4.7: Some common colourants

Organic dyes and their lakes	Inorganic colors	Natural colors
Sunset yellow	Ion oxide red, black	Carmine
Erythrosine	Titanium dioxide	Anthocyanine
tartrazine		ribofloavine

For proper distribution of suspended colourants in the coating solution requires the use of the powdered colourants (<10 microns). Most common colourants in use are certified FD and C or D and C colourants. These are synthetic dyes or lakes. Lakes are choice for sugar or film coating as they give reproducible results. Concentration of colourants in the coating solutions depends on the colour shade desired, the type of dye, and the concentration of opaquant-extenders. If very light shade is desired, concentration of less than 0.01% may be adequate on the other hand, if a dark colour is desired a concentration of more than 2.0% may be required. The inorganic materials (e.g. iron oxide) and the natural colouring materials (e.g. anthocyanins, carotenoids) are also used to prepare coating solution. Magenta red dye is non-absorbable in biologic system and resistant to degradation in the gastro (opaque colour concentrate for film coating) and intestinal track.

Opacifier

These are very fine inorganic powder used to provide more pastel colours and increase film coverage. These inorganic materials provide white coat or mask colour of the tablet core. Colourants are very expensive and higher concentration is required. These inorganic materials are cheap. In presence of these inorganic materials, amount of colourants required decreases. Most commonly used materials are titanium dioxide, silicate (talc and aluminum silicates), carbonates (magnesium carbonates), oxides (magnesium oxide) and hydroxides (aluminum hydroxides).

Miscellaneous Coating Solution Component

Flavors, sweeteners, surfactants, antioxidants, antimicrobials, etc. may be incorporated into the coating solution.

3. Enteric Coating

Enteric coatings are those which remain intact in the stomach (and exhibit low permeability to gastric fluids) but break down readily once the dosage form reaches the small intestine. This type of coating is used to protect tablet core from disintegration in the acid environment of the stomach and is used because of following reasons:

   i. To maintain the activity of drugs that are unstable when exposed to the gastric milieu (e.g. erythromycin and pancreatin).

   ii. To minimize either nausea or bleeding that occurs with those drugs that irritate the gastric mucosa (e.g. aspirin and certain steroids).

   iii. To prevent irritation of stomach by certain drugs like sodium salicylate.

   iv. Delivery of API into intestine.

   v. To provide a delayed release.

   Generally two types of enteric layer systems are used:

One layer system: The coating formulation is applied in one homogeneous layer, which can be whites-opaque or coloured. In this only one application is needed.

Two layer system: To prepare enteric tablets of high quality and pleasing appearance the enteric formulation is applied first, followed by coloured film. Both layers can be of enteric polymer or only the basic layer contains enteric polymer while top layer is fast disintegrating and water-soluble polymer.

Ideal properties of enteric coating material are listed below:

i. Resistance to gastric fluids

ii. Permeable to intestinal fluid

iii. Compatibility with most coating solution components and the drug substance

iv. Formation of continuous film

v. Nontoxic, cheap and ease of application

Polymers used for enteric coating are as follow:

Cellulose Acetate Phthalate (CAP)

It is widely used in industry. It is reconstituted colloidal dispersion of latex particles. It is composed of solid or semisolid polymer spheres of CAP ranging in size from 0.05–3 microns. Cellulose Acetate Trimellitate (CAT) developed as an ammoniated aqueous formulation showed faster dissolution than a similar formulation of CAP. Disadvantages include: It dissolves above pH 6 only, delays absorption of drugs, it is hygroscopic and permeable to moisture in comparison with other enteric polymer, it is susceptible to hydrolytic removal of phthalic and acetic acid changing film properties. CAP films are brittle and usually used with other hydrophobic film forming materials.

Acrylate Polymers

Eudragit L and Eudragit S are two forms of commercially available enteric acrylic resins. Both of them produce films resistant to gastric fluid. Eudragit L and S are soluble in intestinal fluid at pH 6 and 7 respectively. Eudragit L is available as an organic solution, solid or aqueous dispersion. Eudragit S is available only as an organic solution and solid.

Hydroxypropyl Methylcellulose Phthalate

HPMCP 50, 55 and 55-s (also called HP-50, HP-55 and HP-55-s) is widely used. HP-55 is recommended for general enteric preparation while HP-50 and HP-55-s for special cases. These polymers dissolve at a pH 5–5.5.

Polyvinyl Acetate Phthalate

It is similar to HP-55 in stability and pH dependent solubility.

4. Specialized Coating

Compressed Coating

This type of coating requires a specialization tablet machine. Compression coating is not widely used but it has advantages in some cases in which the tablet core cannot tolerate organic solvent or water and yet needs to be coated for taste masking or to provide delayed or enteric properties to the finished product and also to prevent incompatibility by separating incompatible ingredients.

Electrostatic Coating

Electrostatic coating is an efficient method of applying coating to conductive substrates. A strong electrostatic charge is applied to the substrate. The coating material containing conductive ionic species of opposite charge is sprayed onto the charged substrate. Complete and uniform coating of corners and adaptability of this method to such relatively nonconductive substrate as pharmaceutical is limited.

Dip Coating

Coating is applied to the tablet cores by dipping them into the coating liquid. The wet tablets are dried in a conventional manner in coating pan. Alternative dipping and drying steps may be repeated several times to obtain the desired coating. This process lacks the speed, versatility, and reliability of spray-coating techniques. Specialized equipment has been developed to dip-coat tablets, but no commercial pharmaceutical application has been obtained.

Vacuum Film Coating

Vacuum film coating is a new coating procedure that employs a specially designed baffled pan. The pan is hot water jacketed, and it can be sealed to achieve a vacuum system. The tablets are placed in the sealed pan, and the air in the pan is displaced by nitrogen before the desired vacuum level is obtained. The coating solution is then applied with airless spray system. The evaporation is caused by the heated pan, and the vapour is removed by the vacuum system. Because there is no high velocity heated air, the energy requirement is low and coating efficiency is high. Organic solvent can be effectively used with this coating system with minimum environmental or safety concerns.

Factors Affecting Coating

Air Capacity

This value represents the quantity of water or solvent that can be removed during the coating process which depends on the quantity of air flowing through the tablet bed, temperature of the air and quantity of water that the inlet air contains. The coating contains the ingredients that are to be applied on the tablet surface and solvents which act as carrier for the ingredients.

Surface Area of Tablet

It plays an important role for uniform coating. The total surface area for unit weight decreases significantly from smaller to larger tablets. Application of a film with the same thickness requires less coating composition. In the coating process only a portion of the total surface is coated. Continuous partial coating and recycling eventually results in fully coated tablets.

Coating Efficiency of Machine

Tablet coaters use the expression "coating efficiency" a value obtained by dividing the net increase in coated tablet weight by the total nonvolatile coating weight applied to the tablet. Ideally 90–95% of the applied film coating should be on the tablet surface. Coating efficiency for conventional sugar coating is much less and 60% would be acceptable. The significant difference in coating efficiency between film and sugar coating relates to the quantity of coating material that collects on the wall.

Equipment used for coating:
- The standard coating pan
- The perforated coating pan
- The fluidized bed coater
    1. Standard coating pan, e.g. pellegrin pan system, immersion sword system, immersion tube system.
    2. Perforated pan system, e.g. accela-cota system, hicoater system, glattcoater system driacoated system.
    3. Fluidized bed coater.

Conventional Pan System

It consists of a circular metal pan mounted somewhat angularly on a stand and is rotated on its horizontal axis by a motor. Heated air is directed into the pan and onto the tablet bed surface, and is exhausted by means of ducts positioned through the front of the pan.

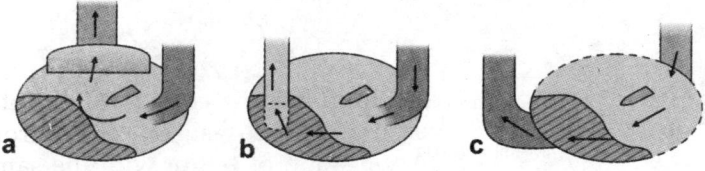

Figs 4.2a to c: (a) Conventional coating pan, (b) Upgraded conventional coating pan, (c) Side vented coating pan

Characteristic features of conventional pan system are: Generally, the energy required for evaporating the moisture from the coating layers is derived from the drying air. The duration of the coating process as well as the quality of the end-product thus crucially depend on the efficiency of heat and mass transfer. Increasing the heat and mass transfer either directly (for example, by increasing temperature and rotation speed or implementation of perforations) or indirectly by improving the drying air supply can improve drying efficiency. With the conventional drying method, the drying air is blown across the surface of the core bed. As only the surface of the core bed is exposed to the drying air, insufficient drying of core materials and impaired spraying processes might occur. Hence, different drying gadgets have been developed, of which the two conventional ones are:

   i. Immersion sword and
  ii. Immersion tube.

Immersion Sword

With the immersion sword system, drying air is introduced through a perforated metal sword device that is immersed in the tablet bed. The drying air flows upward from the sword through the bed. Since the air is more intimately mixed with the wetted tablets, a more efficient drying environment is provided (Fig. 4.3).

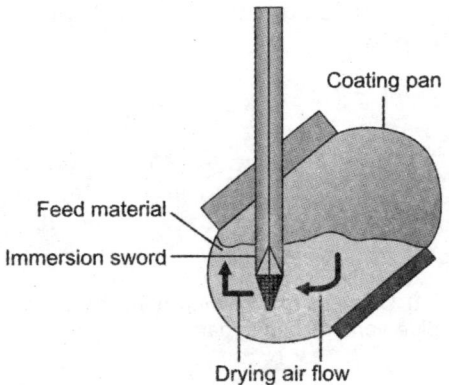

Fig. 4.3: Immersion sword system

Immersion Tube

In this type of system the immersed tube delivers the heated air, and a spray nozzle is built in the tip of the tube. During this operation, the coating solution is applied simultaneously with the heated air from the immersed tube. The drying air flows upward through the tablet bed and is exhausted by a conventional duct. Both the immersion sword and immersion tube systems are adaptable to conventional coating pans. Relatively rapid processing times have been reported for both film and sugar coating with this system (Fig. 4.4).

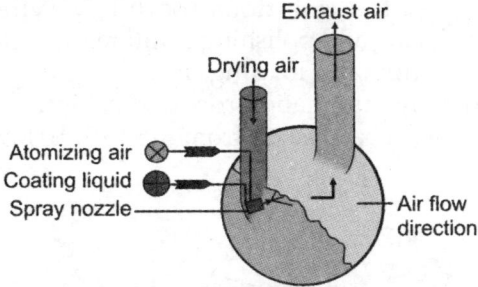

Fig. 4.4: Immersion tube system

Accela-cota and Driacoater Systems

Accela-cota

In Accela-cota and Hi-coater systems, drying air is directed into the drum, is then passed through the tablet bed, and is exhausted through perforation in the drum.

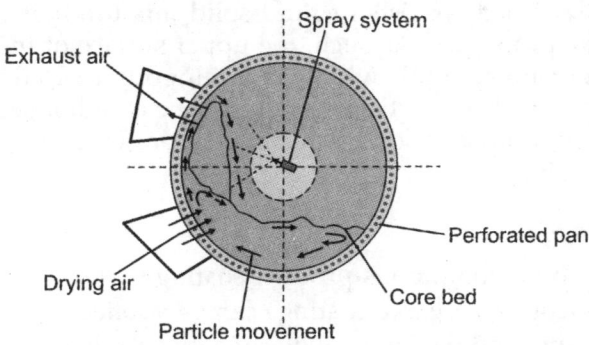

Fig. 4.5: Accela-cota

Driacoater

The driacoater introduces drying air through hollow perforated ribs located on inside periphery of the drum. As coating pan rotates the ribs dip into the tablet bed, and drying air passes through and fluidizes the tablet bed. Air is exhausted from back of the pan. For hard sugar coating, driacoater with perforated multisided drums are used. The machines are capable to handle sugar and sugar free solutions (Sorbitol, Xylitol, Malitol, Isomalt, etc.) glazing and polishing solutions as well as aqueous suspensions. Automatic loading and unloading, inside pan cleaning and fully automatic process capabilities characterize this driacoater with batch sizes from 625 to 3750 litres (Fig. 4.6).

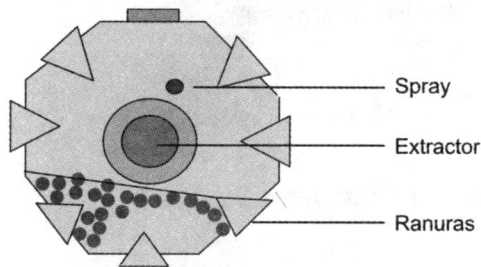

Fig. 4.6: Driacoater

Fluidized Bed Dryer (FBD)

A fluidized bed consists of fluid-solid mixture that exhibits fluid-like properties. As such, the upper surface of the bed is relatively horizontal, which is analogous to hydrostatic behavior. The bed can be considered to be an inhomogeneous mixture of fluid and solid that can be represented by a single bulk density.

Advantages

i. Uniform, continuous product coating.

ii. Aqueous or organic coatings can be applied.

iii. Coating and drying take place in one machine.

iv. The coating process and the filling and emptying of the machine can be carried out in complete isolation and without product spreading into the environment.

v. When using organic solvents, the process machines can be made inert and used with a solvent recovery system.

Principle of Operation

With fluid bed coating, particles are fluidized and the coating fluid sprayed on and dried. Small droplets and a low viscosity

of the spray medium ensure an even product coating. The various types of fluid bed systems (Fig. 4.7) are:
1. Top spray coating
2. Bottom spray coating (wurster coating)
3. Tangential spray coating (rotor pellet coating).

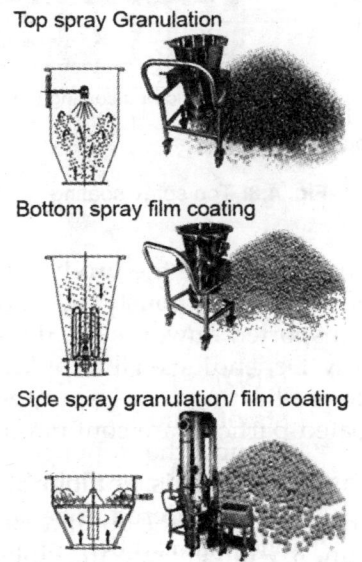

Top spray Granulation

Bottom spray film coating

Side spray granulation/ film coating

Fig. 4.7: Types of fluid bed systems

Top Spray Coating

This process is used for general coatings right up to enteric coating. With top spray coating in the fluid bed (batch and continuous), particles are fluidized in the flow of heated air, which is introduced into the product container via a base plate (Fig. 4.8).

The coating liquid is sprayed into the fluid bed from above against the air flow (countercurrent) by means of a nozzle. Drying takes place as the particles continue to move upwards in the air flow. Small droplets and a low viscosity of the spray medium ensure that the distribution is uniform. Coating in the continuous fluid bed is particularly suitable for protective

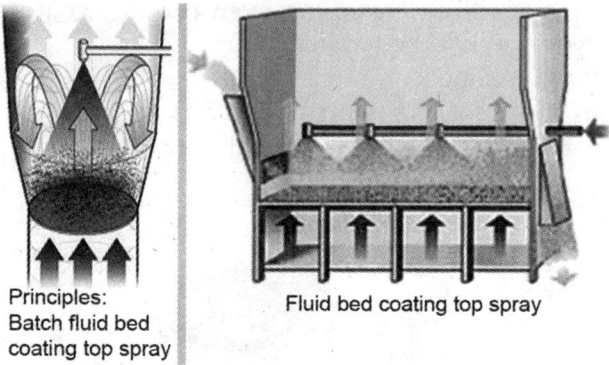

Principles:
Batch fluid bed
coating top spray

Fluid bed coating top spray

Fig. 4.8: Top spray coating

coatings/colour coatings where the product throughput rates are high. The product is continuously fed into one side of the machine and is transported onwards via the sieve bottom by means of the air flow. Depending on the application, the system is sub-divided into pre-heating zones, spray zones and drying zones. The dry coated particles are continuously extracted.

Bottom Spray Coating (Continuous Fluid Bed)

When the hot air flows through the bottom screen of container and coating column, it will generate the siphonage principle. Convection is created through the strong force from bottom toward top. The granules will then fall down and will be sucked into the coating column again, while the bottom spray gun will spray towards top to achieve coating purpose. Particularly suitable for protective coatings/colour coatings where the product throughput rates are high. The product is continuously fed into one side of the machine and is transported onwards via the sieve bottom by means of the air flow (Fig. 4.9).

Depending on the application, the system is sub-divided into pre-heating zones, spray zones and drying zones whereby spraying can take place from below in the form of a bottom spray. The dry, coated particles are continuously extracted.

Tangential Spray Coating (Rotor Pellet Coating)

The cores (seeds) are placed on the turntable and hot air is blown upward between the turntable and the granulation

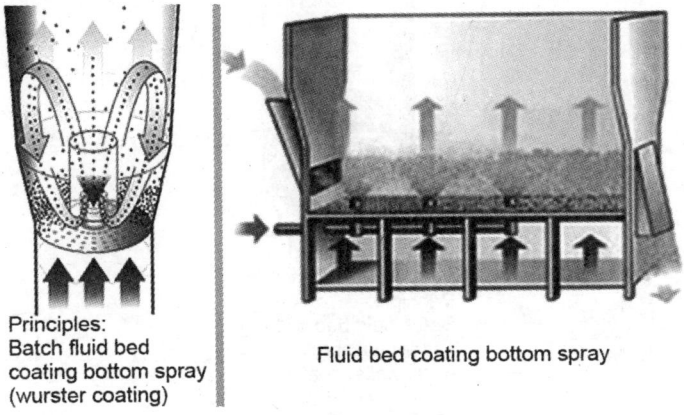

Principles:
Batch fluid bed
coating bottom spray
(wurster coating)

Fluid bed coating bottom spray

Fig. 4.9: Bottom spray coating

area. The passage of air causes the cores to roll on the turntable; at the same time, the coating solution is sprayed on the rolling cores through the pump and spray gun. The process involves simultaneous coating and drying of the cores, layer after layer, until the repeated actions achieve the desired coating thickness or granule size. Powder coating is achieved by charging powder and spray binder at the same time. Powder and binder are combined to form the required layer, thus the repeated layer after layer actions can achieve the desired granule size or coating thickness. Ideal for coatings with high solid content. The product is set into a spiral motion by means of a rotating base plate, which has air fed into the powder bed at its edge. The spray nozzle is arranged tangentially to the rotor disc and also sprays concurrently into the powder bed. Very thick film layers can be applied by means of the rotor method (Fig. 4.10).

Problems in Tablet Coating

Orange Peel Effect

A surface defect resulting in the film being rough and nonglossy. Appearance is similar to that of an orange peel off.

Cause: Inadequate spreading of the coating solution before drying (Table 4.8).

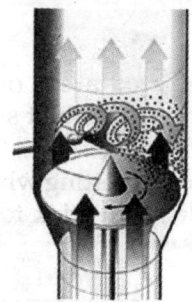

Principle:
Batch fluid bed coating
Tangential spray
(rotor pellet coating)

Fig. 4.10: Tangential spray coating

Table 4.8: Causes and rectification of orange peel/roughness

S. no.	Causes	Rectification
1.	Rapid drying	Optimizing drying conditions
2.	High solution viscosity	Decreasing viscosity of solution

Cratering

It is due to film coating whereby volcanic-like craters appears on the tablet surface.

Cause: The coating solution penetrates into the tablet, generally at the crown where the surface is more porous, causing localized disintegration of the core and disruption of the coating.

Table 4.9: Causes and rectification of cratering

S. no.	Causes	Rectification
1.	Inefficient drying.	By optimizing drying conditions.
2.	Higher rate of application of coating solution.	Increase viscosity of coating solution to decrease spray application rate and decreasing the rate of application.

Picking

It is defined as when isolated areas of film are pulled away from the surface and when the tablet sticks together and then part.

Cause: Due to localize overwetting which produces wet tablet bed where adjacent tablets can stick together and then break apart.

Table 4.10: Causes and rectification of picking

S. no.	Cause	Rectification
1.	Inefficient drying.	Use optimum and efficient drying conditions or increase the inlet air temperature.
2.	Higher rate of application of coating solution.	Decrease the rater of application of coating solution by increasing viscosity of coating solution.

Pitting

It is defect whereby pits occur in the surface of a tablet core without any visible disruption of the film coating.

Cause: Temperature of the tablet core is greater than the melting point of the materials used in the tablet formulation.

Table 4.11: Cause and rectification of pitting

Cause	Rectification
Improper drying (inlet air) temperature.	Changing the drying (inlet air) temperature such that the temperature of the tablet core is not greater than the melting point of the batch of additives used.

Blistering

It is defined as the detachment of film from the substrate forming blister.

Cause: Entrapment of gases in or beneath the film due to overheating either during spraying or at the end of the coating.

Table 4.12: Cause and rectification of blistering

Cause	Rectification
High temperature during drying effecting the strength, elasticity and adhesion of the film.	Use mild drying condition.

Chipping

It occurs when the film becomes chipped and dented, this occurs generally at the edges of the tablet.

Cause: Less fluidizing air or speed of rotation of the drum in pan coating.

Table 4.13: Cause and rectification of chipping

Cause	Rectification
High degree of attrition during coating process.	Increasing hardness of the film by using high molecular weight polymer.

Blooming

In this the coating becomes dull immediately or after prolonged storage at high temperatures.

Cause: Due to collection of low molecular weight ingredients on the surface added in the coating formulation. Generally the ingredient is plasticizer.

Table 4.14: Cause and rectification of blooming

Cause	Rectification
Use of high concentration and low molecular weight plasticizer.	Decreasing plasticizer concentration and increasing molecular weight of plasticizer.

Cracking/Splitting

In this the film either cracks across the crown of the tablet (cracking) or splits around the edges of the tablet (splitting).

Cause: Internal stress in the film exceeds tensile strength of the film.

Table 4.15: Cause and rectification of cracking/splitting

Cause	Rectification
Use of higher molecular weight polymers.	Use lower molecular weight polymers or polymeric blends. Changing the plasticizer and concentration.

Blushing

It is described as whitish specks or haziness in the film.

Cause: It is thought to be due to precipitated polymer exacerbated by the use of high coating temperature.

Table 4.16: Causes and rectification of blushing

S. no.	Causes	Rectification
1.	High coating temperature.	Decrease the drying air temperature.
2.	Use of sorbitol along with hydroxypropyl cellulose, hydroxypropyl methyl. cellulose, methyl cellulose and cellulose ethers, in formulation which causes largest fall in the thermal gelation temperature.	Avoiding use of sorbitol with hydroxypropyl cellulose, hydroxypropyl methylcellulose, methyl cellulose and cellulose ethers.

Colour Variation

There is variation in colour of the film.

Cause: Change of the frequency and duration of appearance of tablets in the spray zone or the size/shape of the spray zone (Table 4.17).

Infilling

It is defect which renders the intagliations indistinctness.

Cause: Inability of foam formed by air spraying of a polymer solution which breaks. The foam droplets on the surface of the

Table 4.17: Cause and rectification of colour variation

Cause	Rectification
Inadequate mixing, uneven spray pattern, insufficient coating, migration of soluble dyes-plasticizers and other additives during drying.	By geometric mixing, using different plasticizers and using mild drying conditions.

tablet breakdown readily due to attrition but the intagliations form a protected area allowing the foam to accumulate and "set". Once the foam has accumulated to a level approaching the outer contour of the tablet surface, normal attrition can occur allowing the structure to be covered with a continuous film.

Table 4.18: Cause and rectification of infilling

Cause	Rectification
Bubble or foam formation because of air spraying of a polymer solution	Add alcohol or use spray nozzle capable of finer atomization.

Twinning

This is the term for two tablets that stick together, and it is a common problem with capsule shaped tablets. It can be solved by balancing the pan speed and spray rate and reducing the spray rate or increasing the pan speed.

EVALUATION OF COATED TABLETS

Evaluation of coated tablets requires evaluation of both the coatings and the coated tablets. Physical characterization of the coating system should include particle size, preparation time and viscosity because each affects the handling and use of the powdered on step coating systems. Large particles minimizes dust and short process time have obvious advantages. Low viscosity enables to create a coating with high ration of solids, which leads to faster tablet coating. Once, tablet are coated they should be evaluated for:

   i. Gloss
  ii. Opacity
 iii. Color uniformity
  iv. Disintegration
   v. Adhesion time
  vi. Logo bridging
 vii. Film strength and flexibility.

ISOLATED KEY POINTS

- The sugar coating involves several steps like, sealing, subcoating, colour coating and printing.
- Sugar coating process yields elegant and highly glossed tablet.
- Film coating is deposition of a thin film of polymer surrounding the tablet core.
- Film coating is more favored than sugar coating because weight increase is 2–3%, single stage process, easily adaptable to controlled release, it retains colour of original core, high adaptability to GMP, automation is possible, etc.
- Accela-cota and fluidized bed equipment are widely used for film coating.
- Materials used in film coating include film formers, solvents, plasticizers, colourants, opaquant-extenders, surfactant, antioxidant, etc.
- Widely used film formers are hydroxypropyl methylcellulose (HPMC), methyl hydroxy ethyl cellulose (MHEC), ethyl cellulose (EC), hydroxy propyl cellulose (four grades available, i.e. K-15, K-30, K-60 and K-90), eudragit® RS, Eudragit® E) are used for film coating. Eudragit® L and S are used for enteric coating. Eudragit®, Eudragit®, eudragit® S are available as organic solution.
- Quality of film can be modified by plasticizer. Commonly used plasticizers include PG, glycerin, low molecular weight PEG, castor oils, etc. castor oil and spans are more used for organic-solvent based coating solution while PE and PEG are used for aqueous coating.
- FD and C or D and C certified colourants are used. Lakes are choice for film coating as they give reproducible results. Colourants are expensive and higher concentration is required. So materials like titanium dioxides, silicates, and

carbonates are used to provide more pastel colours and increase film coverage.

• Enteric coating is used to protect tablet core from disintegration in the acid environment of stomach to prevent degradation of acid sensitive API, prevent irritation to stomach by certain drugs, delivery of API into intestine, to provide a delayed release components for repeat action, etc.

• Polymers used for enteric coating are cellulose acetate phthalate (CAP), acrylates (Eudragit®L and Eudragit®S, hydroxypropyl methylcellulose phthalate (HPMCP 50, HPMCP 55 and HPMCP 55-s) and polyvinyl acetate phthalate.

• Polymers like modified acrylates, ethyl cellulose, etc. are used for the same.

COATING PROBLEMS AND REMEDY

• Blistering is due to entrapment of gases in or underneath the film due to overheating either during spraying or at the end of the coating run. Remedy is by mild drying.

• Chipping is related to higher degree of attrition associated with the coating process. Increase in molecular weight grade of polymer can solve this problem.

• Cratering is related to penetration of the coating solution into the surface of the tablet. Decrease in spray application rate and use of optimum and efficient drying conditions can solve this problem.

• Pitting is defect in which temperature of the tablet core is greater than the melting point of the materials used in tablet formulation. Dispensing with preheating procedures at the initiation of coating and modifying the drying temperature can solve this problem.

• Infilling is because of bubble/foam formation during air spraying of a polymer solution. Addition of alcohol or use of spray nozzle capable of finer atomization can solve this problem.

• Orange peel/roughness is related to inadequate spreading of the coating solution before drying. Remedy is by decrease in viscosity of coating solution.

• Cracking is seen when internal stresses in the film exceeds tensile strength of the film. This is common with higher molecular weight polymers or polymeric blends. Remedy is by using lower molecular weight polymers.

- Colour variation is because of improper mixing, uneven spray pattern, insufficient coating or migration of soluble dyes during drying. Geometric mixing, mild drying conditions and reformulation with different plasticizers can solve this problem.
- Blooming or dull film is generally because of higher concentration and lower molecular weight of plasticizer. Remedy is by using lower concentration and higher molecular grade of plasticizer.

PRACTICE QUESTIONS

1. Define the term tablet coating. Give various advantages of tablet coating.
2. Enumerate the various types of tablet coating technique. Why sugar coating is done?
3. Discuss in detail, the various steps involve in sugar coating with suitable examples of substances use.
4. Write short notes on:
   a. Binder solution used for subcoating.
   b. Dusting powder used for subcoating.
   c. Suspension used for subcoating.
5. What is film coating? Why is it done? Give difference between film coating and sugar coating.
6. Discuss in detail about various materials used in film coating with suitable examples.
7. Write short notes on (with reference to coating of tablets):
   a. Plasticizers
   b. Colorants
   c. Solvents used
   d. Film forming polymers
8. What is enteric coating? Give its significance? How enteric coating is done? Explain it with the help of suitable examples.
9. Write short notes on specialized coating techniques:
   a. Compressed coating
   b. Dip coating
   c. Vacuum film coating

10. Enumerate various factors affecting coating. List at least two equipment used for coating.
11. Discuss in brief about conventional pan coating system with the help of neat and labeled diagram.
12. Discuss in brief about immersion sword and immersion tube coating system with the help of neat and labeled diagram.
13. What is FBD? Give its advantages.
14. Write principle of operation of FBD. Describe top spray, bottom spray and tangential spray FBD in detail with neat and labeled diagram.
15. Enumerate various problems in tablet coating. How these problems can be resolved.
16. Give various methods of evaluation of coated tablets.

OBJECTIVE TYPE QUESTIONS

1. .... coating is used to protect tablet core from disintegration in the acid environment of the stomach.
2. Which of the following is not the property of enteric coating material listed below?
   i. Resistance to gastric fluids
   ii. Permeable to intestinal fluid
   iii. Give immediate release
   iv. Formation of continuous film
3. Which of the following is not a type of fluid bed system?
   1. Top spray coating
   2. Horizontal spray coating
   3. Bottom spray coating (wurster coating)
   4. Tangential spray coating (rotor pellet coating)
4. Match the following:

S. no.	Coating problems		Causes
1.	Blistering	a	Higher degree of attrition during coating process.
2.	Chipping	b	Penetration of the coating solution into the surface of tablet.
3.	Cratering	c	Inadequate spreading of the coating solution before drying.
4.	Orange peel	d	Entrapment of gases in or underneath the film.

5. Match the following:

S. n.o	Sugar coating processes		Functions
1.	Sealing/water proofing	a	Increases the bulk and round off the tablet.
2.	Subcoating	b	Smoothes the subcoated surface and increases the tablet size.
3.	Grossing/smoothing	c	Provides a moisture barrier and harden the tablet surface.
4.	Polishing	d	Give characteristics gloss.

ANSWERS

1. Enteric
2. 3
3. 2
4. 1-d, 2-a, 3-b, 4-c
5. 1-c, 2-a, 3-b, 4-d

5 Sustained and Controlled Release Dosage Forms

DEFINITION

Well-characterized and reproducible dosage form, which is designed to control drug release profile at specified rate to achieve desired concentration either at particular site or blood plasma. In other words control release system provides actual therapeutic control, whether this would be temporal (time related), spatial nature (site related) or both.

Classification

Different authors categorize control release system in different ways but for simple understanding, we have categorized control release form into following headings:

- *Sustained release (or extended release):* Delivers an agent at a controlled rate for an extended time. Few authors have also categorize sustained release into different heading and differentiate it from controlled release by saying that sustained release formulation follows first order release while controlled release follows zero order release Fig. 5.1.
- *Localized drug release:* Might localize drug action by spatial placement near where it is needed, e.g. depots, implants, Patches.
- *Targeted drug delivery:* Might target drug action by using techniques to deliver drug to a particular cell type.
- *Delayed release:* A dosage form to which an enteric or other coating has been applied, thus delaying release of the drug until its passage into the intestines, e.g. enteric-coated tablets of Lansoprazole (Table 5.1).

174

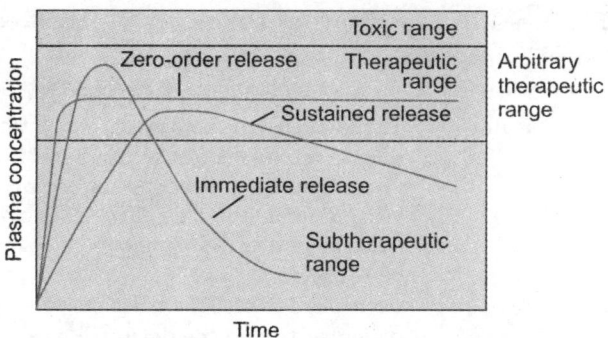

Time

Fig. 5.1: Plasma concentration versus time graph

Table 5.1: Benefits of controlled release system over conventional release system

Advantages of controlled release over conventional release system	
Therapeutic advantage	*Conventional release system:* A typical peak-valley plasma concentration–time profile is obtained which makes attainment of steady-state condition difficult. The unavoidable fluctuations of drug concentration may lead to under medication or over medication (Fig. 5.2). *Controlled release:* Reduction in drug plasma level fluctuation; maintenance of a steady plasma level of the drug over a prolonged time period (Fig. 5.2).
Reduction in adverse side effects and improvement in tolerability	*Conventional release system:* The fluctuations in drug levels may lead to precipitation of adverse effects especially of a drug with small therapeutic index (TI) whenever over medication occur. *Controlled release:* Drug plasma levels are maintained within a narrow window with no sharp peaks.
Patient comfort and compliance	*Conventional release system:* Poor patient compliance, increased chances of missing the dose of a drug with short half-life for which frequent administration is necessary. *Controlled release:* Reduction in dosing frequency enhances compliance.

Contd.

Table 5.1: Benefits of controlled release system over conventional release system (Contd.)

Advantages of controlled release over conventional release system

Reduction in health care cost	The total cost of therapy of the controlled release product could be comparable or lower than the immediate release product. With reduction in side effects, the overall expense in disease management also would be reduced.
Avoid night time dosing:	Controlled release formulations are good for patients to avoid the dosing at night time.

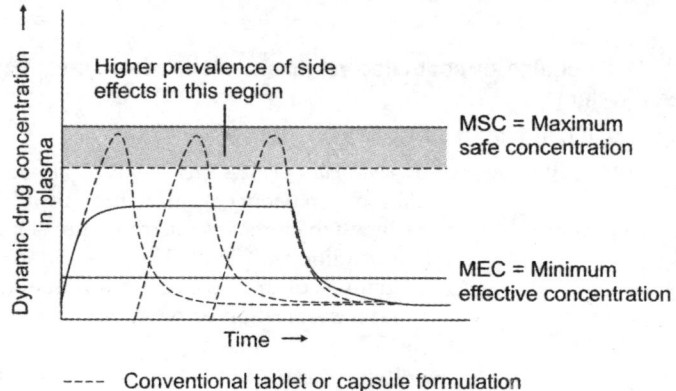

---- Conventional tablet or capsule formulation
——— Zero-order controlled release formulation

Fig. 5.2: Plasma concentration versus time graph

Disadvantages

1. *Dose dumping:* Increase quantity of drug release causes dumping of drug which in turn leads to toxicity.
2. *Reduced potential for accurate dose adjustment:* Administrating a fraction of drug is not possible.
3. *Need for additional patient education:*
   "Do not crush or chew the dosage unit".
   "Tablet residue may appear in stools".
4. *Stability problems:* The complexity of sustained release dosage formulation will lead to stability problem.
5. Retrieval of the drug is difficult in case of toxicity/poisoning/ hypersensitive reaction.

6. Higher cost of the formulation.
7. *Half life:* Drugs having shorter half-life (less than one hour) and drugs having longer half-life (more than twelve hrs) cannot be formulated as sustained release dosage formulation.
8. If a dosage form contains more than 500 mgs of active ingredient formulation of sustained release dosage formulation is difficult.

Factors influencing design of sustained release dosage form:

1. *Physicochemical properties of drug:* Stability, solubility, partition coefficient and protein binding are to be considered.
2. *Route of drug delivery:* Area of the body where drugs are applied or administered plays a vital role.
3. *Biological properties:* Pharmacokinetics and pharmacodynamics.
4. *Acute or chronic dosing:* Cure, control and length of drug therapy must be considered.
5. *The disease:* Pathological conditions play a significant role. The physiological changes in gastrointestinal tract, liver, kidneys, or heart due to diseases often affect absorption, distribution and elimination of drugs and there is a possibility that prolonged release dosage forms are particularly susceptible to the changes. In such cases, the dosing regimen should be studied and established as to reflect the pathological changes.
6. *The patient:* Ambulatory/bedridden, young or old, etc. must be considered.

Physicochemical Properties of Drug (Fig. 5.3)

1. *Aqueous solubility and pKa:* A drug with good aqueous solubility, especially if pH independent, serves as a good candidates. Absorption of poorly soluble drugs is dissolution rate-limited which means that the controlled release device does not control the absorption process (Fig. 5.4).

Drug absorption is governed by two properties, i.e. aqueous solubility and its pKa.

Aqueous solubility influences its dissolution rate, thereby its concentration in solution and hence driving force for diffusion across the membrane. 'Noyes Whitney equation' gives the relation between dissolution rate and the aqueous solubility.

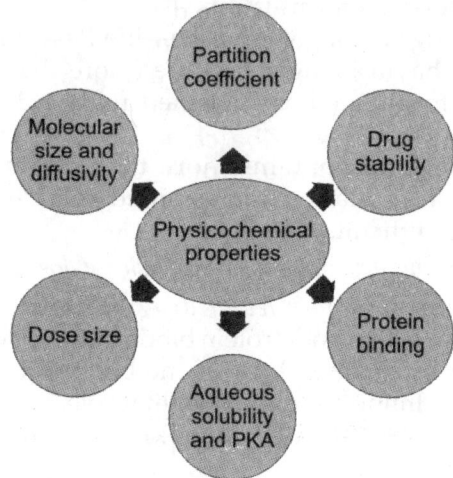

Fig. 5.3: Physiochemical factors influencing design of sustained release dosage form

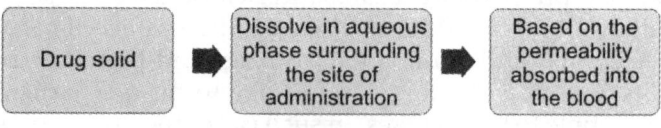

Fig. 5.4

Noyes Whitney equation:

$$dc/dt = K_d \, A \, Cs$$

Where, dc/dt = dissolution rate. K_d = Dissolution rate constant. A = total surface area of drug. Cs = aqueous saturation solubility.

pKa

pKa is – Log (Ka) where Ka is the acid dissociation constant.

Aqueous solubility of weak acids and bases is governed by pKa of compound and the pH of the solution or medium. According to pH theory, the unionized form of a drug will be absorbed preferentially in a passive manner through membranes. Thus, for acidic drugs absorption is favored in acidic environment and for basic drug in basic environment.

Hence, the release of an ionizable drug must be programmed inaccordance with the pH variations across the GIT. Drugs existing largely in ionized forms are poor candidates for sustained release system, e.g. hexamethonium.

The Henderson-Hasselbalch equation describes the ionization of drug in particular pH.

Two equivalent forms of the equation are:

$$pH = pK_\alpha + \log\frac{[A^-]}{[HA]}$$

And

$$pH = pK_\alpha + \log\left(\frac{[conjugate\,base]}{[acid]}\right).$$

Here, pK_a is $-\log(K_a)$ where K_a is the acid dissociation constant, that is:

$$pK_\alpha = -\log(K_\alpha) = -\log\left(\frac{[H_3O^+][A^-]}{[HA]}\right)$$

For the non-specific brønsted acid-base reaction:

$$HA + H_2O \rightleftharpoons A^- + H_3O^+$$

In these equations, A^- – denotes the ionic form of the relevant acid. Bracketed quantities such as [base] and [acid] denote the molar concentration of the quantity enclosed.

2. *Partition coefficient:* Between the time a drug is administered and is eliminated from the body, it must diffuse through a variety of biological membranes. The ability of drug particles to penetrate through these membranes is given by Partition coefficient. According to 'Hanch correlation' a parabolic relationship between the log of its partition coefficient with that of the log of its activity or ability to be absorbed (Fig. 5.5).

3. *Drug stability:* They may be designed considering their transit in the GIT. Drugs with stability problems are poor candidates for sustained release. A different route can be selected for such type of drugs like transdermal route.

4. *Protein binding:* Most part of the blood protein get re-circulated and are not eliminated, drug-protein binding can

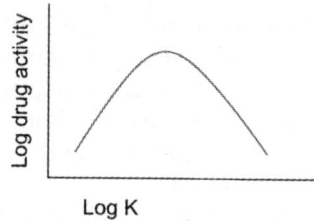

Fig. 5.5: Hanch correlation—log drug activity versus log K

serve as a depot. In general charged compounds have a greater tendency to bind a protein. Example: Diazepam, dicoumarol, novobiocin have 95% plasma protein binding.

5. *Molecular size and diffusivity:* A drug must diffuse through a variety of biological membranes in the body. The ability of a drug to diffuse through membranes is called diffusivity which is a function of molecular weight.

In most polymers it is possible to relate log D to some function of molecular size as,

$$\text{Log D} = -S_v \log V + K_v = -S_m \log M + K_m$$

V – Molecular volume.

M – Molecular weight.

S_v, S_m, K_v and K_m are constants.

The value of D is related to the size and shape of the cavities, as well as the drugs. The drugs with high molecular weight show very slow kinetics.

6. *Dose size:* For oral dosage form a dose size of 0.5 to 1.0 gm is considered maximum. Higher doses have to be given as liquids. Drugs with low therapeutic index needs to be given additional care, if dose size is high.

Route of Drug Delivery

Oral and parenteral (im) routes are the most popular followed by transdermal application. Routes of minor importance in controlled drug delivery are buccal/sublingual, rectal, nasal, ocular, pulmonary, vaginal and intrauterinal. The features desirable for a drug to be given by a particular route are discussed in Fig. 5.6.

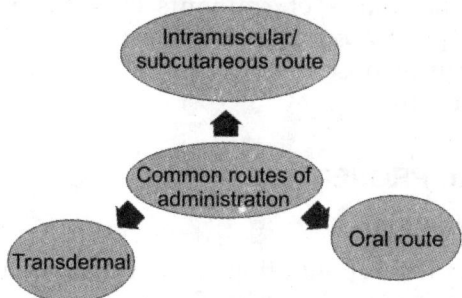

Fig. 5.6: Common route of drug administration

Most Popular Routes of Drug Administration

a. *Oral route:* For a drug to be successful as oral controlled release formulation, it must get absorbed through the entire length of GIT. Since the main limitation of this route is the transit time (a mean of 14 hours), the duration of action can be extended for 12 to 24 hours. The route is suitable for drugs given in dose as high as 1000 mg. A drug whose absorption is pH dependant, destabilized by GI fluids/enzymes, undergoes extensive presystemic metabolism (e.g. nitroglycerine), influenced by GIT motility, has an absorption window and/ or absorbed actively (e.g. riboflavin) is a poor candidate for oral controlled release formulation.

b. *Intramuscular/subcutaneous routes:* These routes are suitable when the duration of action is to be prolonged from 24 hours to 12 months. Only a small amount of drug, about 2 ml or 2 grams, can be administered by these routes. Factors important in drug release by such routes are solubility of drug in the surrounding tissues, molecular weight, partition coefficient and pKa of the drug and contact surface between the drug and the surrounding tissues.

c. *Transdermal route:* Low dose drugs like nitroglycerine can be administered by this route. The route is best suited for drugs showing extensive first-pass metabolism upon oral administration. Important factors to be considered for percutaneous drug absorption are partition coefficient of drug, contact area, skin condition, skin permeability of drug, skin perfusion rate, etc.

In short, the main determinants in deciding a route of administration of a controlled release are physiochemical properties of drug, dose size, absorption efficiency and desired duration of action.

BIOLOGICAL PROPERTIES

Pharmacokinetics

1. *Absorption:* The rate-limiting step in drug delivery from a sustained release product is release, from the dosage form rather than absorption. The rate, extent and uniformity of absorption is an important factor, as here Kr<<<Ka. A drug with slow absorption is a poor candidate for such dosage forms since continuous release will result in a pool of unabsorbed drug, e.g. iron.

2. *Distribution:* It not only lowers the concentration of circulating drug but it also can be rate limiting in its equilibration with blood and extracellular fluid. The V_d and the ratio of drug in tissue to that of plasma at steady state is an important parameters to be considered in determining the release rate.

3. *Metabolism:* Metabolism to other active form can also be considered as sustained effect. The extent of metabolism should be identical and predictable when the drug is administered by different routes. If a drug, upon chronic administration, is capable of either inducing or inhibiting enzyme synthesis, it will be poor candidate.

4. *Elimination half-life:* Smaller the t½, larger the amount of drug to be incorporated in the sustained release dosage form. Drug with the half-life in the range of 2 to 4 hours make good candidate for such a system, e.g. propranolol. Drugs with long half-life need not be presented in such a formulation, e.g. amlodipine.

Pharmacodynamic Characteristics

1. *Side effect:* The incident of side effects can be minimized by controlling the concentration at which the drug exists in plasma at any given time. Hence, sustained release

formulation appear to offer a solution to this problem. For Example:

- Slow release potassium—SR of potassium to prevent gastric irritation.
- Timed release of aspirin—to prevent gastric irritation.

2. *Dosage form index (DI):* It is defined as the ratio of C_{ss} max to C_{ss} min. Since the goal of sustained release formulation is to improve therapy by reducing the dosage form index while maintaining the plasma drug levels within the therapeutic window, ideally its value should be as close to 1 as possible.

3. *Margin of safety:* The most widely used measure for the margin of safety of a drug is its therapeutic index.

$$TI = TD_{50}/ED_{50}$$

TD_{50} = median toxic dose

ED_{50} = median effective dose.

For potent drugs TI value is small. Larger is the value of TI safer is the drug. Drugs with small value of TI are poor candidates for the formulation. A drug is considered to be relatively safe if TI exceeds 10. Some drugs of TI less than 10 are Digitoxin, Digoxin and Phenobarbitone.

Pharmacokinetic Parameters in the Design of Controlled Drug Delivery Systems

The controlled release dosage forms are so designed that they release the medicament over a prolonged period of time usually longer than the typical dosing interval for a conventional formulation. The drug release rate should be so monitored that a steady plasma concentration is attained by reducing the ratio C_{ss} max/C_{ss} min, while maintaining the drug levels within the therapeutic window. The rate-controlling step in the drug input should be determined not by the absorption rate but by the rate of release from the formulation which ideally should be slower than the rate of absorption. In most cases, the release rate is so slow that if the drug exhibits two-compartment kinetics with delayed distribution under normal circumstances, it will be slower than the rate of distribution and one can, thus, collapse the plasma concentration—time profile in such instances into a one-compartment model, i.e. a one-compartment model is suitable and applicable for the design of controlled drug delivery systems. Assuming that the kinetics of ADME of a drug are first-order processes, to achieve a steady, non-fluctuating plasma concentration, the rate of release and hence rate of input of drug from the controlled release dosage form should be identical to that from constant rate intravenous infusion. In other words, the rate of drug release from such a system should ideally be zero-order or near zero-order. One can thus treat the desired release rate R_O of controlled drug delivery system according to constant rate, i.v. infusion. In order to maintain the desired steady-state concentration C_{SS}, the rate of drug input, which is zero-order release rate (R_O), must be equal to the rate of output (assumed to be first-order elimination process). Thus,

$$R_O = R_{output} \qquad (1)$$

The rate of drug output is given as the product of maintenance dose D_m and first-order elimination rate constant Ke.

$$R_{output} = D_M \, Ke \qquad (2)$$

For a zero-order constant rate infusion, the rate of output is also given as:

$$R_{output} = K_e \, C_{ss} \, V_d \qquad (3)$$

Since $Cl_T = K_E \, V_d$, the above equation can also be written as:

$$R_{output} \;=\; C_{ss} \, Cl_T \qquad (4a)$$

Or $\qquad R_O \qquad = C_{SS} \, Cl_T \qquad (4b)$

The bioavailability of a drug from controlled release dosage form cannot be 100% as total release may not be 100% and the drug may also undergo presystemic metabolism. Hence, if F is the fraction bioavailable then:

$$R_O \;=\; C_{ss} \, Cl_T / F \qquad (5)$$

and $\qquad R_O \;=\; D_M / t \qquad (6)$

Substituting equation 6 in equation 5 and rearranging, we get:

$$D_M = C_{ss} \, Cl_T \, t / F \qquad (7)$$

Where t = dosing interval. From above equation, one can calculate the dose drug that must be released in a given period of time in order to achieve the desired target steady-state concentration. It also shows that total systematic clearance is an important parameter in such a computation.

Since attainment of steady-state levels with a zero-order controlled drug release system would require a time period of about 5 biological half-lives, an immediate release dose, D_I, called as 'loading dose', may be incorporated in such a system in addition to the controlled release components. The total dose, D_T needed to maintain therapeutic concentration in the body would then be:

$$D_T = D_I + D_M \tag{8}$$

The immediate release dose is meant to provide the desired steady-state rapidly and can be calculated by equation:

$$D_I = C_{ss} V_d/F = R_O/Ke \tag{9}$$

The above equation ignores the possible additive effect from the immediate and controlled release components. For many controlled release products, there is not built-in loading dose. The dosing interval for a drug following one-component kinetics with linear disposition is related to elimination half-life and therapeutic index TI.

Oral Controlled Release Systems

The oral route is the most popular and successfully used route for controlled delivery of drugs because of convenience and ease of administration, greater flexibility in dosage from design and ease of production and low cost of such a system. The controlled release systems for oral use are mostly solids and based on dissolution, diffusion or a combination of both mechanisms in the control of release rate of drug. Depending upon the manner of drug release, these systems are classified as follows:

a. *Continuous release systems:* These systems release the drug for a prolonged period of time along the entire length of GIT with adequate transit time. The various systems under this category are:

1. Dissolution controlled release systems.
2. Diffusion controlled release systems.
3. Dissolution and diffusion controlled release systems.

4. Ion-exchange resin-drug complexes.
5. Slow dissolving salts and complexes.
6. pH-dependent formulation.
7. Osmotic pressure controlled systems.
8. Hydrodynamic pressure controlled systems.

b. *Delayed transit and continuous release systems:* These systems are designed to prolong their residence in the GIT. Frequently, the dosage form is fabricated to remain in the stomach and hence the drug present therein should be stable to gastric pH. Various systems included in this category are:
1. Altered density
2. Mucoadhesive
3. Size-base

c. *Delayed release systems:* The design of such systems involve release of drug only at a specific site in the GIT. The drugs present in such system are those that are:
i. Destroyed in the stomach or by intestinal enzymes and secretions
ii. Cause gastric distress
iii. Absorbed from a specific intestinal site, or
iv. Meant to exert local effect at a particular GI site.

The two types of delayed release systems are:
1. Intestinal release systems.
2. Colonic release systems.

Dissolution Controlled Release Systems

These types of systems can be easily designed. The drug present in such a system can be any of the one:
• Having slow dissolution rate, e.g. griseofulvin it act as natural prolonged release products.
• Which produce slow dissolving forms on coming in contact with GI fluids, e.g. ferrous sulfate.
• Having high aqueous solubility and dissolution rate, e.g. pentoxifylline.

Matrix Dissolution Controlled Systems

Matrix systems are also called as monoliths because the drug is homogeneously dispersed throughout a rate-controlling medium. They are very common and employ waxes such as beeswax, carnauba wax, etc. which control drug dissolution by controlling the rate of dissolution fluid penetration into the matrix by altering the porosity of tablet, decreasing its wettability or by itself getting dissolved at a slower rate. The wax embedded drug is generally prepared by dispersing the drug in molten wax and congealing and granulating the same. The drug release is often first-order from such matrices.

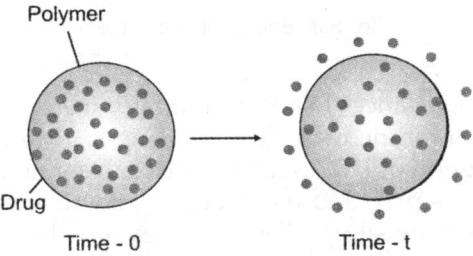

Time - 0   Time - t

Fig. 5.7: Matrix system

Coating Dissolution Controlled Systems

In this type of system the drug particles are coated or encapsulated by one substances like cellulose, PEGs, polymethacrylates, waxes, etc. The resulting pellets may be filled as such in hard gelatin capsules called as spansules or compressed into tablets. The dissolution rate of coat depends upon the solubility and thickness of the coating which may range from 1 to 200 microns (Fig. 5.8).

Diffusion Controlled Release Systems

In this types of systems the rate-controlling step is the diffusion of dissolved drug through a polymeric barrier. The drug release rate is never zero-order since the diffusional path length increases with time as the insoluble matrix is gradually depleted of drug. The two types of diffusion controlled systems are— matrix systems and reservoir devices.

Matrix Diffusion Controlled Systems

In this type of system the drug is dispersed in an insoluble matrix of rigid nonswellable hydrophobic materials or swellable

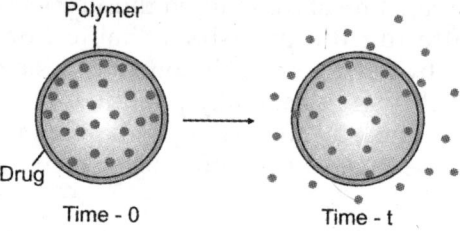

Fig. 5.8: Encapsulated system

hydrophilic substances like PVC and fatty materials like stearic acid, etc. with plastic materials, the drug is generally kneaded with the solution of PVC in an organic solvent and granulated. Waxy matrix is prepared by dispersing the drug in molten fat followed by congealing. The granules are then compressed into tablets. Swellable matrix systems are popular for sustaining the release of highly water-soluble drugs. The material for such matrices are generally hydrophilic gums and may be of natural origin (guar gum, tragacanth), semisynthetic (HPMC, CMC) or synthetic polyacrylamides. The drug and the gum are granulated together with a solvent such as alcohol and compressed into tablets. The release of drug from such initially dehydrated hydrogels involves simultaneous absorption of water (resulting in hydration, gelling and swelling of gum) and desorption of drug via a swelling controlled diffusion mechanism. As the gum swells and the drug diffuses out of it, the swollen mass, devoid of drug appears transparent or glass-like and therefore the system is sometimes called as glassy hydrogel. The drug release follows fickain first-order diffusion under equilibrium conditions.

Reservoir Devices

Also called as laminated matrix devices. These systems are hollow containing an inner core of drug surrounded in a water insoluble polymer membrane. The polymer can be applied by coating or microencapsulation techniques. The drug release mechanism across the membrane involves its partitioning into the membrane with subsequent release into the surrounding fluid by diffusion. The polymers commonly used in such devices are HPC, ethyl cellulose. Major disadvantage of all such microencapsulation drug release systems is a chance of sudden drug dumping which is not common with matrix devices.

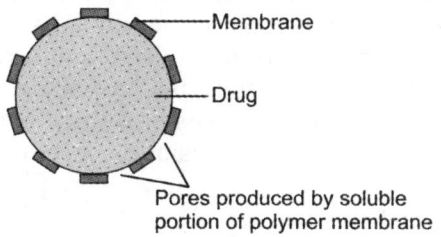

Fig. 5.9: Reservoir devices

Dissolution and Diffusion Controlled Release Systems

In dissolution and diffusion controlled release systems, the drug core are encased in a partially soluble membrane. Pores are thus created due to dissolution of parts of the membrane which:

• Permit entry of aqueous medium into the core
• Facilitate diffusion of dissolved drug out of the system.

An example is mixture of ethyl cellulose with PVP or methyl cellulose; the latter dissolves in water and creates pores in the insoluble ethyl cellulose membrane.

Ion Exchange Resin-drug Complexes

The Controlled delivery of ionizable acidic and basic drugs can be done by complexing them with insoluble nontoxic anion exchange and cation exchange resins respectively. The drug is released slowly by diffusion through the resin particle structure. The following equation represents the release of a drug, NH_2R', from a cation exchange resin RSO_3H when in contact with GI fluid containing an ionic compound $A^+ B^-$ (either gastric HCl or intestinal NaCl):

$$RSO_3 - NH_3^+ R' + A^+ B^- \rightarrow RSO_3^- A^+ + NH_3^+ R' B^-$$

A number of basic drugs like noscapine, phenylpropanolamine and have been retarded by such an approach. The complex can be prepared by incubating the drug-resin solution or passing the drug solution through a column containing ion-exchange resin.

Slow Dissolving Salts and Complexes

Salts or complexes of drugs which are slowly soluble in the GI fluids can be used for controlled release of the active principle. Amine drugs can be reacted with tannic acid to form poorly soluble complexes that can be formulated as long acting tablets. Example is penicillin G which is complexed with N, N′ - dibenzyl ethylenediamine to give benzathine penicillin G that can be formulated as oral suspension.

pH-independent Formulations

Such systems are designed to eliminate the influence of changing GI pH on dissolution and absorption of drugs by formulation them with sufficient amount of buffering agents (salts of phosphoric, citric or tartaric acids) that adjust the pH to the desired value as the dosage form passes along the GIT and permit drug dissolution and release at a constant rate independent of GI pH. The dosage form containing drug and buffer is coated with a permeable substance that allows entry of aqueous but prevents dispersion of tablet.

Osmotic Pressure Controlled Systems

The oral osmotic pump, popularly called as oros, works on the principle of osmotic pressure which release the drug at a constant zero-order rate. A core comprising of drug and an osmotically active substance (also called as osmogen) like mannitol is surrounded by a rigid semipermeable membrane coating such as cellulose ester having an orifice of 0.4 mm diameter produced by laser beam for drug exit. When exposed to GI fluids, water flows through the semipermeable membrane into the tablet due to osmotic pressure which dissolves the drug and pumps it out through the orifice by the osmotic force. Such devices can be used to target specific area of the GIT (Figs 5.10 and 5.11).

The oros principle can be used to design multiunit dosage. Forms consisting of drug core particles coated with a water permeable membrane in which delivery orifice is made by using a channeling agent such as PVP and the coated particles filled in a capsule.

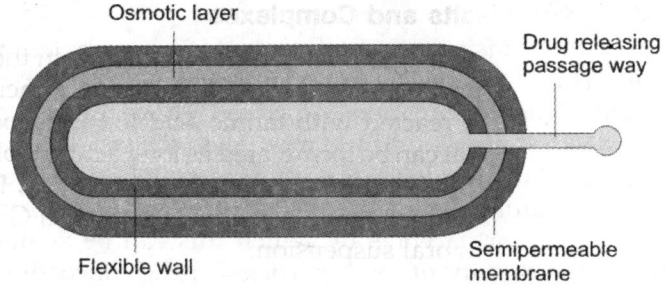

Osmotic layer

Drug releasing passage way

Flexible wall

Semipermeable membrane

Fig. 5.10: Schematic diagram of osmotic pressure controlled systems

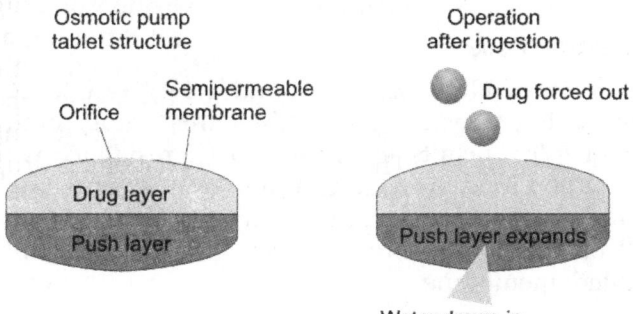

Osmotic pump tablet structure

Operation after ingestion

Orifice

Semipermeable membrane

Drug forced out

Drug layer

Push layer

Push layer expands

Water drawn in

Fig. 5.11: Osmotic pump tablet

Hydrodynamic Pressure Controlled Systems

The hydrodynamic pressure generated by swelling of a hydrophilic gum can also be used to activate the delivery of drugs. The device comprises of a rigid, shape retaining housing enclosing a collapsible, impermeable compartment containing liquid drug. The space between the external housing and the drug compartment contains a layer of swellable, hydrophilic gum such as polyhydroxyalkyl methacrylate. In the GIT, the gum imbibes water through the opening present at the lower side of external housing and sweels creating a hydrodynamic pressure. The pressure thus created squeezes the collapsible drug reservoir to release the medicament through the delivery orifice at a zero-order rate. Such systems are also called as push-pull osmotic pumps.

Changing Density

Generally the transit time of GI contents is usually less than 24 hours. This is the major limiting factor in the design of oral controlled release formulations which can reduce the frequency of dosing to a time period little more than the residence time of drug. But, if the residence time of drug in the stomach and/or intestine is prolonged the frequency of dosing can be further reduced. There are 3 ways by which this can be achieved. Changing the density of drug particles, using mucoadhesive polymers and altering the size of the dosage form. The altered density approach involves use of either high or low density pellets.

High Density Pellets

The density of GI fluids is around 1.4 g/cc. Use of drug pellets having density greater than this value, preferably above 1.6 g/cc, results in prolonged GI residence which is unaffected by food. Iron oxide and barium sulfate have been used to increase the density of drug pellets. The drug is coated on the heavy core and then covered by a diffusion controlled membrane.

Low Density Pellets

These pellets having density less than that of GI fluids, float on the gastric juice for an extended period of time while slowly releasing the drug. Globular shells such as that of poprice and cellulose have been used to lower the density of system. A swellable gum like HPMC can be used for a similar purpose.

Floating or buoyant tablets/capsules: Can be formulated by granulating a drug with 20 to 80% of hydrogel such as HPMC, HEC and HPC. On contact with GI fluids, the tablets swells and forms a diffusible gel barrier that lowers the density of system to less than 1 allowing it to float. Lipophilic polymers such as silicone elastomer can also be modified to have swelling properties. This is achieved by impregnating a water miscible liquid such as glycerol or a water-soluble salt such as sodium chloride in the lipophilic polymer swells due to absorption of water by the hydrophilic additives in the matrix.

Mucoadhesive Systems

A bioadhesive polymer such as cross-linked polyacrylic acid, when incorporated in a tablet, allows it to adhere to the gastric mucosa or epithelium. Such a system continuously releases small amount of drug into the intestine over prolonged periods of time.

Size-based Systems

Gastric emptying of a dosage form can be delayed in the fed state if its size is greater than 2 min. Dosage form if size 2.5 cm or larger can delay emptying long enough to allow once daily dosing. Disadvantage is that they are difficult to swallow.

Intestinal Release Systems

A drug may be enteric coated for intestinal release for several known reasons such as to prevent gastric irritation, prevent destabilization in gastric pH, etc. certain drugs are delivered to the distal end of small intestine for absorption via Peyer's patches or lymphatic system. Peyer's patches are mucosal lymphoid tissues that are known to absorb macromolecules like proteins and peptides and antigens by endocytosis. Selective release of such agents to Pyer's patch region prevents them from getting destroyed/digested by the intestinal enzymes. Such a site can be utilized for oral delivery of insulin. Lymphatic system on the other hand is known to absorb highly lipophilic agents directly into the systemic circulation without their first-pass through liver. The drug is absorbed by two mechanisms-chylomicrons which are fatty vesicles that entrap hydrophobic drugs, and pinocytic uptake of macromolecules.

Colonic Release Systems

Drugs are poorly absorbed through colon but be delivered to such a site for two reasons:
  i. Local action as in the treatment of ulcerative colitis with mesalamine and
  ii. Systematic absorption of protein and peptide drugs like insuline and vasopressin.

Advantage is taken of the fact that pH-sensitive bioerodible polymer like polymethacrylates release the medicament only at the alkaline pH of colon or use of divinylbenzene cross-linked polymers that can be cleaved only by azoreductase of colonic bacteria to release free drug for local effect or systematic absorption.

Parenteral Controlled Release Systems

The parenteral administration route is the most effective and common form of delivery for active drug substances with poor bio-availability and the drugs with a narrow therapeutic index. For this reason, whatever drug delivery technology that can reduce the total number of injection throughout the drug therapy period will be truly advantageous not only in terms of compliance, but also for potential to improve the quality of the therapy. Such reduction in frequency of drug dosing is achieved, in practice, by the use of specific formulation technologies that guarantee that the release of the active drug substance happens in a slow and predictable manner. For several drugs, depending on the dose, it may be possible to reduce the injection frequency from daily to once or twice monthly or even less frequently. In addition to improving patient comfort, less frequent injection of drugs in the form of depot formulation smoothes out the plasma concentration time profiles by eliminating the peaks and valleys. Such smoothing out of the plasma profiles has the potential to not only boost the therapeutic benefit but also to reduce unwanted events and side effects. The development of new injectable drug delivery system has received considerable attention over the past few years. This interest has been sparked by the advantages this delivery system possess, which include ease of application, localized delivery for a site specific action, prolonged delivery periods, decreased body drug dosage with concurrent reduction in possible undesirable side effect common to most forms of systemic delivery and improved patient compliance and comfort. The release can either be continuous or pulsatile depending on the structure of the device and the polymer characteristics, continuous release profiles are suitable to generate on 'infusion like' plasma level time profile in the systemic circulation without the necessity of hospitalization. The prime drawback is that, once administered, the drug cannot be easily removed if an undesirable action is precipitated or if the drug is no longer required.

Parenteral Depot System

Depot: Long acting parenteral drug formulations are designed, ideally to provide slow constant, sustained, prolonged action. Reason for development of PDS (parenteral depot system).

1. No surgical removal of depleted system is required as it is metabolized in non-toxicological by product.
2. The drug release from this system can be controlled by following.
   - Diffusion of drug through the polymer.
   - Erosion of the polymer surface with concomitant release of physically entrapped drug.
   - Cleavage of covalent bond between the polymer bulks or at the surface followed by diffusional drug loss.
   - Diffusion controlled release at the physically entrapped drug with bio-adsorption of the polymer until drug depletion.

Type of Depot

On the basis of different mechanism, depot formulation categories into four types:

1. Dissolution-controlled depot formulation
2. Adsorption-type depot formulation
3. Encapsulation-type depot formulation
4. Esterification-type depot formulation.

Dissolution-controlled Depot Formulations

In this depot formulation the rate limiting step of drug absorption is the dissolution of drug particles in the formulation or in the tissue fluid surrounding the drug formulation. So drug absorption can control by slow dissolution of drug particle. The rate of drug dissolution (Q/t) d under sink conditions is defined by

$$(Q/t)\, d = Sa\, Ds\, Cs/hd$$

Where Sa is the surface area of the drug particles in contact with the medium; Ds is the diffusion coefficient of drug molecules in the medium; Cs is the saturation solubility of drug in the medium; and hd is the thickness of the hydrodynamic diffusion layer surrounding each of the drug particle.

Basically, two approaches can be utilized to control the dissolution of drug particle to prolong the absorption and hence the therapeutic activity of the drug.

I. Formation of salt or complexes with low aqueous solubility. Typical examples are preparations of penicillin G procaine (Cs = 4 mg/ml) and penicillin G benzathine (Cs = 0.2 mg/ml) from the highly water-soluble alkali salts of penicillin G and preparations of naloxone pamoate and naltrexone-Zn-tannate from the water-soluble hydrochloride salts of naloxone and naltrexone, respectively.

II. Suspension of macrocrystals. Macrocrystals (large crystals) are known to dissolve more slowly than micrcrystals (small crystals). This is called the macrocrystal principle (from equation stated above, surface area of drug particle is directly proportional to dissolution) and can be applied to control the rate of drug dissolution. Typical example is the aqueous suspension of testosterone isobutyrate for intramuscular administration.

Adsorption-type Depot Preparation

This depot preparation is formed by the binding of drug molecules to adsorbents. In this case only the unbound, free species of the drug is available for absorption. As soon as the unbound drug molecules are absorbed a fraction of the bound drug molecules is released to maintain equilibrium. This depot preparation is exemplified by vaccine preparations in which the antigens are bound to highly dispersed aluminum hydroxide gel to sustain their release and hence prolong the duration of stimulation of antibody formation.

Encapsulation-type Depot Preparations

This depot preparation is prepared by encapsulating drug solids within a permeation barrier or dispersing drug particles in a diffusion matrix. The release of drug molecule is controlled by the rate of permeation across the permeation barrier and the rate of biodegradation of the barrier macromolecules. Both permeation barrier and diffusion matrix are fabricated from biodegradable or bioabsorbable macromolecules, such as gelatin, dextran, polylactic acid, lactide-glycolide copolymers, phospholipids, and long-chain fatty acids and glycerides.

Typical examples are naltrexone pamoate-releasing bio-degradable microcapsule, liposomes, and norethindrone-releasing biodegradable lactide-glycolide copolymer beads.

Esterification-type Depot Preparations

This depot preparation is produced by esterifying a drug to form a bioconvertible prodrug-type ester and then formulating it in an injectable formulation. This chemical approach depends upon number of enzyme (esterase) present at the injection site. This formulation forms a drug reservoir at the site of injection. The rate of drug absorption is controlled by the interfacial partitioning of drug esters from the reservoir to the tissue fluid and the rate of bioconversion of drug esters to regenerate active drug molecules. It is exemplified by the fluphenazine enanthate, nandrolone decanoate in oleaginous solution.

Injectable Drug Delivery System

a. In situ forming drug delivery systems (ISFD)
b. Microsphere
c. Liposomes
d. Suspension
e. Solid lipid nanoparticle.

A. In Situ Forming Drug Delivery Systems (ISFD)

Injectable in situ forming implants are classified into five categories, according to their mechanism of depot formation:
  i. Thermoplastic pastes.
  ii. In situ cross-linked systems.
  iii. In situ polymer precipitation.
  iv. Thermally induced gelling system.
  v. In situ solidifying organogels.

i. Thermoplastic Pastes (TP)

Thermoplastic pastes are semisolid polymers, which injected as a melt and form a depot upon cooling to body temperature. They are characterized as having a low melting point or Tg (glass transition temperature) in the range of 25–65°C and an intrinsic viscosity in the range of 0.05–0.8 dl/g. Below the viscosity of 0.05 dl/g, no delayed release could be observed, where as above 0.8 dl/g the ISFD was no longer injectable using a needle. At injection temperature above 37°C but below 65°C these polymers behave like viscous fluids which solidify to highly viscous depots. Drugs are incorporated into the molten polymer by mixing without the application of solvents. Bioerodible thermoplastic pastes could be prepared from monomers such as D, L-lactide, glycolide, E-caprolactone, dioxanone and orthoesters. Polymers and copolymers of these monomer have been extensively used in surgical sutures, ocular implants, soft tissue repair, etc. but disadvantage associated with this polymeric system was the high melting temperature of thermoplastic pastes requiring injection temperature at least 60°C. This led to very painful injections and necrosis at the injection site resulting in the encapsulation of the depot by scar tissue, which again inhibited drug diffusion. Poly (orthoesters), POE have well-suited properties for TP due to their good biocompatibility, relatively low softening temperatures in the range of 35–45°C and degradation by surface erosion.

ii. *In Situ Cross-linked Polymer Systems*

The formation of a cross-linked polymer network is advantageous, to control the diffusion of the hydrophilic macromolecules. Cross-linked polymer network can be found in situ by free radical reactions initiated by heat (thermosets) or absorption of photon or ionic interactions between small cation and polymer anions, e.g. biodegradable copolymers of D, L-lactide or L-lactide with E-caprolactone to prepare a thermosetting system for prosthetic implants and slow release drug delivery systems. The disadvantage of this system is it requires free radical producing agents such as benzoyl peroxide into the body which may induce tumor promotion.

iii. *In Situ Polymer Precipitation*

The concept ISFD based on polymer precipitation was first developed by Dunn and coworkers in 1990. A water-insoluble and biodegradable polymer is dissolved in a biocompatible organic solvent to which a drug is added forming a solution or suspension after mixing. When this formulation is injected into the body, the water miscible organic solvent dissipates and water penetrates into the organic phase. This leads to phase separation and precipitation of the polymer forming the depot at the site of injection. This method has been designed as Atrigel™ technology, which used as a drug carrier for eligard, contains the leuteinizing hormone releasing hormone (LHRH) agonist leuprolide acetate (7.5, 22.5 or 30 mg) and poly (lactide-co-glycolic acid) (PLGA) 75/25 dissolved in N-methyl-2-pyrrolidone (NMP) in a 45 : 55 (m/m) polymer:NMP ratio. This system led to suppression of testosterone levels in dogs for approximately 91 d. One of the problem with these system is the possibility of a burst in drug release especially during the first few hours after injection into the body. In order to control the burst effect, four factors have been examined:

1. The concentration of polymer in the solvent
2. The molecular weight of the polymer
3. The solvent used
4. The addition of surfactant.

Also the drug burst is directly related to the dynamics of the phase inversion. Carbopol is another polymer, which can be used to prepare such type of systems. It is a pH dependent polymer, which forms a low viscosity gel in alkaline environment (e.g. pH-7.4) and stays in solution in acidic pH. The addition of HPMC, a viscosity inducing agent, to carbopol reduces the carbopol concentration and hence the solution acidity while preserving the viscosity of the in situ gelling system. This system gels upon an increase in pH when injected.

iv. Thermally Induced Gelling System

Many polymers undergo abrupt changes in solubility as a function of environmental temperature. The thermosensitive polymer, poly (N-isopropylacrylamide) [poly (NIPAAM)] exhibit sharp lower critical solution temperature, LCST at about 32°C, which can be shifted to body temperature by formulating poly NIPAAM based gels with salt and surfactant. Unfortunately, poly NIPAAM is not suitable for biomedical applications due to its well-known cytotoxicity (activation of platelets) and non-biodegradability. Triblock poly (ethylene oxide) - poly (propylene oxide) - poly (ethylene oxide) copolymer, PEO-PPO-PEO (pluronics or poloxamers), have shown gelation at body temperature when highly concentrated polymer solution >15% w/w were injected. These polymer concentration shown disadvantage of changing the osmolarity of the formulation, kinetics of the gelation, and causes discomfort in ophthalmic applications due to vision blurring and crusting.

v. In Situ Solidifying Organogels

Organogels are composed of water insoluble amphiphilic lipids, which swell in water and forms various types of lyotropic liquid crystals (A material is called lyotropic if it forms liquid crystal phases because of the addition of a solvent.). The amphiphilic lipids examined for drug delivery are glycerol monooleate, glycerol monopalmitostearate, glycerol monolinoleate, sorbitan monostearate (SMS) and different gelation modifiers (polysorbates 20 and 80) in various organic solvents and oils. These compound forms a cubic liquid crystal phase upon injection into an aqueous medium which is gel like and highly viscous. SMS organogels containing w/o emulsion were investigated *in vivo* as delivery vesicles for vaccines using albumin (BSA) and haemagglutin (HA) as model anigens (An antigen is a substance or molecule that when introduced into the body triggers the production of an antibody by the immune system which will then kill or neutralize the antigen that is recognized as a foreign and potentially harmful invader).

B. Microspheres

Microsphere and microcapsules of these polymers are generally prepared by three methods:

1. Solvent evaporation
2. Phase separation
3. Fludized bed coating.

1. Solvent Evaporation

The solvent evaporation method particularly developed for biodegradable polymers involves, dissolving the polymer in a volatile organic solvent, containing drug, emulsified and finally removing the solvent under vacuum to form discrete monolithic microspheres.

2. Phase Separation

Phase separation microencapsulation procedures are suitable for entraping water soluble agents in lactide/glycolide excipients. These processes involve coacervation of polymers from an organic solvent by addition of a non-solvent such as silicone oil.

3. Fludized Bed Coating

In the fludized bed coating technique the bioactive agent is dissolved in the organic solvent along with the polymer. The solution is then processed in Wurster air suspension coating apparatus to form microcapsules.

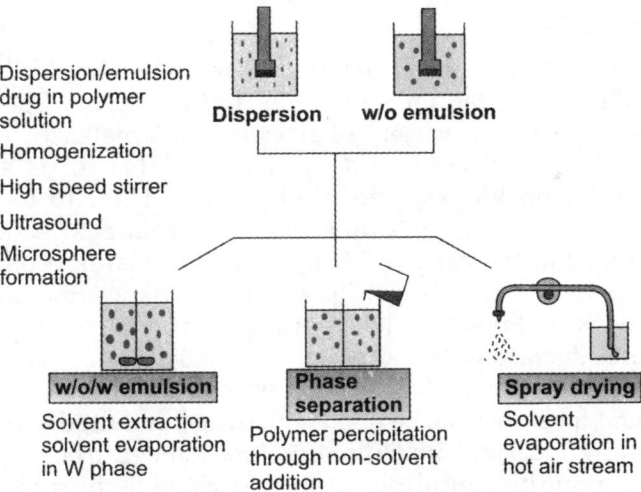

Dispersion/emulsion drug in polymer solution

Dispersion   **w/o emulsion**

Homogenization

High speed stirrer

Ultrasound

Microsphere formation

w/o/w emulsion
Solvent extraction solvent evaporation in W phase

Phase separation
Polymer percipitation through non-solvent addition

Spray drying
Solvent evaporation in hot air stream

Fig. 5.12: Microcapsules preparation technique

Numerous biodegradable polymers have been investigated for preparation of microspheres as depot formulation. The application of biodegradable microspheres to deliver small molecules, proteins, and macromolecules using multiple routes of administration has been widely investigated and several products have been brought to market in the listed 10–20 years. A list of marketed injectable products is listed in Table 5.2.

Microspheres had been discussed in previous chapter of this book under microencapsulation.

Table 5.2: Examples of marketed microsphere drug product

Drug	Commercial name	Company
Risperidone	Risperdal	Janseen/alkermes, inc.
Naltrexone	Vivitrol	Alkermes
Leuprolide	Lupron depot	Tap
	Enantone depot	Takeda
	Trenantone	Takeda
	Enantone Gyn	Takeda
Minocycline	Arestin	Orapharma

C. Liposomes

The name liposome is derived from two Greek words: 'Lipos' meaning fat and 'Soma' meaning body. A liposome can be formed at a variety of sizes as uni-lamellar or multi-lamellar construction, and its name relates to its structural building blocks, phospholipids, and not to its size. In contrast, the term Nanosome does relate to size and was coined in the early 1990s to denote special liposomes in the low nanometer range; liposome and nanosome are not synonyms. A liposome does not necessarily have lipophobic contents, such as water, although it usually does.

Liposomes are artificially prepared vesicles made of lipid bilayer. Liposomes can be filled with drugs, and used to deliver drugs for cancer and other diseases. Liposomes can be prepared by disrupting biological membranes, for example, by sonication. Liposomes can be composed of naturally-derived phospholipids with mixed lipid chains (like egg phosphatidylethanolamine) or other surfactants. Liposomes should not be confused with micelles and reverse micelles composed of monolayers.

Application

Liposomes are used for drug delivery due to their unique properties. A liposome encapsulates a region on aqueous solution inside a hydrophobic membrane; dissolved hydrophilic solutes cannot readily pass through the lipids. Hydrophobic chemicals can be dissolved into the membrane, and in this way liposome can carry both hydrophobic molecules and hydrophilic molecules. To deliver the molecules to sites of action, the lipid bilayer can fuse with other bilayers such as the cell membrane, thus delivering the liposome contents. By making liposomes in a solution of DNA or drugs (which would normally be unable to diffuse through the membrane) they can be (indiscriminately) delivered past the lipid bilayer. There are three types of liposomes:

1. MLV (multilamellar vesicles).
2. SUV (Small unilamellar vesicles).
3. LUV (Large unilamellar vesicles).

These are used to deliver different types of drugs.

Liposomes are used as models for artificial cells. Liposomes can also be designed to deliver drugs in other ways. Liposomes that contain low (or high) pH can be constructed such that dissolved aqueous drugs will be charged in solution. As the pH naturally neutralizes within the liposome (protons can pass through some membranes), the drug will also be neutralized, allowing it to freely pass through a membrane. These liposomes work to deliver drug by diffusion rather than by direct cell fusion. Another strategy for liposome drug delivery is to target endocytosis events. Liposomes can be made in a particular size range that makes them viable targets for natural macrophage phagocytosis. These liposomes may be digested while in the macrophage's phagosome, thus releasing its drug. Liposomes can also be decorated with opsonins and ligands to activate endocytosis in other cell types.

Applications in Medicine

Table 5.3: List of clinically-approved liposomal drugs

Name	Trade name	Company	Indication
Liposomal amphotericin B	Abelcet	Enzon	Fungal infections
Liposomal amphotericin B	AmBisome	Gilead Sciences	Fungal and protozoal infections
Liposomal cytarabine	DepoCyt	Pacira (formerly Skye Pharma)	Malignant lymphomatous meningitis

Contd.

Table 5.3: List of clinically-approved liposomal drugs (Contd.)

Name	Trade name	Company	Indication
Liposomal daunorubicin	DaunoXome	Gilead Sciences	HIV-related Kaposi's sarcoma
Liposomal doxorubicin	Myocet®	Zeneus	Combination therapy with cyclophosphamide in metastatic breast cancer
Liposomal IRIV vaccine	Epaxal®	Berna biotech	Hepatitis A
Liposomal IRIV vaccine	Inflexal® V	Berna biotech	Influenza
Liposomal morphine	DepoDur	SkyePharma, Endo	Postsurgical analgesia
Liposomal verteporfin	Visudyne	QLT, novartis	Age-related macular degeneration, pathologic myopia, ocular histoplasmosis
Liposome-PEG doxorubicin	Doxil/Caelyx	Ortho Biotech, Schering-Plough	HIV-related Kaposi's sarcoma, metastatic breast cancer, metastatic ovarian cancer
Micellular estradiol	Estrasorb	Novavax	Menopausal therapy

Targeting Cancer

Another interesting property of liposomes are their natural ability to target cancer. The endothelial wall of all healthy human blood vessels is encapsulated by endothelial cells that are bound together by tight junctions. These tight junctions stop any large particles in the blood from leaking out of the vessel. Tumour vessels do not contain the same level of seal between cells and are diagnostically leaky. This ability is known as the enhanced permeability and retention effect. Liposomes of certain sizes, typically less than 200 nm, can rapidly enter tumour sites from the blood, but are kept in the bloodstream by the endothelial wall in healthy tissue vasculature. Anti-cancer drugs such as doxorubicin (Doxil), Camptothecin and Daunorubicin (Daunoxome) are currently being marketed in liposome delivery systems.

New liposomal drugs targeting cancer like liposomal cisplatin (Lipoplatin) has received orphan drug designation for pancreatic cancer from EMEA.

Manufacturing

The correct choice of liposome preparation method depends on the following parameters:

1. The physicochemical characteristics of the material to be entrapped and those of the liposomal ingredients.
2. The nature of the medium in which the lipid vesicles are dispersed.
3. The effective concentration of the entrapped substance and its potential toxicity.
4. Additional processes involved during application/delivery of the vesicles.
5. Optimum size, polydispersity and shelf-life of the vesicles for the intended application.
6. Batch-to-batch reproducibility and possibility of large-scale production of safe and efficient liposomal products.

Formation of liposomes and nanoliposomes is not a spontaneous process. Lipid vesicles are formed when phospholipids such as lecithin are placed in water and consequently form one bilayer or a series of bilayers, each separated by water molecules, once enough energy is supplied. Liposomes can be created by sonicating phospholipids in water. Low shear rates create multilamellar liposomes, which have many layers like an onion. Continued high-shear sonication tends to form smaller unilamellar liposomes. In this technique, the liposome contents are the same as the contents of the aqueous phase. Sonication is generally considered a "gross" method of preparation as it can damage the structure of the drug to be encapsulated.

Prospect

Further advances in liposome research have been able to allow liposomes to avoid detection by the body's immune system, specifically, the cells of reticuloendothelial system (RES). These liposomes are known as **stealth liposomes**, and are constructed with PEG (Polyethylene glycol) studding the outside of the membrane. The PEG coating, which is inert in the body, allows for longer circulatory life for the drug delivery mechanism. However, research currently seeks to investigate at what amount of PEG coating the PEG actually hinders binding of the liposome to the delivery site. In addition to a PEG coating, most stealth liposomes also have some sort of biological species attached as a ligand to the liposome in order to enable binding via a specific expression on the targeted drug delivery site. These targeting ligands could be monoclonal antibodies (making an immunoliposome), vitamins, or specific antigens. Targeted liposomes can target nearly any cell type in the body and deliver drugs that would naturally be systemically delivered. Naturally toxic drugs can be much less toxic if delivered only to diseased tissues. Polymersomes, morphologically related to liposomes can also be used this way.

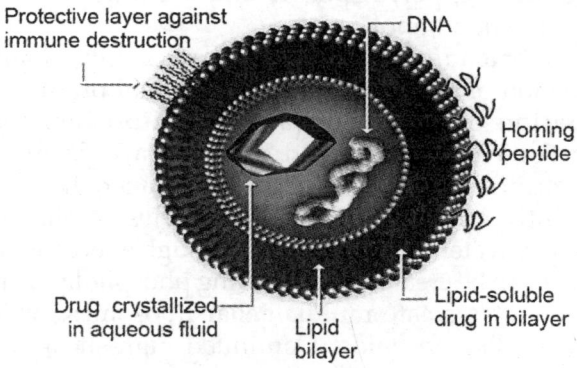

Protective layer against immune destruction
DNA
Homing peptide
Drug crystallized in aqueous fluid
Lipid bilayer
Lipid-soluble drug in bilayer

Fig. 5.13: Liposomal drug delivery system

Liposomes are composite structures made of phospholipids and may contain small amounts of other molecules. Though liposomes can vary in size from low micrometer range to tens of micrometers, unilamellar liposomes, as pictured here, are typically in the lower size range with various targeting ligands attached to their surface allowing for their surface-attachment and accumulation in pathological areas for treatment of disease.

D. Suspensions

A suspension is a widely used pharmaceutical dosage form which offers a potential use as a parenteral sustained release system. Subcutaneous administration of a drug as an aqueous or oil suspension results in the formation of a depot at the injection site. The depot act as a drug reservoir, slowly releasing the drug continuously at a rate dependent upon both the intrinsic aqueous solubility of the drug and the dissolution of the drug particles into tissue fluid surrounding the drug particle in the subcutaneous tissue. Oleaginous suspension of micronized crystal of penicillin procaine in vegetable oil, such as peanut or sesame oil, gelled with 2% aluminum monostearate was reported to produce therapeutic blood level of penicillin in both animal and human for 162 hr.

E. Solid Lipid Nanoparticle (SLN)

SLN are colloidal particles composed of a biocompatible/biodegradable lipid matrix that is solid at body temperature and exhibit size range in between 100 and 400 nm. Upon parenteral administration SLN shows excellent physical stability, protection of incorporated labile drugs from degradation, controlled drug release (fast or sustained) depending on the incorporation of model, good tolerability and site specific targeting. Techniques utilized for preparation of SLN are high pressure homogenization (HPH), microemulsion, solvent emulsification-evaporation or diffusion, w/o/w double emulsion method and high speed stirring and/or ultrasonication. SLN loaded with prednisolone by HPH, released the drug *In vitro* (i.e. in absence of enzyme) over a period of more than 5 weeks.

In Vitro Testing of Parenteral Depot Formulation

Modified release dosage forms are typically designed to release their contents over periods of weeks, months or even years, it becomes impractical to wait for a realtime test for batch release of product. Therefore, accelerated methods are often developed to assist in batch release of product. Accelerated tests, by their nature, (e.g. elevated temperature or use of solvents) can change not only the rate of drug release but also the mechanism of release. Consequently care needs to be taken in selecting an accelerated release method. However, the development of an additional realtime test will still be needed if the intent is to develop an *In vitro* test that is predictive of *in vivo* product performance. Success has been reported with the use of a modified rotating paddle for suspensions, Franz cell diffusion system for gels, flow-through cell for implants, and floatable dialysis bag for microspheres or nanoparticles. Important factor to be consider while selecting apparatus are its agitation characteristics, flow rate and choice of medium (the medium should mimic the physiological conditions of target animal).

F. Transdermal Drug Delivery Systems

Transdermal delivery systems are typically administered medicaments in the form of patches that deliver drugs for systemic effects at a predetermined and controlled rate. Some of the advantages of these systems over other controlled release formulations are:

1. Drugs with very short half-lives, e.g. nitroglycerine when administered as transdermal patches, release medicaments at a constant rate for a time period more than that obtainable with oral formulations.
2. Drugs with narrow therapeutic indices can be safely administered since better control of release is possible.
3. The noninvasive nature of these systems permits easy removal and termination of drug action in situations of toxicity.
4. Problems encountered with oral administration like degradation gastric irritation, first-pass effect, etc. are avoided.
   The route is unsuitable when:
1. The drug dose is large.
2. The drug has large molecular size (makes absorption difficult; should ideally be below 800–1000 unit.
3. The dose is skin sensitizing and irritating.
4. The drug is metabolized in skin.
5. The drug undergoes protein binding in skin.
6. The drug is highly lipophilic or hydrophilic (should be moderately soluble in both oil and water).
   Other disadvantages of such systems include variation in absorption efficiency at different sites of skin, difficulty of

adhesion to certain skin types and length of time for which a patch can be left on any area due to permeability changes (usually not more than 7 to 10 days).

Several types of transdermal drug delivery devices are available but they can be basically divided into two broad categories based on the mechanism by which drug release in controlled:

1. Monolithic (or matrix) systems.

2. Reservoir (or membrane) systems.

All such devices are fabricated as multilayer laminate structures in which the drug-polymer matrix or a drug reservoir is sandwiched between two polymeric layers. The inner layer, called as backing layer, is impermeable and meant to prevent drug loss through it. It is generally composed of metallized plastic. The outer layer which contacts the device with the skin is adhesive layer. It is permeable and in some cases, may act as rate-limiting membrane. It is generally made of pressure sensitive adhesive materials like acrylic copolymers, polyisobutylene, polysiloxane or contact adhesives.

The choice of monolithic or reservoir type of system for controlling drug release depends upon the major rate-limiting step in the absorption of drug from such devices. The two rate-limiting steps are:

1. Rate of drug diffusion from the device, R_1, and

2. Rate of drug permeation through the stratum corneum, R_2.

The overall rate of drug transport is proportional to the sum $(R_1 + R_2)$.

Monolithic (or Matrix) Devices

These devices are used when R_2 is the rate-controlling step ($R_2 < R_1$) and the drug has a large therapeutic index so that overdosing does not precipitate toxic reactions. The two categories of matrix devices are—one in which the drug is dissolved (usually below saturation levels) in the polymer matrix and the other in which the drug is dispersed (generally much above saturation level). The polymers employed for matrix systems may be hydrophilic or lipophilic and includes PVC, PVP, polysaccharides, polyesters, microporous polypropylene and ethylene vinyl acetate copolymers. The drug release rate from matrix systems is rapid initially and falls as the matrix gets depleted of drug. The rate is thus proportional to the square root of time.

Reservoir (or Membrane) Devices

These devices are used when drug permeation rate is rapid and absorption should therefore be controlled by controlling drug release ($R_1 < R_2$). It is also suitable for potent drugs with low therapeutic index where monitoring drug levels in a narrow range is essential. The drug is usually contained within the reservoir as a suspension in a liquid (such as silicone) or gel carrier. The rate-controlling thin polymeric membrane is made of olefinic polymers and copolymers, cellulosic esters, polyamides or PVC. When applied on skin, the device shows a rapid release as long as the solution inside the reservoir is saturated.

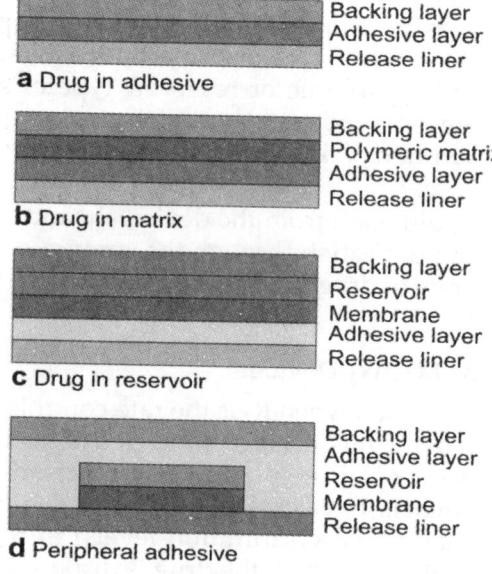

Fig. 5.14: Transdermal system design

Mixed Monolithic-reservoir Devices

A third type of system, it is basically a device having drug release kinetics intermediate between monolithic and reservoir systems. Here the drug-polymer matrix is layered by a rate of controlling membrane. Release is controlled initially by the membrane but as the drug gets depleted, the rate is controlled by diffusion of drug through a thicker layer of polymer matrix.

A major limitation of transdermal therapy is poor skin penetrability of several drugs. This problem can be overcome by use of penetration enhancers such as glycerol, propylene, glycol, DMSO, SLS, etc.

Drugs commonly presented in such systems are nitroglycerine, clonidine, scopolamine and estradiol.

G. Ophthalmic Drug Delivery Systems

Absorption of ophthalmic drugs across the corneal membrane is a diffusion process and depends to a large extent on:

1. Physicochemical properties of the permeating molecule, and
2. Drainage and output of tears.

Most drugs for ophthalmic use like pilocarpine, epinephrine, local anesthetics, atropine, etc. are weak bases which are generally formulated at acidic pH to enhance stability. But due to their highly ionized form, ocular diffusion is poor. This, coupled with tear drainage, further reduces the rate and extent of absorption. Moreover, if the drug has short half-life, the problems become more complicated. Frequent dosing of large doses of such drugs becomes necessary to achieve the therapeutic objective which often results in corresponding increase in local (e.g. irritation) and systemic side effects. One of the approaches to improve drug effectiveness is to prolong its contact with corneal surface. Highly viscous preparations like suspensions and ointments are intended to achieve this purpose but do not offer the amount of control desired. Continuous delivery of drugs in a controlled manner can overcome most of these problems. A number of ocular drug delivery systems have been developed for providing zero-order input. The best known system is ocular insert or ocusert developed to deliver pilocarpine in the treatment of glaucoma. Available in two release forms -20 and 40 mcg/hour, the system provides relief for 7 days (following insertion in the cul-de-sac, just below the cornea) in contrast to eyedrops which are required to be instilled 3 to 4 times daily. The system is basically a thin, flexible wafer, composed of a drug reservoir core surrounded on either side of rate-controlling membranes of ethylene-vinyl acetate copolymer.

H. Intravaginal and Intrauterine Drug Delivery Systems

Controlled release intravaginal systems are used for delivery of contraceptive steroid hormones. The advantage of this route includes—no first-pass effect, improved bioavailability and lesser drug dose in comparison to that required by oral route. Two types of devices have been developed—a matrix diffusion controlled device, e.g. medroxyprogesterone acetate dispersed in viscous silicone elastometer, and the other, dissolution controlled device, e.g. dispersion of a progestin and an estrogen in an aqueous solution of PEG 400 to form microscopic drug reservoir in a mixture of silicone elastometers. The device is generally prepared by extrusion of the resultant composition into a doughnut shaped vaginal ring. The system releases the medicament for 21 days to achieve a cyclic intravaginal contraception.

Intrauterine route is also used for fertility control. Two types of medicated intrauterine devices (IUDs) have been developed to produce effective contraception for 12 months or more.

1. *Copper medicated IUD:* It consists of a polypropylene or polyethylene plastic support of number 7 or letter T with certain amount of copper wire wound around them. T shape IUD is popular since its shape conforms to the uterine cavity and resists displacement and rotation within the cavity as well as expulsion from the cavity. The copper wire of surface area 200 mm shows maximum contraceptive activity. Oxidation of copper in the body fluids releases its ion slowly and exerts its effect locally. The device is effective for more than 3 years.

2. *Progesterone releasing IUD (progestasert):* It is also a T shaped polyethylene device with a progesterone reservoir dispersed in a silicone polymer placed in the vertical arm which is enclosed in a sleeve of rate-controlling membrane of ethylene-vinyl acetate copolymer. The device releases progesterone at a rate of 65 mcg/day for a period of one year.

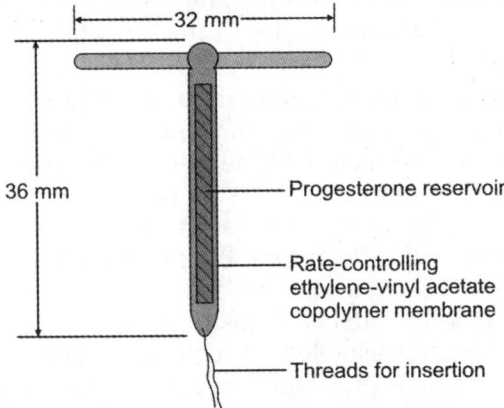

Fig. 5.15: Progesterone releasing IUD (progestasert)

Evaluation of the Controlled Release Dosage Formulation

In a conventional oral delivery system, drug content is released within short period of time and plasma drug levels peak usually reach within a few hours after dosing. Since, the dosage form will encounter gastric content proximal duodenal content, *in vivo* disintegration and dissolutions are relatively well defined. In such a case, *In vitro* dissolution is based on the fastest possible dissolution rate, and can have a direct correlation with *in vivo* bioavailability. But this kind of arrangement is simply not possible with CR systems. For oral CR products, *in vitro* testing is not aimed at how fast, but how uniformly the drug released. A variety of *in vitro* dissolution characteristics of CR dosage forms set them apart from conventional formulation. These include the following:

1. Dissolution is measured in terms of optimum drug release, not the fastest release rate.
2. The optimum release rate is related to the required biologic input function.
3. Dosage forms are designed for different release patterns, e.g. first order versus zero order, both with and without a rapid release component.
4. Disintegration may or may not precede the process of dissolution.

5. *In vitro* medium may not adequately mimic the pH, motility and viscosity variation of the GI tract to which dosage form is exposed.

Considering that the release of the active ingredient from the preparation in the gastrointestinal tract is affected by many physiological factors including the mechanical force exerted by the digestive tract in relation to its movement, and the volume, composition, pH, surface tension, and viscosity of the gastrointestinal fluid. Therefore, the *In vitro* release behaviors should be investigated under as many conditions as possible to understand possible effects of gastrointestinal variables on *in vivo* release. To achieve stable blood concentrations, it is generally desirable to prepare prolonged release dosage forms whose release rates are minimally pH dependent. Therefore, release of the active ingredient should be evaluated at multiple levels of pH, such as 1.2, 4.0 and 6.8, representing typical gastrointestinal pH variation. Considering the variation in gastrointestinal motility; agitation rates should also vary more than 2 levels among 50, 100 and 200 rpm, when the paddle method is used, at an appropriate pH. If it is anticipated that the release rate is influenced by the wettability, ionic strength and composition of the test medium, their effects should also be investigated. It is also desirable to perform release tests using different kind of apparatus. Current USP guideline for *In vitro* dissolution tests for CR products are limited. CR products are referred to the USP as modified-release dosage form and further classified as sustained-release and delayed release products. Dissolution testing of extended release dosage forms (USP, IP, JP, BP, EP (dissolution testing for sustained dosage formulations).

These include sustained release or controlled release dosage forms which reduces the frequency of dosing compared to conventional dosage forms. The dissolution is done to study the effect of pH on release profile of dosage form when it passes through GIT. Test is carried out at temperature of 37 + 0.5°C.

Apparatus 1 (Basket) or Apparatus 2 (Paddle): Are used at higher rotational frequencies (according to USP, IP, BP, JP, EP).

Apparatus 2 (Reciprocating cylinder): Is used for testing bead type formulations (according to USP, IP, BP).

Apparatus 3 (Flow cell): Is used for dosage forms containing limited solubility of API (according to USP, IP, BP, JP, EP).

Apparatuses 4 and 6 (Paddle over disk and cylinder) are used for evaluating transdermal dosage forms (according to USP)

Apparatus 5 (Reciprocating disk): It is used for evaluating Transdermal as well as non-disintegrating oral dosage forms (according to USP).

The test is done over a wide pH range of 0.1 N HCl to 7.5 pH over 22 hours (according to USP). Physiological pH of 0.8–2 (stomach); pH 5–6.5 (jejunum), pH 6–7.5 (ileum) are used according to EP. Three test time points will be specified in monographs.

Early time point of 1–2 hours is established to prove that there is no probability of dose dumping of drug. Intermediate time point is established to study the *In vitro* release profile of drug and final time point is chosen to show the complete release of drug. The acceptance criteria for sustained release formulation as per USP is listed in Table 5.4.

Time: The test-time points, generally three, are expressed in terms of the labeled dosing interval, D, expressed in hours. Specimens are to be withdrawn within a tolerance of ± 2% of the stated time.

Dissolution testing of delayed release dosage forms (USP, IP (dissolution testing for prolonged dosage forms), BP, JP, EP).

According to US regulatory guidelines delayed release dosage forms are "the products that release the drugs at a time later than immediately after administration (i.e. these drug products exhibit a lag time in quantifiable plasma concentrations)". So, the dissolution is done to show that they are intact in stomach pH and release the drug only in intestinal region. Test is carried out at temperature of 37 ± 0.5°C.

Basket, paddle, reciprocating cylinder and flow-through cell are used for dissolution testing of delayed release dosage forms (By USP, BP, IP and EP uses paddle, basket and flow through apparatuses while JP recommends only flow through cell apparatus for dissolution testing). The dissolution is done in two stages one in acid stage to show the intactness of dosage form and in buffer stage to evidence the drug release in specific region. Two methods are used for testing of delayed release formulation.

Method A: The test is carried out by placing the dosage form in 750 ml of 0.1N HCl. The sample was withdrawn after two hours and analyzed. Immediately within 5 minutes 250 ml of

Table 5.4

Level	Number tested	Criteria
L_1	6	No individual value lies outside each of the stated ranges and no individual value is less then the stated amount at the final test time.
L_2	6	The average value of the 12 units $(L_1 + L_2)$ lies within each of the stated ranges and is not less then the stated amount at the final test time; none is more then 10% of labeled content outside each of the stated ranges; and none is more then 10% of labeled content below the stated amount at the final test time.
L_3	12	The average value of the 24 units $(L_1 + L_2 + L_3)$ lies within each of the stated ranges, and is not less then the stated amount at the final test time; not more the 10% of labeled content outside each of the stated ranges; not more than 2 of the 24 units are more then 10% of lebeled content below the stated amount at the final test time; and none of the unit is more than 20% of labeled or more than 20% of labeled content below the stated amount at the final test time.

phosphate buffer is added and contents are mixed thoroughly and final pH of buffer is adjusted to 6.8 ± 0.05. The test is run for another 45 minutes or as specified in individual monographs and the sample is analyzed.

Method B: Here the test is initially carried out by placing the dosage form in 1000 ml of 0.01 N HCl and sample is analyzed after two hours and the medium is discarded and 1000 ml of 6.8 ± 0.05 buffer is added and the test is run for 45 minutes more or as specified in individual monographs.

Basket, paddle, flow through cell make use of method A, B while reciprocating cylinder make use of method B with 300 ml of dissolution medium.

Unless otherwise specified in the individual monograph, the requirements of this portion of the test are met if the quantities, based on the percentage of the labeled content, of active ingredient dissolved from the tested conform the acceptance criteria tabulated below:

Stage	Number tested	Acceptance criteria
A_1	6	No individual value exceeds 10% dissolved.
A_2	6	Average of $A_1 + A_2$ (12 units) is NMT 10% dissolved and no individual unit is greater than 25% dissolved.
A_3	12	Average of $A_1 + A_2 + A_3$ (24 units) is NMT 10% dissolved, and no individual unit is greater than 25% dissolved.

ISOLATED KEY POINTS

- Control release (CR) system provides actual therapeutic control, whether this would be temporal (time related), spatial nature (site related) or both.
- CR system reduces adverse reaction, increase patient compliance and reduces cost but it needs special precaution during administration and involves risk of dose dumping.
- Factors influencing CR dosage forms are—physiochemical properties, route of delivery, biological properties, duration of treatment and pathological condition of patient.
- Pharmacokinetic principle involved in CR system – The rate of drug release is controlling factor and it should be such that it maintains desired concentration at specified site.
- CR dosage form can be administered through oral route or parenteral route but basic priciples involved for control release system are usually smae, i.e. diffusion controlled, dissolution controlled or both.
- Unlike convention system, for oral CR products, *In vitro* testing is not aimed at how fast, but how uniformly the drug released.

PRACTICE QUESTIONS

1. Define an ideal controlled drug delivery system. How does it differ from targeted and sustained release systems?

2. What is the major objective of controlled release formulation? List the advantages and disadvantages of such a system.
3. Define the term sustain release. Give classification of sustain release dosage form.
4. Give advantages and disadvastages of controlled release dosage from over conventional dosage from.
5. Enumerate various factors affecting sustain release dosage form in brief.
6. Discuss in brief about pharmacokinetic parameters in the design of controlled release.
7. What criteria are necessary for the selection of a drug as candidate for formulation of a controlled release dosage from? Explain giving optimum ranges for the biopharmaceutic and pharmacokinetic properties/parameters of the drug.
8. Classify the oral controlled release formulations.
9. The drug release from diffusion controlled matrix can never be a zero-order process. Explain.
10. Why are reservoir device susceptible to dose dumping.
11. What are the various approaches by which the gastric transit of a dosage form can control delivery.
12. What are the various ways by which controlled drug release through inject able solutions can be attained.
13. What are the advantages and disadvantages of transdermal drug delivery systems? What criteria are necessary for a drug to be given by such a route?
14. Give classification of oral controlled release system, with suitable examples.
15. Differentiate between dissolution and diffusion controlled release systems.
16. Give construction working of osmotic pump with a neat labeled diagram.
17. Write short notes on:
    a. Low density pellets.
    b. Floating tablets.
    c. Mucoadhesive system.
    d. Colonic release system.
18. Discuss in brief about parenteral controlled release system.
19. Discuss in brief about transdermal drug delivery system.

OBJECTIVE TYPE QUESTIONS

1. Dosage form index (DI) is defined as the ratio of ....
2. The major disadvantage of SR dosage form is ....
   ....
3. Drugs having shorter and longer .... cannot be formulated as sustained release dosage formulation.
4. Noyes Whitney equation is ....
5. Acidic drugs absorption is favored in .... environment and for basic drug in .... environment.
6. .... routes are the most popular routes for preparation of sustain release dosage forms.
7. By .... the duration of action can be extended for 12 to 24 hours, while by .... routes the duration of action can be prolonged from 24 hours to 12 months.
8. The .... works on the principle of osmotic pressure which release the drug at a constant .... order rate.
9. In Hydrodynmic pressure controlled systems the hydrodynamic pressure generated by swelling of .... which is used to activate the delivery of drugs.
10. .... delivery systems are typically administered medicaments in the form of patches that deliver drugs for systemic effects at a predetermined and controlled rate.

ANSWERS

1. Css.max to Css.min
2. Dose dumping
3. Half-life
4. $Dc/dt = K_d \, A \, Cs$
5. Acidic, basic
6. Oral and parenteral (i.m)
7. Oral route, intramuscular/subcutaneous
8. Oral osmotic pump, zero
9. Hydrophilic gum
10. Transdermal

6

Ophthalmic Products

Eye is unique and very precious organ. It is considered as window of the soul. We can enjoy and view the whole world only with this organ. There are many eye ailments which affect this organ and one can loss the eyesight also. Therefore, many ophthalmic drug delivery systems are available. These are classified as conventional and novel drug delivery systems. Most commonly available ophthalmic preparations are eye drops and ointments. But these preparations when instilled into the cul-de-sac are rapidly drained away from the ocular cavity due to tear flow and lachrymal nasal drainage. Only a small amount is available for its therapeutic effect resulting in frequent dosing. Thus, inefficient drug delivery into the eye occurs due to rapid tear turn over, lachrymal drainage and drug dilution by tears.

Topical administration for ocular therapeutics is ideal because of smaller doses required compared to the systemic use, its rapid onset of action and freedom from systemic toxicity. Topically applied ocular drugs have to reach the inner parts of the eye and transcorneal penetration is believed to be the major route for drug absorption. Corneal absorption is much slower process than elimination. For many drugs K loss (first order elimination rate) is approximately 0.5–0.7/min and K absorption (first order absorption rate) is about 0.001/min. The sum of these two rate constants control the fraction of the applied dose absorbed into the eye. So the ocular bioavailability can be increased by decreasing K loss or by increasing K absorption. The former can be achieved by modifying the ocular dosage forms and the latter by formulating ocular dosage forms containing lipophilic prodrugs or by adding penetration enhancers. Therefore, to optimize topical ocular drug delivery system prolonged contact time with the corneal surface and better penetration through cornea is necessary. A considerable amount of effort has been made in ophthalmic drug delivery since 1970s. The two main approches attempted are improvement in bioavailability and controlled release drug delivery.

Physiology of Eye (Fig. 6.1)

The eyeball has three regions namely outer most core which comprises of transparent cornea and white opaque scelra, middle which contains iris anteriorly, the choroids and the cilliary body posterioirly and the inner layer contains retina which is an extention of central nervous system. Ophthalmic preparations generally act at cornea and this region acts as the gate way for these formulations. The penetration of drus through the cornea is dependent on the stroma epithelium of the cornea. This layer is of bilipid layer, i.e. fat-water-fat structure and thus control passage of drugs. The aqueous humor and the vitreous humor constitute fluid systems in the eye. This fluid escapes through the posterior part and anterior part.

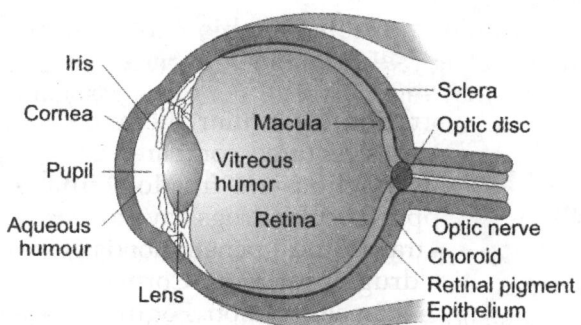

Fig. 6.1: Physiology of eye

The ocular drugs applied topically are intended for the local action or for penetration into the anterior chamber and thus distributes to whole tissues of the eye. Some of the characters required for optimizing the ocular drug delivery system are:

- Good corneal penetration.
- Prolong contact time with corneal tissue.
- Simplicity of instillation for the patient.
- Sterility of the product.
- Non-irritative and comfortable form (viscous solution should not provoke lachrymal secretion and reflex blinking).
- Appropriate rheological properties and concentrations of the viscous system.

Ideal Ophthalmic Formulations

- Ophthalmic solutions should be free from foreign particles.
- Insoluble drug particles are made in the form of suspensions. They should be redispersed on shaking the container.
- There should not be any leakage from the finished dosage form of ointment and it should be free from larger particles and it must meet the requirements of metal particles.

For achieving the drug delivery through the eye, different methods were followed like:

1. Using different grades of polymers
2. Preparation of viscous gels
3. Colloidal preparations
4. Using erodible and non-erodible ocular inserts which prolong the drug retention time at cornea.

It is found that the cornea offers more resistance to the negatively charged compounds.

Important Characteristics Required for Ophthalmic Preparation

An ophthalmic preparations should have the following desired characteristics:

1. *Foreign substances:* The ophthalmic products should be clear and free from foreign particles, fibers and filaments. They should be clarifield by passing through bacteria proof filters, such as, membrane subdivision to minimize irritation. A separate filter should be used for different ophthalmic products in order to avoid the contamination.
2. *Adequate viscosity:* To increase the contact time of the drug in the eye, various thickening agents are added in the

ophthalmic preparations. Polyvinyl alcohol (1–4%), polyethylene glycol, methylcellulose are some of the commonly used thickening agents. These agents gives desired viscosity to the preparation. An ideal viscosity enhancer should have the following properties:

- It can be filter easily.
- It can be sterilize easily.
- It should be compatible with other ingredients.
- It should have adequate clarity.

3. *Isotonicity:* Ophthalmic products must be isotonic with lachrymal secretions to vaoid discomfort and irritation. A 0.9% solution of sodium chloride is isotonic with lachrymal secretion and eye can tolerate a range of tonicity from 0.5 to 2% sodium chloride solution. Other isotonic vehicles used are like 1.9% boric acid and sodium acid phosphate buffer.

4. *pH of the preparation:* pH plays an important role in therapeutic activity, solubility, stability and comfort to the patient. Tears have a pH of about 7.4. Eye can tolerate solution having wide range of pH provided they are not strongly buffered, since the tears will rapidly restore the normal pH is irritate to the eye.

5. *Sterility:* Ophthalmic preparation must be sterile when prepared. *Pseudomonas aeruginosa* is very common gram negative bacteria if present may cause serious infection of cornea and can lead to complete loss of eyesight in 24–48 hours.

To maintain sterility in multidose container containing ophthalmic products, a suitable preservative is added. The preservative should be non-toxic, non-irritant and should be well-suited with midicament (s). The ophthalmic products are sterilized by autoclaving, filtration, though bacteria proof filters and addition of bactericide at low temperature.

6. *Wetting ability:* Vehicles used in ophthalmic preparation must have good wetting ability to penetrate cornea and other tissue. The wetting agents are choosen which should not cause any damage to tissues of eye. Some commonly used wetting agents are polysorbate 20, polysorbate 80, dioctyl sodium sulphosuccinate, etc.

Various Types of Ophthalmic Products

Ophthalmic products include:

1. Eye drops
2. Eye lotions
3. Contact lens solution
4. Eye ointments.

Eye Drops

Eye drops are sterile aqueous or oily solutions of drugs that are installed into the eye with a dropper. They usually contain drugs having antiseptic, analgesic, anti-inflammatory effects.

An ideal eye drop should have following characteristics:

1. It should be sterile.
2. It should be iso-osmotic with lachrymal secretions.
3. It should be free from foreign particles, fiber and filaments.
4. It should have pH more or less equivalent to lachrymal secretions.
5. It can be preserved with a suitable preservative.
6. It should remain stable during its entire shelf life.

Formulation of Eye Drops

The eye drops are prepared in 4 stages. These stages are as under:

1. *Preparation of bactericidal and fungicidal vehicle:* The equeous or oily vehicle is used in the preparation of eye drops. The equeous vehicle may support bacterial or fungal growth, so one of the following bactericide may be used preserve the eye drops:

    i. Phenylmercuric nitrate/acetate   0.002%
    ii. Benzalkonium chloride   0.01%
    iii. Chlorohexidine acetate   0.01%

Phenylmercuric nitrate should not be used in eye drops which are intened for prolonged treatment. Similarly benzalkonium chloride is not suitable as preservative for eyedrops containing local anaesthetics.

2. *Preparation of solution of medicament (s) and excients:* The medicaments are dissolved in the aqueous vehicle containing

suitble antimicrobial agent. The excipient are also dissolved in the vehicle at this stage to form a stable preparation.

3. *Clarification:* The eye drops are cleared by passing the solution through bacteria proof filter and immediately transferred into final containers and sealed to exclude micro-organism.

4. *Sterilization:* The eye drops are sterilized by autoclaving or heating with bactericide at 98° to 100° C for 30 minutes or filtration through bacteria proof filter.

5. *Container:* The eye drops should be packed in neutral glass containers or in a suitable plastic containers. The bottle must conform to limit test for alkalinity of glass. Nowadays, neutral glass small bottle having capacity of 4 ml to 8 ml are used. It has two polypropylene screw caps, one for attacking a silicon rubber teat to the container and the other for covering the teat. The plastic squeeze bottles having rigid plastic cap and polythene friction plug containing baffle that produces uniform drops are also used these days.

Excipients used in Eye Drops

The following excipients are used in the preparation of eye drops:

1. *Thickening agent:* The thickening agents, like methylcellulose, polyvinyl alcohol, polyethylene glycol are used to increase the viscosity of eye drops, they help to prolong the contact time of the drug in the eye.

2. *Buffers:* Buffers like sodium citrate are added to adjust and maintain the pH of the eye drops.

3. *Antioxidants:* They are added in several eye drops to provide protection from oxidation. Sodium metabisulphite (0.05 to 0.5%) and sodium thiosulphate (0.1 to 0.2%) are commonly used as antioxidants. Sometimes the eye drops are protected from oxidation by replacing the air in the eye drops with an inert gas.

4. *Wetting agents:* These are used for increasing the penetration of eye drops into the corner of the eye. Polysorbate 20 and polysorbate 80 are used as wetting agent.

5. *Isotonicity:* Eye drops are made isotonic with the lachrymal secretion with help of various buffers and other solution.

Precaution Used in Handling Eye Drops

The following precautions are required to be observed while using eye drops:

1. Do not touch the dropper surface.
2. Do not rinse the dropper.
3. Do not use eye drops that have changed colour.
4. After instillation of drops, do not close eyes tightly or blink more often than usual as this may remove the medicine from the place where it is needed.

Example: To prepare and dispense 1000 ml of atropine eye drops BPC

Rx

Atropine sulphate	10 g
Phenylmercuric nitrate	500 ml
Solution	0.002%
Purified water, add up to	1000 ml

Make an eye drops

Direction: To be used as directed by the physician.

Eye-lotions

These are sterile aqueous solutions used for washing the eyes. The eyes-lotions are supplied in concentrated form and are required to be diluted with warm water immediately before use. Eye-lotions should be isotonic and free from foreign particles to avoid irritation to the eye. They are required to be prepared fresh and should not be stored for more then two days as the lotion may get contaminated with mirco-organisms. The drugs used for preparing eye solutions include sodium bicarbonate, boric acid, borax or zinc sulphate.

Formulation of Eye-lotion

They are prepared iso-osmotic with because they are used in large quantity and if not properly formulated may cause discomfort in the eye. The eye lotion are sterile by autocalving or by passing through bacteria proof filter. Sodium chloride eye-lotion and sodium bicarbonate eye-lotion are commonly used to remove foreign substances from the eye.

Example: Prepare and disoense 100 ml or sodium chloride eye-lotion BPC

Rx

Sodium chloride	0.9 g
Purified water to produce	100 ml

Method: Weigh the requied of sodium chloride. Dissolve sodium chloride in purified water and made the final volume by adding more of purified water, filter it and transfer it to a bottle, sterilize it by autoclaving and finally seal it.

Storage: Eye-lotions are supplied in amber coloured screw caped fluted bottled. The containers must be labelled clearly "for external use only" "sterile solution not for injection".

Eye Ointments

Eye ointments are sterile preparations meant for application to the eye. These are prepared under aseptic conditions and packed in sterile collapsible tubes which keep the preparation sterile until whole of it is consumed.

Formulation of Eye Ointments

The ointments base selected for an eye ointment must be non-irritating to the eye. The eye ointment base should melt near the body temperature. So as to permit the diffusion of the drug threw the lachrymal secretions of the eye. For the preparation of eye ointments the following base is used.

Yellow soft paraffin	80 g
Liquid paraffin	10 g
Wool fat	10 g

Method: Melt wool fat, yellow soft paraffin on a water bath and liquid paraffin. Filter through coarse filter paper placed in heated funnel. It is sterilized by dry method (160°C for 2 hours) add the medicament with the eye ointment base. Pack in sterile containers.

Wool fat is used in order to ensure satisfactory emulsification of the solution and helps in the absorption of active ingredients. Liquid paraffin is incorporated to reduced the viscosity of the base, so that it can easily expelled from the collapsible tube and applied to the eye.

Example: Prepare and dispense 100 g of atropine eye ointment BP

Rx

Atropine sulphate	1 g
Sterile base	100 g

Prepare an eye ointment

Sterile base is prepared by using the following ointment base:

Yellow soft paraffin	80 g
Liquid paraffin	10 g
Wool fat	10 g

Contact Lens Solutions

A contact lens (also known simply as contact) is a corrective, cosmetic, or therapeutic lens usually placed on the cornea of the eye. Some soft contact lenses are tinted a faint blue to make them more visible when immersed in cleaning and storage solution. Some cosmetic lenses are deliberately colored to alter the appearance of the eye. Some lenses now have a UV protection surface treatment to reduce UV damage to the eye's natural lens. Generally two solutions are used for hard contact lenses:

1. *Wetting liquid:* These solutions are used primarily for treating the lenses before insertion. Due to its hydrophobic nature, polymethyl methacrylate is poorly wetted by the lachrymal fluid of the eye. Hence, the contact lenses required moistening with a wetting agent to make the insertion easy and comfortable. Since, the contact lenses solutions are required to be used daily for eyes together, therefore, they should be prepared carefully and all the ingredient used should be of good quality. The formulation of contact lenses solution contain a wetting agent, thickening agent, antimicrobial agent and an isotonicity adjuster.

2. *Storage liquid:* Storage solutions are used for overnight cleansing soaking, and storage. The contact lenses after its removal from the eye are cleaned with wetting solution and rinsed with purified water. Then they are stored in a storage solution to prevent dehydration. The formulation of storage solution contains a nonionic surface active agent which will help in cleaning the contact lenses, preservative are also added to prevent the microbial growth. The solution should be changed after every few days because the preservatives

may be practically inactivated by the organic material present on the form of debris. Contact lens solutions should be sterile. The label should warn against contamination during used.

Soft Contact Lens Liquid

Certain medicaments from eye drops and preservatives from wetting and storage solutions are strongly absorbed by the soft contact lenses hence soft contact lenses should be remove before instilling eye drops. For cleaning, soft contact lenses are heated in 0.9% sodium chloride solution. The wetting and storage solution used to hard contact lenses should not be used. Special proprietary storage solution are available. The wetting of soft contact lenses is not a problem because of hydrophilic nature of the lens and they should be stored in sterile solutions.

Enhancement in bioavailability: Topical bioavailability can be improved by maximizing precorneal drug absorption and minimizing precorneal drug loss.

1. Viscosity Improver

In order to prolong precorneal residence time and to improve bioavailability attempts were made to increase the viscosity of the formulation. The viscosity enhancers used were hydrophilic polymers such as cellulose, polyalcohol and polyacrylic acid. Sodium carboxymethylcellulose is one of the most important mucoadhesion polymers having monoadhesive strength. The effects of polyacrylic acid and polyacrylamide based hydrogels are tested on miotic response of pilocarpine. Carbomer were used in liquid and semisolid formulations as suspending or viscosity increasing agents. Formulations including creams, gels and ointments were used as ophthalmic products. Polycarbophil is water insoluble cross-linked polyacrylic acid helps in the retention of the drug delivery system in the eye due to the formation of hydrogel bonds and mucoadhesive strength. Hyaluronic acid offers a biocompatible and biodegradable matrix for fabrication of ocular sustained release dosage form-dosage forms based on the benzyl esters of hyaluronic acid were used for ophthalmic sustained release of methyl prednisolone. Films and microspheres were also prepared from hyaluronic acid. Polysaccharide such as xanthan gum was found to increase the viscosity. Today, hydrophilic polymers continue to be used in formulation of ophthalmic products outs the lunotions are mere for patient comfort and for bioadhesion rather than viscosity enhancement. Viscosity vehicles increases the contact time and no marked sustaining effect is seen.

2. Gels

Gel formation is an extreme case of viscosity enhancement through the use of viscosity enhancers. So the dosing frequency can be decreased to once a day. Cellulose acetate phthalate dispersion constituted a microreservoir system of high viscosity. Poloxamer 407 is used as an ophthalmic vehicle for pilocarpine delivery and found that the gel formation enhances the activity of pilocarpine 10. Timolol maleate form thermogelling drug delivery system composed of cellulose ether ethylhydroxyethyl cellulose. The effect of flurbiprofen a nonsteroidal anti-inflammatory, formulated in carbopol 940 and pluronic F 127 hydrogels were compared in ocular hypertension. Gelrite is a polysaccharide (gellen gum), which forms a clear gel in the presence of mono or divalent cation. The high viscosity of the gel, however, results in blurring of vision and malted eyelids which substantially reduce patient acceptability. Sterilization is another drawback for large-scale production.

3. Penetration Enhancers

They act by increasing corneal uptake by modifying the integrity of corneal epithelium. Chelating agents, pre-servatives, surfactants and bile salts were studied as possible penetration enhancers. But the effort was diminished due to the local toxicity associated with enhancers. Penetration enhancers have also been reported to reduce the drop size of conventional ophthalmic solutions especially if they do not elicit local irritation.

4. Prodrugs

Prodrugs enhance corneal drug permeability through modification of the hydrophilic or lipophilicity of the drug. The method includes modification of chemical structure of the drug molecule, thus making it selective, site specific and a safe ocular drug delivery system. Drugs with increased penetrability through prodrug formulations are epinephrine, timolol, pilocarpine and albuterol.

5. Cyclodextrins

Cyclodextrins act as carriers by keeping the hydrophobic drug molecules in solution and delivering them to the surface of the biological membrane, where the relatively lipophilic membrane has a much lower affinity for the hydrophilic cyclodextrin molecules WO, therefore, they remain in the aqueous vehicle system. Optimum bioavailability can be achieved when just enough cyclodextrin (<15%) is added to the aqueous eye drops solution to solubilize the lipophilic water insoluble drug. But increased concentration will result in decrease in bioavailability.

6. Bioadhesive Polymers

The bioadhesive polymers adhere to the mucin coat covering the conjunctiva and the corneal surfaces of the eye, thus prolonging the residence time of a drug in the conjunctival sac. These polymers can be neutral, synthetic or semisynthetic. Polyacrylic acid, polycarbophil and hyaluronic acid are synthetic polymers commonly used. Chitosan is a bioadhesive vehicle suitable for ophthalmic formulation since it exhibits general biological properties such as biodegradability, nontoxicity and biocompatibility. Due its positive charge at neutral pH and ionic interaction with the negative charges of sialic acid occurs. Xanthan and carrageenan are also described as bioadhesive polysaccharides.

Enhancement in Controlled Drug-delivery

It is realized that the preferred system of ophthalmic delivery would provide improved bioavailability, site-specific delivery and with continuous drug release. So achievements have been made in the following areas (Fig. 6.2).

1. In Situ Forming Gels

The progress has been made in gel technology with the development of droppiable gel. They are liquid upon instillation and undergo phase transition in the ocular cul-de-sac to form viscoelastic gel and this provides a response to

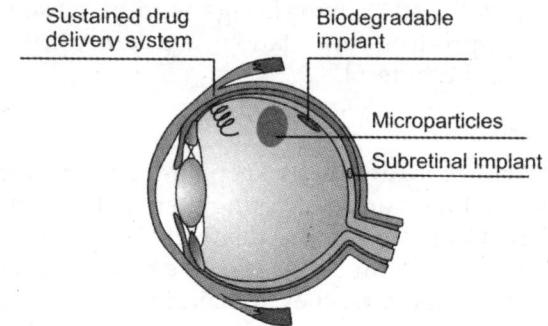

Sustained drug
delivery system

Biodegradable
implant

Microparticles

Subretinal implant

Fig. 6.2: Representing the ophthalmic drug delivery platforms

environmental changes. Three methods have been employed to cause phase transition in the eye surface. These are change in pH, change in temperature and ion activation:

- *pH:* In this method gelling of the solution is triggered by a change in the pH. CAP latex (cross-iinked polyacrylic) acid and derivatives such as carbomers are used. They are low viscosity polymeric dispersion in water which undergoes spontaneous coagulation and gelation after instillation in the conjunctival cul-de-sac.

- *Temperature:* In this method gelling of the solution is triggered by change in the temperature. Sustained drug delivery can be achieved by the use of a polymer that changes from solution to gel at the temperature of the eye. But disadvantage of this is characterized by high polymer concentration (25% Poloxamers). Methyl cellulose and smart hydrogels are other examples.

- *Ionic strength:* In this method gelling of the solution instilled is triggered by change in the ionic strength. Example is Gelrite. Gelrite is a polysaccharide, low acetyl gellan gum, which forms a clear gel in the presence of mono or divalent cations. The concentration of sodium in human tears is 2.6 g/l is particularly suitable to cause gelation of the material when topically installed into the conjunctival sac.

2. Oil in Water Emulsions

Phospholipids and pluronics were used as the emulsifiers. Antioxidants were added to improve their shelf-life. The intra-

ocular pressure reducing effect of a single, topically administered dose of a Pilocarpine emulsion lasted for 29 h in
rabbits compared to generic Pilocarpine solution which
lasted only for 5 h. Oil in water emulsion is useful for
delivery of water insoluble drugs, which is solubilised in
the internal oil phase.

3. Colloidal Particles

The potential use of polymeric colloidal particles as ophthalmic
drug delivery systems started in late 1970s.The first two
systems studied in this area were pilocarpine cellulose acetate
hydrogen phthalate latex systems and piloplex. But both the
system could not enter commercial development because of
various issues, like local toxicity, non-biodegradable polymer
and large scale sterilization.

4. Liposomes

The use of liposomes as a topically administered ocular drug
delivery system began in the early stage of research into
ophthalmic drug delivery. But the results were favorable for
lipophilic drugs and not for hydrophilic drugs. It was
concluded that liposomes must be suitable for ocular drug
delivery, provided, they had an affinity for, and were able to
bind to ocular surfaces, and release contents at optimal rates.
Positively charged liposomes have a greater affinity, to increase
both precorneal drug retention and drug bioavailability. The
addition of stearylamine to a liposomal preparation enhanced
the corneal absorption of dexamethyl valerate. The corneal
epithelium is thinly coated with negatively charged mucin to
which the positive surface charge of the liposome may absorb
more strongly. Coating with bioadhesive polymers to
liposomes, prolong the precorneal retention of liposomes.
Carbopol 1342-coated pilocarpine containing liposomes were
shown to produce a longer duration of action. Liposomal
preparation of acetazolamide, hydrocortisone and tropicamide
has been reported. Coating the liposome with bioadhesive
polymer like carbopol increased the corneal retention followed
by sustained action cyclosporine applied topically to the *eye* in
the olive oil drops in a liposome encapsulated form and in a
cellophane shield showed slow releasing property.

5. Nanoparticles

Nanoparticles provide sustained release and prolonged therapeutic activity when retained in the cul-de-sac after topical administration and the entrapped drug must be released from the particles at an appropriate rate. To enhance particle retention, it is desirable to fabricate the particles with bioadhesive materials. Biodegradation is also a highly desirable property for the fabrication of nanoparticles. Most commonlyused polymers are venous poly (alkyl cyanoacrylates), poly S-caprolactone and poly (lactic-co-glycolic acid), which undergo hydrolysis in tears. Coating of nanoparticles with bioadhesive polymers improves the bioavailability. Chitosan coated nanocapsules improve the bioavailability. Nanoparticles as an ophthalmic drug delivery have been demonstrated for both hydrophilic and hydrophobic drugs (Fig. 6.3).

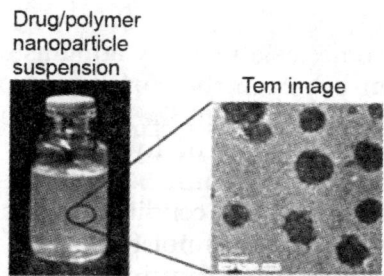

Drug/polymer
nanoparticle
suspension

Tem image

Fig. 6.3: Vial containing nanoparticle suspension

6. Micro Particulates

There are drug containing, micron sized polymeric particles suspended in a liquid medium. Drugs can be physically dispersed in the polymer backbone. The drug is released in cul-de-sac through diffusion, chemical reaction, and polymer degradation and microparticles are larger than nanoparticles. Acyclovir loaded chitosan microspheres and pilocarpine loaded albumin or gelatin microspheres are available. Microparticulate technology has the advantage of better patient acceptability, since they can be topically administered as an eye drop. But the manufacture and control of large scale manufacturing of sterile microparticulates is very challenging and expensive.

7. Inserts

These are were membrane controlled reservoir system for the treatment of glaucoma. Iris, cilliary body and the trabecular meshwork are the organs which are directly affected by these ocuserts. Ethylene vinyl acetate is the main polymer used in these ocuserts (Fig. 6.4). In pilocarpine ocuserts, pilocarpine is placed between the two polymers. Alginic acid which is extracted from seaweed acts as carrier for the pilocarpine. A white annular border mixed with titanium dioxide is present and acts a border. This makes the patients visibility clear. This device is placed in cul-de-sac of the eye.

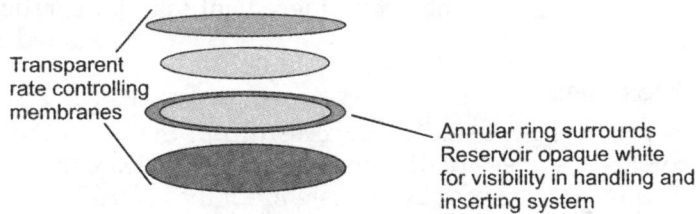

Transparent rate controlling membranes

Annular ring surrounds Reservoir opaque white for visibility in handling and inserting system

Fig. 6.4: Ocusert of pilocarpine

Keratitis sicca is a dry eye condition of the eye, where the tear production of the eye is not functioning properly. For correcting this condition, liquid tear substitutes were developed, which replace the aqueous component of tears, thus maintaining the tear film on the eye. Merck has developed Lacrisert as substitute for artificial tears. This was inserted in conjunctival sac of eye with special reusable applicator. It softens with in an hour and dissolves within 14–18 hours thus maintaining the tear film on the eye.

8. Implantable Systems

The poly lactic acid and its copolymers with glycolic acid have been used extensively as implants. An ocular implant for delivering ganciclovir for the treatment of cytomegalovirus has also been developed. This delivers drug directly to the retina for over 5 months. These systems are less popular as they require minor surgery.

9. Minidisc

Minidisc is a controlled release monolithic matrix type device consisting of a contoured disc with a convex front and a concave back surface. The principal component is bis (4-methacryloxybutyl)-polydimethyl siloxane. They can be made hydrophilic and hydrophobic to permit extended release of both water soluble and water insoluble drugs.

10. Soft Contact Lenses

The most widely used material is poly-2-hydroxyethylmethacrylate. Its copolymers with PVP are used both to correct eyesight and hold and deliver drugs. Controlled release can be obtained by binding the active ingredient via biodegradable covalent linkages.

11. Niosomes

Niosomes are reported as successful ophthalmic carriers. Discoidal niosomes are discomes of timolol maleate that have been reported to be promising systems for the controlled ocular administration of water soluble drugs. The disc shape provides for a better fit in the cul-de-sac of the eye and then large size may prevent their drainage into the systemic pool.

12. Pharmacosomes

They are the vesicles formed by the amphiphilic drugs. Any drug possessing a free carboxyl group or an active hydrogen atom (–OH, –NH$_2$) can be esterifies to the hydroxyl group of a lipid molecule, thus, generating an amphiphilic prodrug. These are converted to pharmacosomes on dilution with water. They show greater stability, facilitated transport across the cornea and a controlled release profile.

13. Collagen Shields

They are manufactured from porcine scleral tissue, which bears a collagen composition similar to that of human cornea. They are hydrated before being placed on the eye and the drug is loaded with the collagen shield simply by soaking it in the drug solution. They provide a layer of collagen solution that lubricates the eye. Collagen shields presoaked in tobramycin were used to treat *Pseudomonas aeruginosa* infected cornea excoriation. But shield are not fully transparent and thus reduce visual activity. But they are appropriate delivery systems for both hydrophilic and hydrophobic drugs with poor penetration properties.

Recent Advances

New ophthalmic delivery system includes ocular inserts, collagen shields, ocular films, disposable contact lens and other Novel drug delivery systems like liposomes and nanoparticles. Newer trend is a combination of drug delivery technologies for improving the therapeutic response of a nonefficacious drug. This can give a superior dosage forms for topical ophthalmic application.

Examples of different ophthalmic products (Table 6.1)

Table 6.1: Development status of different ophthalmic products

Product	Development status	Brand name (generic name, firm)
Contact lenses	Clinical	–
Collagen shields	Preclinical	–
Gellan gum	Marketed	Timoptic-XE (timolol maleate, merck)
Polycarbophil	Marketed	Azasite (azithromycin, Insite/Inspire)
Cationic exchange resin	Marketed	Betoptic-S (betaxolol, Alcon)
Prodrug	Marketed	Betagan (levobunolol, Allergan) Lumigan (Bimatoprost, Allergan) Propine (dipivefrin, Allergan) Travatan (travoprost, Alcon) Xalatan (latanoprost, Pfizer)
Soft drug	Marketed	Lotemax, Alrex (loteprednol etabonate, Bauch and Lomb)
Lyophilized teflon strips	Clinical	–
Plastic rods	Clinical	Allergan
Nonerodible implants	Marketed	Vitrasert (ganciclovir, bausch and lomb); Retisert

Contd.

Table 6.1: Development status of different ophthalmic products *(Contd.)*

Product	Development status	Brand name (generic name, firm)
		(fluocinolone acetonide, Bausch and Lomb)
	Marketed	Ocusert (pilocarpine, Alza)
	Clinical	Iluvien (fluocinolone acetonide, Alimera)
	Clinical	Ivation (triamcinolone acetonide SurModics)
	Preclinical	Subretinal implant, SurModics
	Preclinical	Subretinal injector, SurModics
Cell based	Clinical	Encapsulated cell technology (human ciliary neurotrophic factor, neurotech); human umbilical tissue–derived cells (Centocor)
Erodible implants	Approved	Surodex (dexamethasone, allergan) Posurdex
	Clinical	(dexamethasone, Allergan)
Iontophoresis	Preclinical aciont	IOMED (now ReAble Empi), and clinical EyeGate

Evaluation tests for ophthalmic preparations:
- Particle size determination
- Test for clarity of ophthalmic solutions
- Test for pH of the solution
- Test for particulate matter
  - Light obscuration particle count test
  - Microscopic particle count test
- Test for sterility of ophthalmic products
- Pyrogen test

1. Particle Size Determination

The desired particle size of the suspension is 5–10 µm or less. Eyes show sensitivity to the particle size of 20 µm or more. The particle size of the ophthalmic suspension is to be determined as it affects the drug absorption and larger size of the particles cause irritation to the ocular tissue.

Optical microscopy: Particle size can be measured microscopically by sizing against a graticule and counting, but for a statistically valid analysis, millions of particles must be measured. This is impossibly arduous when done manually, but automated analysis of electron micrographs is now commercially available. Instruments such as the retsch Camsizer can perform this analysis on the run using standard camera technology.

Sieve analysis: In this the particles of a powder mass are placed on screen made of uniform apertures. By the application of some type of motion to the screen the particles of larger size retain on the screen and smaller ones pass through other screens. Sieves measuring particle size of 5 µ are available now with the introduction of electroformed screens.

Coulters Counter Method (Electroresistance Counting Methods)

In this the momentary changes in the conductivity of a liquid passing through an orifice is measured when individual non-conducting particles pass through. The particle count is obtained by counting pulses, and the size is dependent on the size of each pulse.

Technique advantages: Very small sample aliquots can be examined.

Technique disadvantages: Sample must be dispersed in a liquid medium as some particles may (partially or fully) dissolve in the medium altering the size distribution. The results are only related to the projected cross-sectional area that a particle displaces as it passes through an orifice. This is a physical diameter, not really related to mathematical descriptions of particles (e.g. terminal settling velocity).

Acoustic Spectroscopy or Ultrasound Attenuation Spectroscopy

In this method ultrasound is employed for collecting information on the particles that are dispersed in fluid. Dispersed particles absorb and scatter ultrasound similarly to light. It turns out that instead of measuring scattered energy versus angle, as with light, in the case of ultrasound, measuring the transmitted energy versus frequency is a better choice. The resulting ultrasound attenuation frequency spectra are the raw data for calculating particle size distribution. It can be measured for any fluid system with no dilution or other sample preparation. Calculation of particle size distribution is based on theoretical models that are well verified for up to 50% by volume of dispersed particles.

Laser diffraction methods: These depend upon analysis of the "halo" of diffracted light produced when a laser beam passes through a dispersion of particles in air or in a liquid. The angle of diffraction increases as particle size decreases. This method is particularly good for measuring sizes between 0.1 and 3,000 µm. A particular advantage is that the technique can generate a continuous measurement for analyzing process streams.

2. Tests for Ophthalmic Solutions

Clarity of the solution: Retention of clarity of solution is a main concern regarding stability of solution. In this a microscopic light is projected though a diaphragm into the solution. The solution will remain clear if there are no undissolved particles. If not the solution appears hazy due to the scattering of light by undissolved particles. Light scattering instruments are most widely used to test the clarity of the solution.

Test for Particulate Matter in Ophthalmic Solutions

Ophthalmic solutions should be essentially free from particulate matter which can be observed on visual inspection. This test describes the physical tests performed to enumerate extraneous particles with specific size ranges. Particulate matter includes mobile, randomly sourced, extraneous substances, other than gas bubbles that cannot quantified by chemical analysis due to less amount and of their heterogeneous compositions.

Methods:
- Light obscuration method
- Microscopic method

Light Obscuration Method

This method applies for ophthalmic solution including solutions constituting from sterile solids, for which the test for particulate matter is specified in the individual monograph.

The ophthalmic product meets the requirements of the test if the average numbers of particles present in the units tested does not exceed the appropriate value listed in Table 6.2.

Table 6.2: Light obscuration particle count test

	Diameter	
	≥10 µm	≥25 µm
Number of particles	50 per ml	5 per ml

If the average number of particles exceeds this limit, the test article is subjected to microscopic method.

Microscopic Method

This method is performed when some particles are not exactly detected by the light obscuration method. This test enumerates the subvisible particles essentially solid, particulate matter present in the ophthalmic solutions. The test sample is collected on a micro porous membrane filter. The ophthalmic product meets the requirements of the test if the average number of particles present in the units tested does not exceed the appropriate value listed in Table 6.3.

Table 6.3: Microscopic method particle count test

	Diameter		
	≥10	≥25	≥50
Number of particles	50 per ml	5 per ml	2 per ml

3. Test for Sterility

This is used to test the presence of microorganisms in the test solution. It is done by 2 methods.

- Membrane filtration method
- Direct inoculation (immersion) method.

Membrane filtration method: In this the test solution is first passed through size exclusion membrane capable of retaining the microorganisms. The concept is that the microorganisms will collect on the surface of a 0.45 micron pore size filter. The filter is rinsed and then the membrane is transferred to appropriate test medium as specified in the monograph.

Direct inoculation (immersion) method: In this the test article is directly inoculated into the test medium and then the medium is incubated for the growth of microorganisms, if present.

Test media: The test media are fluid thioglycollate medium (FTM) and soybean casein digest medium (SCDM). FTM is selected based upon its ability to support the growth of anaerobic and aerobic microorganisms. SCDM is selected based upon its ability to support a wide range of aerobic bacteria and fungi (i.e. yeasts and molds).

Incubation time: In both the methods the test medium after the transferring of the test solution is to be incubated for 3 days in case of bacteria and 5 days in case of fungi and then the growth is compared with that of standard. If no growth is observed then the sample passes the test and it meets the GMP requirements. The following Table 6.4 outlines the requirement for sterility testing as per USP. The requirement for sterility testing as per USP.

Table 6.4: The requirement for sterility testing as per USP

Volume/container	Minimum quantity to test in each media
<1 ml	The entire contents of each container
1–40 ml	Half the contents of each container but not <1 ml
41–100 ml	20 ml
>100 ml	10% of the contents of the container, but not <20 ml

4. Test for Pyrogens

It is used to check for the presence of pyrogens in the ophthalmic formulation. Two general tests are performed.
- Rabbit test and
- LALs test

Rabbit Test

The pyrogen test is designed to limit to an acceptable level the risks of febrile reaction in the patient to the administration, by injection, of the product concerned. Unless otherwise specified in the individual monograph, inject into an ear vein of each of three rabbits 10 ml of the test solution per kg of body weight, completing each injection within 10 minutes after start of administration. The test solution is *either* the product, constituted if necessary as directed in the labeling, *or* the material under test treated as directed in the individual monograph and injected in the dose specified therein. Assure that all test solutions are protected from contamination. Perform the injection after warming the test solution to a temperature of 37 ± 2°. Record the temperature at 30 minute intervals between 1 and 3 hours subsequent to the injection.

Test Interpretation

Consider any temperature decreases as zero rise. If no rabbit shows an individual rise in temperature of 0.5° or more above its respective control temperature, the product meets the requirements for the absence of pyrogens. If any rabbit shows an individual temperature rise of 0.5° or more, continue the test using five other rabbits. If not more than three of the eight rabbits show individual rises in temperature of 0.5° or more and if the sum of the eight individual maximum temperature rises does not exceed 3.3°, the material under examination meets the requirements for the absence of pyrogens.

LALs test: Limulus amoebocyte lysate (LAL) is an aqueous extract of blood cells (amoebocytes) from the horseshoe crab, Limulus polyphemus. LAL reacts with bacterial endotoxin or lipopolysaccharide (LPS), which is a membrane component of gram-negative bacteria. This reaction is the basis of the LAL test.

Method: Blood is removed from the horseshoe crab's pericardium and the blood cells are separated from the serum using centrifugation and are then placed in distilled water, which causes them to swell up and burst ("lyse"). This releases the chemicals from the inside of the cell (the "lysate"), which is then purified and freeze-dried. To test a sample for endotoxins, it is mixed with lysate and water; endotoxins are present if coagulation occurs.

5. Test for Ophthalmic Gels, Suspensions and Ointments

Viscosity measurement: Brook-field viscometer, cone and plate viscometer. The flow of fluids through the dropper or tube is influenced by viscosity of the product. In order to have a better flow and to maintain residence time in the eye, the viscosity of the formulation should be checked under controlled temperature. Brook-field viscometer: it measures the shearing stress on a spindle rotating at a definite, constant speed while immersed in the sample. The degree of spindle lag is indicated on a rotating dial. This reading multiplied by a conversion factor based on spindle size and rotational speed, gives a value for viscosity in centipoise (Fig. 6.5).

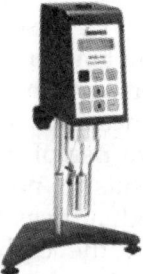

Fig. 6.5: Brook-field viscometer

Cone and plate viscometer: It used a cone of very shallow angle in bare contact with a flat plate. With this system the shear rate beneath the plate is constant to a modest degree of precision and deconvolution of a flow curve; a graph of shear stress (torque) against shear rate (angular velocity) yields the viscosity in a straight forward manner (Fig. 6.6).

Consistency measurement: It is the measure of penetration of an object into the product to be examined in a container with a specified shape and size. In this the test sample is placed on the base of the Penetrometer such that its surface is perpendicular to the vertical axis of penetrating object. The temperature of the penetrating object is maintained at 25 +/ –0.5°C and then its tip is adjusted such that it just touches the surface of the sample. The penetrating object if released and hold it for 5 sec. then the penetrating object is clamped and

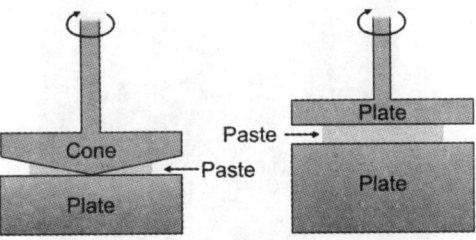

Fig. 6.6: Representation of cone and plate, plate and plate viscometers

the depth of penetration is measured. The test is repeated for 2 remaining containers (Fig. 6.7).

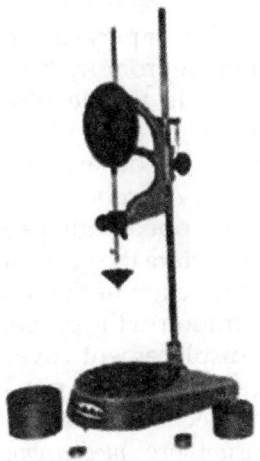

Fig. 6.7: Penetrometer

Texture analysis: It is primarily concerned with the evaluation of mechanical characters when the material is subjected to controlled force which cause deformation of the sample.

Ointment flow characteristic: For example, brook-field CT_3 texture analyser. In this the sample is subjected to controlled forces in compression using a probe or in tension using grips. The resistance of the sample material to these forces is measured by a calibrated load cell. These forces are a function of the properties of the sample and the parameters of the test method.

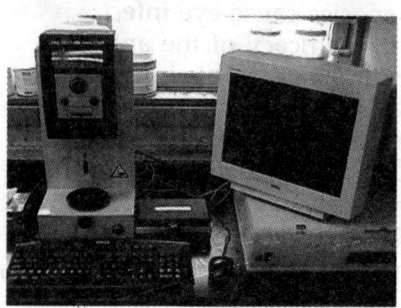

Fig. 6.8: Brook-field CT_3 texture analyser

Gel strength: Gels have gained wide acceptance as semisolid dosage forms. It has been postulated that the strength rather than the viscosity of a gel layer plays a major role in determining the amount of drug release from hydrophilic matrices. Recent advances have occurred in the development of an optimal apparatus to characterize gel strength. The apparatus consists of a sample holder placed on an electronic microbalance connected to a computer. A probe is lowered into the sample by means of a motor equipped with a speed transformer, and the force required to penetrate the gel is measured. The increase in force with time is a function of the mechanical resistance of the sample to the penetration of the probe. Because the lowering speed is known, the displacement covered by the probe as a function of time is calculated and used to compute the gel-strength parameter or mechanical resistance of the gel system.

Sachet or tube extrusion force measurement: In this the device quantifies the force required to extrude the contents from either tube or sachet style packaging that allows the manufacturers to tests the force required to extrude the content of a sachet or tube at regular intervals over a long period of time, throughout its shelf-life.

6. Test for Antimicrobial Effectiveness

Generally an antimicrobial agent is used in multiple dose units of ophthalmic products for protection from microbial contamination that may occur during the suck protection back of an unreleased drop, when the pressure is released after withdrawal of the product. Organisms like *Pseudomonas* and

Staphylococcus species cause eye infections mostly. So there is need to check the efficacy of the antimicrobial agent against these microorganisms. In this cultures of *Candida albicans, Aspergillus niger, Escherichia coli, Pseudomonas aeuroginosa, Staphylococcus aureus* are used. In this a standardized inocula of microorganisms is prepared with a count of 10^5–10^6 per ml. This is used to test the preserved formula. They are incubated for 28 days at 20–25°C and observed for the preservative action at 7, 14, 21 and 28 days. The products preservative action is found to be effective if it satisfies the following:

- There should be reduction of no more than 0.1% of viable bacteria with that of initial concentrations by day 14th.
- There should be decrease in concentration of viable yeasts and molds when compared to initial by day 14th.
- The concentration of remaining viable organisms should be lower as designated at the end of 28th day.

Cidal test: This is another test employed to determine antimicrobial agent efficacy. In this the formulation is tested against 5–14 species of microorganisms including gram –ve, gram + ve, yeast, and fungi in previously standardized inoculums. Cidal times (growth of microorganisms) are measured within 24, 48 and 72 hours of contact.

Conclusion

An ideal system should have effective drug concentration at the target tissue for a tended period of time with minimum systemic effect. Patient acceptance is very important for the design of any comfortable ophthalmic drug delivery system. Major improvements are required in each system like improvement in sustained drug release, large scale manufacturing and stability. Combination of drug delivery systems could open a new direction for improving the therapeutic response of a non-efficacious system. They can overcome the limitations and combine the advantages of different systems.

ISOLATED KEY POINTS

- The ocular drug delivery offers pathway to deliver variety of drugs to treat variety of eye disorders.
- The present study includes different dosage forms available for ocular drug delivery that includes:

Conventional dosage forms: Eye drops, eye solutions and eye suspensions, eye gels, eye ointments.

Novel dosage forms: Polymeric nanoparticles, microspheres, ocular implants, and occuserts, soft drug, prodrug approach, erodible implants and nonerodible implants.

- Different evaluations parameters are performed that include particle size detemination, clarity of the solution, viscosity of the suspensions, test for sterility pyrogen testing, and test for antimicrobial effectiveness.
- Many new approaches are being under development for drug delivery through ocular route that include contact lenses, collagen shields, lyophilized teflon strips, etc.

PRACTISE QUESTIONS

1. What are ophthalmic products? What should be the characteristics of an idea ophthalmic product?
2. Give physiology of eye with the help of a heat and labeled diagram.
3. Enlist the various types of ophthalmic products, give their examples.
4. How ophthalmic products bioavailability can be increase by controlled drug delivery system?
5. What are the recent advancement in ophthalmic products? Give their examples?
6. What are the various evaluation test employed for ophthalmic solutions?

OBJECTIVE TYPE QUESTIONS

1. Ophthalmic preparations are generally act at .... which acts as the gate way for these formulations.
2. Soft contact lenses are made up of the most widely used Material ....
3. The desired particle size of the suspension for the preparation of ophthalmic preparation is ....
4. To check for the presence of pyrogens in the ophthalmic formulation the two general tests done are......................
5. LAL stands for .... and it is an aqueous extract of blood cells (amoebocytes) from ....
6. Pyrogens are .... they are .... In nature, which is a membrane component of gram ...... bacteria.

7. Which of the following is not the characters required for optimizing the ocular drug delivery system?
   i. Good corneal penetration.
   ii. Prolong contact time with corneal tissue.
   iii. Hypertonicity of the the solution.
   iv. Sterility of the product.
8. Which of the following is not an ophthalmic product?
   i. Spects and sunglasses
   ii. Eye-lotions
   iii. Contact lens solution
   iv. Eye ointments
9. Which of the following are the evaluation tests for ophthalmic preparations?
   i. Particle size determination and test for clarity of ophthalmic solutions.
   ii. Test for pH of the solution and test for particulate matter.
   iii. Test for sterility of ophthalmic products and pyrogen test
   iv. All of the above.

ANSWERS

1. Cornea
2. Poly (2-hydroxyethylmethacrylate)
3. 5–10 μm or less
4. Rabbit test and LALs test
5. Limulus amoebocyte lysate, horseshoe crab, limulus polyphemus.
6. Bacterial endotoxin, lipopolysaccharide, negative
7. iii
8. i
9. iv

7

Nasal Products

Treatment of aliments by nasal administration is gaining its importance from past few decades due to the ease of administration and vascularity of the mucosa present in nasal cavity which prevents the first pass metabolism. Drugs which are potent and required in lower doses, whose activity is required faster with fewer side effects, can be delivered through the nasal route.

Drugs are administered through nasal route for several years for both topical effect and systemic effect. Topical administration includes delivery of drug to treat rhinitis, nasal congestion, sinusitis, and other related allergies. The drugs include corticosteroids, anticholinergics, antihistamines, etc. It is considered as one of the major route of drug administration to achieve faster and greater bioavailability of drug, as the nasal mucosa has high vasculature and high permeation of drugs. This route is used to administer drugs that are ineffective orally, chronically administered, small dose requirement and need rapid systemic absorption. It is potential route for admi-nistration of proteins and peptides, vaccines and it shows enhanced efficacy and better patient acceptance of drugs.

Advantages

- Noninvasive route
- High permeability of nasal mucosa compared with epithelial tissue of GIT
- Rapid onset of action

- No first pass metabolism
- Potential for direct delivery to CNS
- Avoidance of gastric irritation and vomiting
- Higher bioavailability of drugs than that of GIT
- Most feasible route for delivery of peptides

Disadvantages

- Sterility and stability problems.
- Design of the device is difficult.
- Difficult to use by pediatric and geriatric patients.
- Time available for absorption is less.
- Dose is limited due to less available surface area.
- Disease conditions of nose results in impaired absorption.

Limitations

- Risk of local side effects and irreversible damage of mucosa due to drug or excipients used.
- Low bioavailability due to enzymatic degradation and poor residence time.

Approaches to overcome limitations:

- Use of bioadhesive formulations that increase nasal residence time.
- Use of absorption enhancers that increase membrane permeability.
- Use of protease and peptidase inhibitors (Fig. 7.1).

To achieve nasal delivery the following are considered:

- Physicochemical properties of drug.
- Delivery system—nasal emulsions and ointments, nasal sprays, nasal drops, nasal microspheres, nasal gels.
- *Nasal physiology:* The nose is a complex organ from a kinetic point of view as three different processes: deposition, clearance or translocation and absorption of drugs take place inside the nose. For effective administration of therapeutic drugs through the nasal route, its anatomy and related physiological features must be taken into consideration. The nasal septum divides the nasal cavity into two unequal cavities. The septum consists mostly of cartilage and skin, and therefore, the penetration of drugs is low. The most

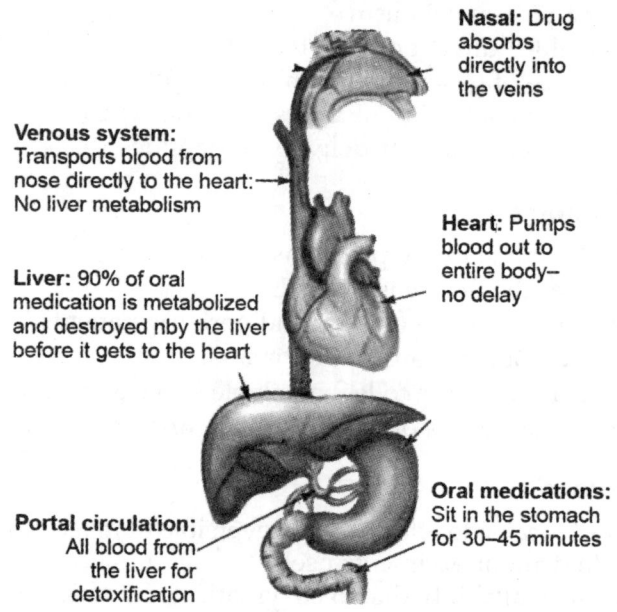

Nasal: Drug absorbs directly into the veins

Venous system: Transports blood from nose directly to the heart: No liver metabolism

Heart: Pumps blood out to entire body– no delay

Liver: 90% of oral medication is metabolized and destroyed nby the liver before it gets to the heart

Oral medications: Sit in the stomach for 30–45 minutes

Portal circulation: All blood from the liver for detoxification

Fig. 7.1: Nasal route of drug delivery – avoid first pass metabolism

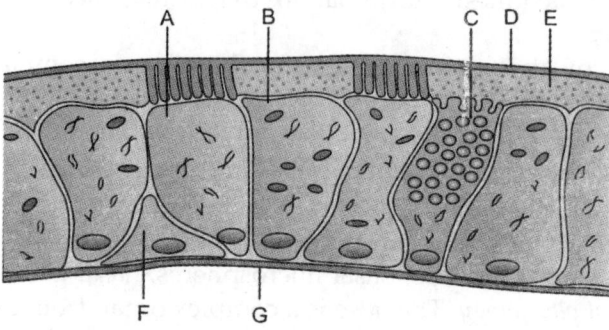

Fig. 7.2: Nasal epithelium showing ciliated cell: Cell types of the nasal epithelium showing ciliated cell (A), non-ciliated cell (B), goblet cells (C), gel mucus layer (D), sol layer (E), basal cell (F) and basement membrane (G)

efficient area for drug absorption is the highly vascularized lateral wall of the nasal cavity: the mucosa lined over the turbinates or conchae.

- *Effect of absorption:* Deposition of the formulation in the anterior portion of the nose provides a longer nasal residence time. The anterior portion of the nose shows low permeability. On the other hand, depositing a drug in the posterior portion of the nose, where the drug permeability is generally higher, provides shorter residence time. The method of administration and properties of the formulation determine the deposition site.

- *Effect of nasal enzymes:* Several enzymes that are present in the nasal mucosa might affect the stability of drugs. For example, proteins and peptides are subjected to degradation by proteases and amino-peptidase at the mucosal membrane. The level of amino-peptidase present is much lower than that in the gastrointestinal tract. Peptides may also form complexes with immunoglobulins (igs) in the nasal cavity leading to an increase in the molecular weight and a reduction of permeability.

- *Rate of nasal secretion:* More the nasal secretion decrease in bioavailability of the drug.

- *Mucociliary clearance:* It is important that the integrity of the nasal clearance mechanism is maintained to perform normal physiological functions such as the removal of dust, allergens and bacteria. The ciliary activity is the driving force of the secretory transport in the nose to constantly remove particles that are trapped on the mucus blanket during inhalation.

The absorption of drugs is influenced by the residence (contact) time between the drug and the epithelial tissue. The mucociliary clearance is inversely related to the residence time, and therefore, inversely proportional to the absorption of drugs administered. A prolonged residence time in the nasal cavity may also be achieved by using bioadhesive polymers, microspheres, chitosan or by increasing the viscosity of the formulation. Nasal mucociliary clearance can also be stimulated or inhibited by drugs, excipients, preservatives and/or absorption enhancers and thus affect drug delivery to the absorption site (Fig. 7.3).

Physicochemical properties of the drug molecules:

- *Chemical form:* The chemical form of a drug is important in determining absorption. For example, conversion of the drug into a salt or ester form can alter its absorption, e.g. it

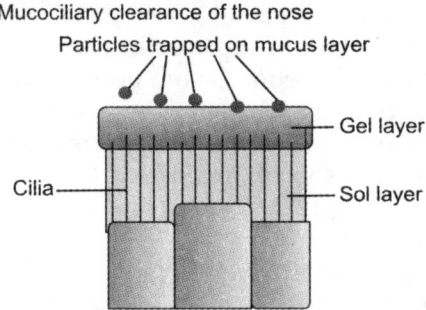

Fig. 7.3: Mucociliary clearance of the nose

was observed that *in situ* nasal absorption of carboxylic acid esters of L-tyrosine was significantly greater than that of L-tyrosine.

- *Polymorphism:* Polymorphism is known to affect the dissolution rate and solubility of drugs and thus their absorption through biological membranes. It is therefore advisable to study the polymorphic stability and purity of drugs for nasal powders and/or suspensions.

- *Molecular weight:* A linear inverse correlation has been reported between the absorption of drugs and molecular weight up to 300 Daltons. Absorption decreases significantly, if the molecular weight is greater than 1000 Daltons except with the use of absorption enhancers.

- *Particle size:* It has been reported that particle sizes greater than 10 μm are deposited in the nasal cavity. Particles that are 2 to 10 μm can be retained in the lungs, and particles of less than 1 μm are exhaled.

- *Solubility and dissolution rate:* Drug solubility and dissolution rates are important factors in determining nasal absorption from powders and suspensions. The particles deposited in the nasal cavity need to be dissolved prior to absorption. If a drug remains as particles or is cleared away, no absorption occurs.

Drug Concentration, Dose and Dose Volume

Drug concentration, dose and volume of administration are three interrelated parameters that impact the performance of the nasal delivery performance. Nasal absorption of L-tyrosine was shown to increase with drug concentration in nasal perfusion experiments. It was shown that aminopyrine was found to absorb at a constant rate as a function of concentration. In contrast, absorption of salicylic acid was found to decline with concentration. This decline is likely due to nasal mucosa damage by the permeant.

Formulation pH

The pH of a nasal formulation is important for the following reasons:

- To avoid irritation of nasal mucosa.
- To allow the drug to be available in unionized form for absorption.
- To prevent growth of pathogenic bacteria in the nasal passage.
- To maintain functionality of excipients such as preservatives.
- To sustain normal physiological ciliary movement.

Lysozyme is found in nasal secretions, which is responsible for destroying certain bacteria at acidic pH. Under alkaline conditions, lysozyme is inactivated and the nasal tissue is susceptible to microbial infection. It is therefore advisable to keep the formulation at a pH of 4.5 to 6.5.

Buffer Capacity

Nasal formulations are generally administered in small volumes ranging from 25 to 200 µl with 100 µl being the most common dose volume. Hence, nasal secretions may alter the pH of the administrated dose. This can affect the concentration of unionized drug available for absorption. Therefore, an adequate formulation buffer capacity may be required to maintain the pH *in situ*.

Osmolarity

Drug absorption can be affected by tonicity of the formulation. Shrinkage of epithelial cells has been observed in the presence of hypertonic solutions. Hypertonic saline solutions also inhibit or cease ciliary activity. Low pH has a similar effect as that of a hypertonic solution.

Formulation Ingredients

Gelling/Viscofying Agents or Gel-forming Carriers

Increasing solution viscosity may provide a means of prolonging the therapeutic effect of nasal preparations. It was showed that a drug carrier such as hydroxypropyl cellulose was effective for improving the absorption of low molecular weight drugs but did not produce the same effect for high molecular weight peptides. Use of a combination of carriers is often recommended from a safety (nasal irritancy) point of view.

Solubilizers

Aqueous solubility of drug is always a limitation for nasal drug delivery in solution. Conventional solvents or co-solvents such as glycols, small quantities of alcohol, transcutol (diethylene glycol monoethyl ether), medium chain glycerides and labrasol (saturated polyglycolyzed C_8–C_{10} glyceride) can be used to enhance the solubility of drugs. Other options include the use of surfactants or cyclodextrins such as HP-β-cyclodextrin that serve as a biocompatible solubilizer and stabilizer in combination with lipophilic absorption enhancers. In such cases, their impact on nasal irritancy should be considered.

Preservatives

Most of the nasal formulations are aqueous based and need preservatives to prevent microbial growth.
- Parabens
- Benzalkonium chloride
- Phenyl ethyl alcohol
- EDTA and
- Benzoyl alcohol

Note: It was reported that mercury containing preservatives have a fast and irreversible effect on ciliary movement and should not be used in nasal systems.

Antioxidants: Used in small quantity to prevent drug oxidation of the drug formulation, e.g. sodium metabisulfite, sodium bisulfite, butylated hydroxytoluene and tocopherol. Usually, antioxidants do not affect drug absorption or cause nasal irritation. Chemical/physical interaction of antioxidants and preservatives with drugs, excipients, manufacturing equipment and packaging components should be considered as part of the formulation development program.

Humectants

Usually drying of mucous membrane and crusts cause many allergic and chronic diseases. Certain preservatives/ antioxidants among other excipients are also likely to cause nasal irritation especially when used in higher quantities. Humectants are added especially in gel-based nasal products to prevent dehydration of nasal mucosa. They avoid nasal irritation and are not likely to affect drug absorption, e.g. glycerin, sorbitol and mannitol.

Role of Absorption Enhancers

Absorption enhancers are used when it is difficult for a nasal product to achieve desirable absorption profile. The selection is based upon their acceptability by regulatory agencies and their impact on the physiological functioning of the nose. They may be required when a drug exhibits poor membrane permeability, large molecular size, lack of lipophilicity and enzymatic degradation by amino peptidases. Generally, the absorption enhancers act via one of the following mechanisms:

- Inhibit enzyme activity;
- Reduce mucus viscosity or elasticity;
- Decrease mucociliary clearance;
- Open tight junctions; and
- Solubilize or stabilize the drug.
  Types of absorption enhancers: Two types
  1. *Chemical enhancers:* Chelating agents, fatty acids, bile acid salts, surfactants, and preservatives.
  2. *Physical enhancers:* Osmotic agents and buffers.

Effect of Pathological Condition

Intranasal pathologies such as allergic rhinitis, infections, or previous nasal surgery may affect the nasal mucociliary transport process and/or capacity for nasal absorption. During the common cold, the efficiency of an intranasal medication is often compromised. Nasal clearance is reduced in insulin-dependent diabetes. Nasal pathology can also alter mucosal pH and thus affect absorption of drugs.

Mechanism of drug absorption:
- *Para cellular route:* Passive absorption-depends on mol wt of drugs. Up to 300 Daltons show good absorption. Molecular weight > 1000 D shows poor absorption.
- *Transcellular route:* Lipophilic drugs-depends on lipophilicity of drugs
- *Active transport:* Carriers are involved in opening of tight junction opening, e.g. chitosan

Nasal Dosage Forms

Nasal Drops

Most simple and convenient systems, but shows low dose precision. These are usually isotonic and slightly buffered to maintained a pH of 5.5 to 6.5. in addition appropriate anti-microbials and drug stabilizers are added if required. They spread more extensively than the spray, e.g. Otrivine Adult nasal drops 10 ml, fenox nasal drops 15 ml, ephedrine nasal drops 0.5%.

Nasal Sprays

Includes both solution and suspension forms. Delivers exact dose of drug (25–200 µl) through metered dose pumps and actuators. Choice of pump and actuator assembly depends on particle size and viscosity of formulation. Although delivery methods vary, most nasal sprays function by instilling a fine mist into the nostril by action of a hand-operated pump mechanism, e.g. calpol saline nasal spray 15 ml, salclear sinazo hay fever and decongestant nasal spray, nasaleze nasal powder spray, pollenase allergy nasal spray (Fig. 7.4).

Antihistamine nasal sprays: Excessive histamine function is the primary cause of allergic reactions in people. Histamine is a chemical naturally produced by the body which creates an inflammatory effect to help the immune system remove foreign substances. Antihistamines work by competing for receptor sites to block the function of histamine, thereby reducing the inflammatory effect.

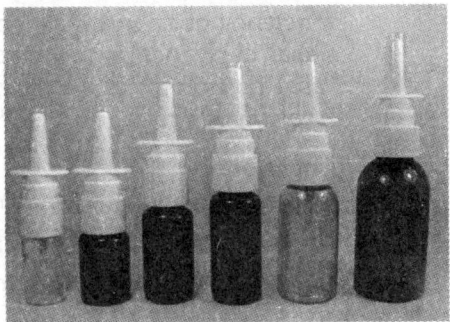

Fig. 7.4: Nasal spray bottles

Astelin (azelastin hydrochloride) and patanase (olopatadine hydrochloride) are the only local antihistamines available as a nasal spray. They are available by prescription only and have gained popularity with sufferers of allergic rhinitis.

Topical decongestant nasal spray: Oxymetazoline hydrochloride decongestant nasal sprays such as afrin and vicks sinex, along with phenylephrine hydrochloride nasal sprays such as neo synephrine and dristan, which are available over-the-counter in the United States and the UK, work to very quickly open up nasal passages by constricting blood vessels in the lining of the nose.

Prolonged use of these types of sprays can damage the delicate mucous membranes in the nose. This causes increased inflammation, an effect known as rhinitis medicamentosa, or the "rebound effect". As a result, decongestant nasal sprays are advised for short-term use only. However, a recent clinical trial has shown that fluticasone which is a corticosteroid nasal spray may be useful in reversing this condition. Natural nasal sprays may also be helpful in this regard however no clinical trials have been carried out to date.

Corticosteroid nasal spray: Corticosteroid nasal sprays such as nasonex and rhinocort can be used to relieve the symptoms of sinusitis, hay fever, allergic rhinitis and non-allergic (perennial) rhinitis. They can reduce inflammation and histamine production in the nasal passages thereby relieving nasal congestion, runny nose, sneezing, sinus pain, headaches, etc. They have been clinically proven however they can cause side effects such as headaches, nausea and nose bleeds.

Nasal Gels

High viscosity solutions or suspensions, e. g. vitamin B_{12} gel., secaris lubricating nasal gel, neilmed nasogel drip free gel spray for nasal dryness.

Main advantages include:

- Reduction of post-nasal drip
- Reduction of taste impact due to reduces swallowing
- Reduction of anterior leakage of the formulation
- Reduction of irritation by using soothing/emollient excipients.

Nasal powders: These are developed for drugs that show poor stability in solution or suspension dosage forms. The main advantages are:

- No preservative
- Superior stability of the formulation
- Local application of the drug.

Note: Particle size, solubility, aerodynamic properties, nasal irritancy, metered dose delivery systems are considered while designing the powder formulation.

Nasal Emulsions and Ointments

They can be applied locally, but they show poor patient acceptability. Physical stability of emulsion is also considered. Intranasal route is gaining a lot of interest for delivery of products like vaccines, hormones and peptides as they can bypass the first pass metabolism and gut wall metabolism or destruction due to GI fluids. The circulatory and the secretary systems in nasal mucosa influence the drug absorption.

When drug is introduced into the nose in the form of liquid or aerosol or powder, it has to pass through nasal valve for which the air should flow at high linear velocity and change direction. Instead of deposition in the cavity and carried back to stomach by mucocillary system, if the drug is delivered in vapour or soluble form, it pass through the surface secretions and thus finally reach the systemic circulation.

Drug delivery devices: These are the devices intended to deliver the drug into nasal route.

Requirements of Drug Delivery Devices

The delivery systems are designed in such a way that they have to dispense exact dose of the drug at every time of delivery and there is need to optimize the drug delivery of individual formulations.

The key requirements include:

- Accuracy after repeated dosing
- Consistent delivery to optimum site of action
- Protection of the formulations which are preservative free
- Patient independent actuation
- Patient compliance and minimal risks.

The drug delivery through the nasal route is achieved by two important devices:

1. Mechanical pump system and
2. Pressurized aerosol system.

1. *Mechanical pump system:* These systems may be of single dose capsule based delivery systems (rota healer) or multiple dose healers (disk healer). The usage is very patient friendly and can deliver biotherapeutics. Patient requires very less training for its usage. But these require high inspirational rates and there is every chance of drug deposition in the oropharynx. Large doses cannot be delivered.

2. *Pressurized aerosol system:* This system helps in dispensing the specific amount of medication into the lungs. Asthma, chronic obstructive pulmonary disease and other respiratory diseases are treated through this delivery system. These types of delivery systems are portable and can be made available in various doses.

The use of inhaler is easy and patients can simply press down with their thumb. The propellant provides the force to generate the aerosol cloud and is also the medium in which the active component must be suspended or dissolved. By actuating the device the drug is released as single metered dose of formulation. The volatile propellant is broken into the droplets and results in aerosol containing micrometer sized particles which are inhaled (Fig. 7.5).

Vehicle systems like solution, suspension or emulsion are used for nasal drug delivery. The use of mechanical pump is

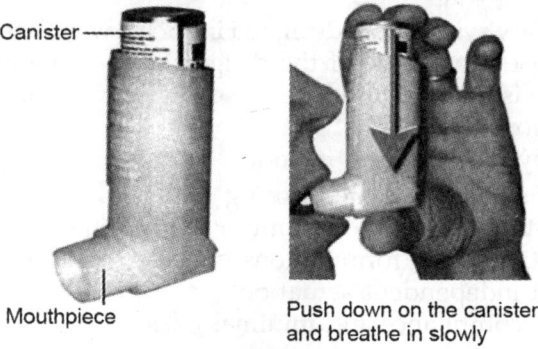

Canister

Mouthpiece

Push down on the canister and breathe in slowly

Fig. 7.5: Pressurized aerosol system

straighter forward when compared with the aerosol systems as these require propellants.

Two types of devices are widely used to deliver drug through nasal cavity:
- Multidose systems
- Unit/bi-dose systems.

Multidose Systems

This system consists of a container that is mounted with a mechanical pump dispenser that is designed to deliver drug in multiple doses from one container.

Unit Dose/Bi-dose Systems

These are used in particular therapies to deliver precise amount of drug in particular therapies and are becoming more attractive to the pharmaceutical industry.

Metered Dose Inhalers

A metered-dose inhaler (MDI) is a device that delivers a specific amount of medication to the lungs, in the form of a short burst of aerosolized medicine that is inhaled by the patient. It is the most commonly used delivery system for treating asthma, chronic obstructive pulmonary disease (COPD) and other respiratory diseases. The medication in a metered dose inhaler is most commonly a bronchodilator, corticosteroid or a combination of both for the treatment of asthma and COPD.

Other medications less commonly used but also administered by MDI are mast cell stabilizers, (such as cromoglicate or nedocromil).

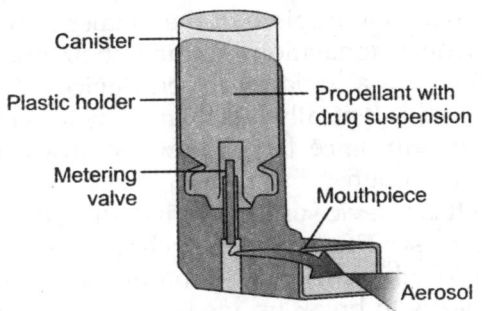

Canister

Plastic holder — Propellant with drug suspension

Metering valve

Mouthpiece

Aerosol

Fig. 7.6: Metered-dose inhalers

Metered-dose inhalers are only one type of inhaler, but they are the most commonly used type. The replacement of chlorofluorocarbons propellants with hydrofluoralkanes resulted in the redesign of metered-dose inhalers in the 1990s. For one variety of beclomethasone inhaler, this redesign resulted in considerably smaller aerosol particles being produced, and led to an increase of potency by a factor of 2.6.

Uses

• Asthma inhalers contain a medication that treats the symptoms of asthma.

• A nicotine inhaler allows cigarette smokers to get nicotine without using tobacco, much like nicotine gum or a nicotine patch. Nicotine inhalers that are marketed for nicotine replacement therapy should not be confused with electronic cigarettes, which produce vapour and which are marketed mainly as devices that smokers can use in nonsmoking areas.

Dry powder inhaler: It is a device that delivers medication to the lungs in the form of a dry powder. DPIs are commonly used to treat respiratory diseases such as asthma, bronchitis, emphysema and COPD although DPIs have also been used in the treatment of diabetes mellitus. DPIs are an alternative to the aerosol based inhalers MDI. The DPIs may require some procedure to allow a measured dose of powder to be ready for the patient to take. The medication is commonly held either in a capsule for manual loading or a proprietary form from inside the inhaler. Once loaded or actuated, the operator puts the mouthpiece of the inhaler into their mouth and takes a deep inhalation, holding their breath for 5–10 seconds. There are a variety of such devices. The dose that can be delivered is typically less than a few tens of milligrams in a single breath since larger powder doses may lead to provocation of cough.

Nebulizer: It is a device used to deliver drug into the lungs in the form of mist. The common technical principal for all nebulizers is to either use oxygen, compressed air or ultrasonic power, as means to break up medical solutions/suspensions into small aerosol droplets, for direct inhalation from the mouthpiece of the device. Nebulizers are commonly used for treatment of cystic fibrosis, asthma, COPD and other respiratory diseases (Fig. 7.7).

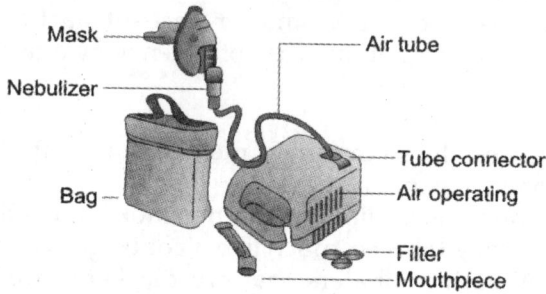

• Mouthpiece • Adult mask • Bag • Nebulizer
• Connecting tube • 5 Air filter

Fig. 7.7: Nebulizer kit

Evaluation Tests

Physical Tests

1. Tests for Nasal Powders

Particle size determination by:

Optical microscopy: Particle size can be measured microscopically by sizing against a graticule and counting, but for a statistically valid analysis, millions of particles must be measured. This is impossibly arduous when done manually, but automated analysis of electron micrographs is now commercially available. Instruments such as the retsch Camsizer can perform this analysis on the run using standard camera technology.

Sieve analysis: In this the particles of a powder mass are placed on screen made of uniform apertures. By the application of some type of motion to the screen the particles of larger size retain on the screen and smaller ones pass through other screens. Sieves measuring particle size of 5 μ are available now with the introduction of electroformed screens.

Coulters Counter Method
(Electroresistance Counting Methods)

In this the momentary changes in the conductivity of a liquid passing through an orifice is measured when individual non-conducting particles pass through. The particle count is obtained by counting pulses, and the size is dependent on the size of each pulse.

Technique advantage: Very small sample aliquots can be examined.

Technique disadvantages: Sample must be dispersed in a liquid medium as some particles may (partially or fully) dissolve in the medium altering the size distribution. The results are only related to the projected cross-sectional area that a particle displaces as it passes through an orifice. This is a physical diameter, not really related to mathematical descriptions of particles (e.g. terminal settling velocity).

Acoustic Spectroscopy or Ultrasound Attenuation Spectroscopy

In this method ultrasound is employed for collecting information on the particles that are dispersed in fluid. Dispersed particles absorb and scatter ultrasound similarly to light. It turns out that instead of measuring scattered energy versus angle, as with light, in the case of ultrasound, measuring the *transmitted energy versus frequency* is a better choice. The resulting ultrasound attenuation frequency spectra are the raw data for calculating particle size distribution. It can be measured for any fluid system with no dilution or other sample preparation. Calculation of particle size distribution is based on theoretical models that are well-verified for up to 50% by volume of dispersed particles.

Laser diffraction methods: These depend upon analysis of the "halo" of diffracted light produced when a laser beam passes through a dispersion of particles in air or in a liquid. The angle of diffraction increases as particle size decreases. This method is particularly good for measuring sizes between 0.1 and 3, 000 μm. A particular advantage is that the technique can generate a continuous measurement for analyzing process streams.

2. Tests for Nasal Solutions and Nasal Drops

Clarity of the solution: Retention of clarity of solution is a main concern regarding stability of solution. In this a microscopic light is projected though a diaphragm into the solution. The solution will remain clear if there are no undissolved particles. If not the solution appears hazy due to the scattering of light by undissolved particles. Light scattering instruments are most widely used to test the clarity of the solution.

Test for Sterility

This is used to test the presence of microorganisms in the test solution. It is done by 2 methods:

- Membrane filtration method
- Direct inoculation (Immersion) method.

Membrane filtration method: In this the test solution is first passed through size exclusion membrane capable of retaining the micro-organisms. The concept is that the micro-organisms will collect on the surface of a 0.45 micron pore size filter. The filter is rinsed and then the membrane is transferred to appropriate test medium as specified in the monograph.

Direct inoculation (Immersion) method: In this the test article is directly inoculated into the test medium and then the medium is incubated for the growth of microorganisms, if present.

Test media: The test media are fluid thioglycollate medium (FTM) and soybean casein digest medium (SCDM). FTM is selected based upon its ability to support the growth of anaerobic and aerobic microorganisms. SCDM is selected based upon its ability to support a wide range of aerobic bacteria and fungi (i.e. yeasts and molds).

Incubation time: In both the methods the test medium after the transferring of the test solution is to be incubated for 3 days in case of bacteria and 5 days in case of fungi and then the growth is compared with that of standard. If no growth is observed then the sample passes the test and it meets the GMP requirements.

Volume/container	Minimum quantity to test in each media
<1ml	The entire contents of each container
1–40 ml	Half the contents of each container but not <1 ml
41–100 ml	20 ml
>100 ml	10% of the contents of the container, but not <20 ml

The following table outlines the requirement for sterility testing as per USP.

Product flush sterility testing: This is the method of choice for devices featuring hollow tubes, such as transfusion and infusion assemblies. Easy to perform, this sterility testing process consists of placing the sample device into a specific bacteriological growth medium selected for products with such small lumens or hollows, and monitoring any subsequent bacteria growth. It requires standard 14 day incubation period.

Test for Pyrogens

It is used to check for the presence of pyrogens in the test formulation. Two general tests are there:
• Rabbit test and
• LALs test

Rabbit Test

The pyrogen test is designed to limit to an acceptable level the risks of febrile reaction in the patient after the administration, by injection, of the product concerned. Unless otherwise specified in the individual monograph, inject into an ear vein of each of three rabbits 10 ml of the test solution per kg of body weight, completing each injection within 10 minutes after start of administration. The test solution is *either* the product, constituted if necessary as directed in the labeling, *or* the material under test treated as directed in the individual monograph and injected in the dose specified therein. Assure that all test solutions are protected from contamination. Perform the injection after warming the test solution to a temperature of 37 ± 2°. Record the temperature at 30-minute intervals between 1 and 3 hours subsequent to the injection.

Test Interpretation

Consider any temperature decreases as zero rise. If no rabbit shows an individual rise in temperature of 0.5° or more above its respective control temperature, the product meets the requirements for the absence of pyrogens. If any rabbit shows an individual temperature rise of 0.5° or more, continue the test using five other rabbits. If not more than three of the eight rabbits show individual rises in temperature of 0.5° or more and if the sum of the eight individual maximum temperature rises does not exceed 3.3°, the material under examination meets the requirements for the absence of pyrogens.

LALs test: Limulus amebocyte lysate (LAL) is an aqueous extract of blood cells (amoebocytes) from the horseshoe crab, Limulus polyphemus. LAL reacts with bacterial endotoxin or lipopolysaccharide (LPS), which is a membrane component of gram-negative bacteria. This reaction is the basis of the LAL test.

Method: Blood is removed from the horseshoe crab's pericardium and the blood cells are separated from the serum using centrifugation and are then placed in distilled water, which causes them to swell up and burst ("lyse"). This releases the chemicals from the inside of the cell (the "lysate"), which is then purified and freeze-dried. To test a sample for endotoxins, it is mixed with lysate and water; endotoxins are present if coagulation occurs.

3. Test for Nasal Gels, Suspensions, Emulsions and Ointments

Viscosity measurement—Brook-field viscometer, cone and plate viscometer. The flow of fluids through pipes is influenced by viscosity of the fluid. In order to have a better flow the viscosity of the formulation should be checked under controlled temperature.

Consistency measurement: Penetrometer. It is the measure of penetration of an object into the product to be examined in a container with a specified shape and size. In this the test sample is placed on the base of the penetrometer such that its surface is perpendicular to the vertical axis of penetrating object. The temperature of the penetrating object is maintained at 25 + /– 0.5°C and then its tip is adjusted such that it just touches the surface of the sample. The penetrating object if released and hold it for 5 sec then the penetrating object is clamped and the depth of penetration is measured. The test is repeated for 2 remaining containers.

Texture analysis: It is primarily concerned with the evaluation of mechanical characters when the material is subjected to controlled force which cause deformation of the sample. Texture analyzer which is used to detect.

Ointment flow characteristic, e.g. brook-field texture analyser.

Ointment consistency: this can be measured by using penetrometry technique.

Gel strength: Gels have gained wide acceptance as semisolid dosage forms. It has been postulated that the strength rather than the viscosity of a gel layer plays a major role in determining the amount of drug release from hydrophilic matrices. Recent advances have occurred in the development of an optimal apparatus to characterize gel strength. The apparatus consists of a sample holder placed on an electronic microbalance connected to a computer. A probe is lowered into the sample by means of a motor equipped with a speed transformer, and the force required to penetrate the gel is measured. The increase in force with time is a function of the mechanical resistance of the sample to the penetration of the probe. Because the lowering speed is known, the displacement covered by the probe as a function of time is calculated and used to compute the gel-strength parameter or mechanical resistance of the gel system.

Flavour release: In this, the driving force for flavor release is shown to depend on the bulk melting temperature of the gel. For gels possessing melting points below the mouth temperature, the driving force for flavor release is the rate at which heat can diffuse into the gels matrix and initiate melting. For harder gels with melting points above mouth temperature the diffusion of gelling agent from the surface of the gel into the adjacent saliva phase is the rate limiting step for flavor release, because this lowers the melting temperature of the surface layer, e.g. the theoretical model gives good agreement with in vitro release experiments using gelatin gels containing sucrose and dye.

Sachet or tube extrusion force measurement: In this the device quantifies the force required to extrude the contents from either tube or sachet style packaging that allows manufacturers to tests the force required to extrude the content of a sachet or tube at regular intervals over a long period of time, throughout its shelf-life.

4. Tests for Aerosols

Delivery Rate and Delivered Amount

These tests are performed only on containers fitted with continuous valves.

Delivery rate: Select not fewer than four aerosol containers, shake, if the label includes this directive, remove the caps and covers, and actuate each valve for 2 to 3 seconds. Weigh each container accurately, and immerse in a constant-temperature bath until the internal pressure is equilibrated at a temperature of 25° as determined by constancy of internal pressure, as directed under the pressure test below. Remove the containers from the bath, remove excess moisture by blotting with a paper towel, shake, if the label includes this directive, actuate each valve for 5.0 seconds (accurately timed by use of a stopwatch), and weigh each container again. Return the containers to the constant-temperature bath, and repeat the foregoing procedure three times for each container. Calculate the average delivery Rate, in g per second, for each container.

Delivered amount: Return the containers to the constant-temperature bath, continuing to deliver 5 second actuations to waste, until each container is exhausted. [Note—ensure that sufficient time is allowed between each actuation to avoid significant canister cooling]. Calculate the total weight loss from each container. This is the delivered amount.

Pressure Test

Select not fewer than four aerosol containers, remove the caps and covers, and immerse in a constant-temperature bath until the internal pressure is constant at a temperature of 25°. Remove the containers from the bath, shake, and remove the actuator and water, if any, from the valve stem. Place each container in an upright position, and determine the pressure in each container by placing a calibrated pressure gauge on the valve stem, holding firmly, and actuating the valve so that it is fully open. The gauge is of a calibration approximating the expected pressure and is fitted with an adapter appropriate for the particular valve stem dimensions. Read the pressure directly from the gauge.

Minimum Fill

Select a sample of 10 filled containers, and remove any labeling that might be altered in weight during the removal of the container contents. Thoroughly cleanse and dry the outsides of the containers by suitable means, and weigh individually. Remove the contents from each container by employing any safe technique (e.g. chill to reduce the internal pressure, remove the valve, and pour). Remove any residual contents with suitable solvents, and then rinse with a few portions of methanol. Retain as a unit the container, the valve, and all associated parts, and heat them at 100° for 5 minutes. Cool, and again weigh each of the containers together with its corresponding parts. The difference between the original weight and the weight of the empty aerosol container is the net fill weight. Determine the net fill weight for each container tested. The requirements are met if the net weight of the contents of each of the 10 containers is not less than the labeled amount.

Leakage Test

Perform this test only on topical aerosols fitted with continuous valves.

Select 12 aerosol containers, and record the date and time to the nearest half-hour. Weigh each container to the nearest mg, and record the weight, in mg, of each as W_1. Allow the containers to stand in an upright position at a temperature of 25.0 ± 2.0° for not less than 3 days, and again weigh each container, recording the weight, in mg, of each as W_2, and recording the date and time to the nearest half-hour. Determine the time, T, in hours, during which the containers were under test. Calculate the leakage rate, in mg per year, of each container taken by the formula:

$$\text{Leakage rate} = (365) \times (24/T) \, (W_1 - W_2)$$

Where plastic-coated glass aerosol containers are tested, dry the containers in a desiccator for 12 to 18 hours, and allow them to stand in a constant-humidity environment for 24 hours prior to determining the initial weight as indicated above. Conduct the test under the same constant-humidity conditions. Empty the contents of each container tested by employing any safe technique (e.g. chill to reduce the internal pressure, remove the valve, and pour). Remove any residual contents by rinsing with suitable solvents, then rinse with a few portions of methanol. Retain as a unit the container, the valve, and all associated parts, and heat them at 100° for 5 minutes. Cool, weigh, record the weight as W_3, and determine the net fill weight $(W_1 - W_3)$ for each container tested. [Note–if the average net fill weight has been determined previously, that value may be used in place of the value $(W_1 - W_3)$ above.] The requirements are met if the average leakage rate per year for the 12 containers is not more than 3.5% of the net fill weight, and none of the containers leaks more than 5.0% of the net fill weight per year. If 1 container leaks more than 5.0% per year, and if none of the containers leaks more than 7.0% per year, determine the leakage rate of an additional 24 containers as directed herein. Not more than 2 of the 36 containers leak more than 5.0% of the net fill weight per year, and none of the 36 containers leaks more than 7.0% of the net fill weight per year. Where the net fill weight is less than 15 g and the label bears an expiration date, the requirements are met if the average leakage rate of the 12 containers is not more than 525 mg per year and none of the containers leaks more than 750 mg per year. If 1 container leaks more than 750 mg per year, but not more than 1.1 g per year, determine the leakage rate of an additional 24 containers as directed herein. Not more than 2 of the 36 containers leak more than 750 mg per year, and none of the 36 containers leaks more than 1.1 g per year. This test is in addition to the customary in-line leak testing of each container.

Number of Discharges per Container

Perform this test only on topical aerosols fitted with dose-metering valves, at the same time as, and on the same containers used for, the test for delivered-dose uniformity. Determine the number of discharges or deliveries by counting the number of priming discharges plus those used in determining the spray contents, and continue to fire until the label claim number of discharges. The requirements are met if all the containers or inhalers tested contain not less than the number of discharges stated on the label.

Delivered Dose Uniformity

Unless otherwise directed in the individual monograph, the drug content of the minimum delivered doses (minimum number of sprays per nostril as described on the label, or instructions for use) collected at the beginning of unit life (after priming as described on the label, or instructions for use) and at the label claim number of metered sprays, from each of 10 separate containers, must meet the following acceptance criteria: not more than 2 of the 20 doses are outside the range of 80 to 120% of label claim, and none are outside the range of 75 to 125% of label claim, while the mean for each of the beginning and end doses falls within the range of 85 to 115% of label claim. If 3–6 doses of the 20 doses collected are outside of 80 to 120% of the label claim, but none are outside of 75 to 125% of label claim, and the means for each of the beginning and end doses fall within 85 to 115% of label claim, select 20 additional containers for second-tier testing. For second-tier testing, the requirements are met if not more than 6 of the 60 doses collected are outside the range of 80 to 120% of label claim, none are outside the range of 75 to 125% of label claim, and the means for each of the beginning and end doses fall within the range of 85 to 115% of label claim.

Chemical Tests

Chemical tests to be performed include:

a. *Chemical potency test:* Potency of the formulation is checked such that the dose delivered shows optimum therapeutic efficiency or not.

b. *PH measurement:* The pH of the formulation is checked as the drug is absorbed only in the ionized form and any change in pH may lead to damage of lysozyme enzyme in the nasal cavity. It is measured by using pH meter.

In Vitro Drug Release Studies

Modified USP type-II dissolution apparatus: A USP Type II dissolution apparatus was modified for studying the in vitro release of drug from ointment. It comprised a 200 ml vessel, 2.5 × 1.5 cm paddle, and an enhancer diffusion cell. The cell contained an adjustable-capacity sample reservoir, a washer for controlling the exposure of the surface area, and an open screw-on cap to secure the washer and membrane over the sample reservoir. The water bath is maintained at 37°C. Filled cells were placed in the bottom of the vessels, and the paddles were lowered to 1 cm above the sample surface. 50 ml of high-performance liquid chromatography-grade filtered water, degassed and prewarmed to 37°C, is used as the dissolution medium.

Advances in Nasal Drug Delivery Systems

Naso-mucoadhesive drug delivery: Mucoadhesives have been used to improve local and systemic delivery of therapeutic compounds. This section examines specific applications of mucoadhesive compounds with respect to nasal administration of small organic molecules, antibiotics, vaccines, DNA, proteins and other macromolecules.

Small organic molecules: Due to the rapid therapeutic action that can be achieved, medications used in emergency medical situations make ideal candidates for nasal drug delivery. One such drug, apomorphine is the drug of choice for treatment of on/off-syndrome in patients suffering from Parkinson's disease. Aqueous solution of the compound is reasonably well absorbed following nasal administration with a relative bioavailability of 45%.

Mucoadhesive delivery with hyaluronic acid and chitosan, HPMC, HEC, MC, etc. are used to deliver antibiotics like gentamicin, vancomycin, tobramycin, ciprofloxacin. Delivery of macromolecules like vaccines, proteins, DNA, in diseased states like influenza, meningitis, pertussis, diphtheria, tetanus, measles, e.g. administration of PEG coated tetanus toxoid nanospheres show promising results in the treatment of tetanus.

Microsphere Technology

- Shows prolonged contact with the nasal mucosa and enhanced absorption.
- Starch, dextran, albumin, gelatin are used to formulate microspheres.
- They cause reversible shrinkage of cells due to moisture uptake form mucosa (e. g. starch microspheres), that cause separation of the tight junctions thereby increase in drug absorption.
- Toxicity and irritancy of microspheres are to be evaluated. Protein drug delivery through stealth nanoparticles.

Peptide and protein drug delivery:

- Localized delivery of cyclosporines A, interferon, deoxyribonuclease, vasoactive intestinal peptides.
- Systemic delivery of insulin, LHRH, growth hormone, calcitonin, somatostatin, THSH, FSH.,
- Administration of peptide hormones: Peptide oxytocin was the first hormone to be administered through nasal route which is used in uterine contraction and lactation.

Drug delivery through micro emulsion:

- The intranasal delivery of clonazepam shows rapid drug delivery to brain and it shows a 2-fold increase when compared to drug administered through IV route.
- Intranasal administration of sumatriptan, used in treatment of migrane shows enhanced rate and extent of drug transport that decreases in dose and dosing frequency.
- Intranasal delivery of eucalyptus oil microemulsion shows rapid soothing effect and antidepressant action.
- Intranasal administration of nimodipine, used in treatment of neurodegenerative diseases shows three-folds increase of drug uptake when compared to intravenous administration.

Conclusion

With the advancement of technology and drug delivery systems the nasal route of drug administration is growing as a promising route of drug administration. It improves the patient compliance providing a noninvasive route. In order to obtain a nasal formulation with good performance, the drug properties, nasal physiology, patient pathological condition, drug delivery system are all considered. Not only locally acting formulations, systemically administered formulations are also developed, while some are in developing stage. In future this route will represent a viable route of drug administration both locally and systemically for a wide range of drugs.

ISOLATED KEY POINTS

- Delivery of drugs through nasal route, which is a non-invasive method, plays an important role of drug delivery to systemic circulation within a short period of time. These drugs are used in the treatment of asthma, COPD, allergic rhinitis, influenza, migraine, and osteoporosis.
- The present study consists of different dosage forms including nasal solutions, suspensions, nasal powders which are mostly administered in the form of aerosol formulations.
- The commonly used devices include MDIs, DPls, and nebulizers.
- Different evaluation parameters are performed to minimize the errors and to meet the requirments of specified properties of the nasal dosage forms that include particle size determination, clarity of the solution, viscosity of the suspensions, drug delivery rate, delivered dose uniformity, etc.
- Many new delivery devices are being developed to deliver accurate dose of drug in easy manner, which improves patient compliance.
- Many new drugs are also being formulated such that they are delivered through nasal route to treat Prakinson's disease and Alzheimer's disease.

PRACTICE QUESTIONS

1. What are nasal products? Give their advantages and disadvantages.
2. Enumerate various physicochemical properties of an drug moiety for designing an nasal product.
3. Discuss in brief about various formulation ingredients required for nasal products.

4. What are the various nasal dosage form? Explain it with the help of suitable exemples.
5. Discuss in brief about mechanical pump system used for nasal drug delivery.
6. Explain the construction working of pressurized nasal system used for nasal drug delivery.
7. What are the various evaluation test done for nasal dosage form?
8. What are the various evaluation test done for nasal solution and nasal drops?

OBJECTIVE TYPE QUESTIONS

1. Nasal formulations are generally administered in volumes ranging from ....
2. .... is a device used to deliver drug into the lungs in the form of mist.
3. Viscosity of nasal formulation is measured with the help of ....
4. Which of the following is not true for nasal drug delivery system
   i. Drugs are administered for both topical effect and systemic effect.
   ii. Drugs administer include corticosteroids, anticholinergics, antihistamines, etc.
   iii. Drug administer give fastest and highest bioavailability
   iv. Used to administer drugs that are ineffective orally, small dose requirement and need rapid systemic absorption
5. Which of the following is advantage in respect to nasal drug delivery system
   i. No first pass metabolism
   ii. No sterility and stability problems
   iii. Design of the device is easy
   iv. Easy-to-use by pediatric and geriatric patients
6. The pH of a nasal formulation is important for the following reasons
   i. To avoid irritation of nasal mucosa.
   ii. To allow the drug to be available in unionized form for absorption.
   iii. To prevent growth of pathogenic bacteria in the nasal passage.

iv. To sustain normal physiological ciliary movement.

v. All of the above

7. Match the following

S.no.	Formulation ingredient		Example
1.	Solubilizers	a	BHT
2.	Preservatives	b	Glycerin
3.	Antioxidants.	c	Cyclodextrins such as HP-β-cyclodextrin
4.	Humectants	d	Benzalkonium chloride

ANSWERS

1. 25 to 200 µL
2. Nebulizer
3. Brook-field viscometer, cone and plate viscometer
4. iii
5. i
6. v
7. 1-c, 2-d, 3-a, 4-b

8

Otic (Ear) Products

Ear plays a major role in hearing and maintenance of postural equilibrium. Drugs products applied through ear are intended for local effect and not for systemic effect for various types of ear disorders. Various new drug delivery devices are also being developed along with the conventional dosage forms like ear drops, ear ointments. Disorders of ear: Infection, inflammation, irritation, earache, cerumen (ear wax) accumulation, hearing loss and tinnitus. In order to understand the methods of drug administration to ear, physiology of ear is to be known.

Anatomy of Ear

The ear is divided into three parts:

- Outer or external ear
- Middle ear and
- Inner ear

External or Outer Ear

The external ear consists of:

- Pinna or auricle—the outside part of the ear.
- Ear canal—it connects the outer ear to the inside or middle ear.
- Tympanic membrane is also called the eardrum. The tympanic membrane divides the external ear from the middle ear.

279

Middle ear (Tympanic Cavity)

The middle ear consists of:

- A cavity that usually contains air
- Ossicles—it consists of three small bones which are connected with each other. They transmit the sound waves to the inner ear. The bones are called:
  - Malleus
  - Incus
  - Stapes
- Eustachian tube—it is a canal like structure which links the middle ear with throat area. It helps to equalize the pressure between the middle ear and the air around you that allows for the proper transfer of sound waves. The middle ear cavity and Eustachian tube are lined with mucous membrane, just like the inside of the nose and throat.

Inner ear

The inner ear consists of:

- Cochlea (contains the receptors for hearing)
- Vestibule (contains the receptors for balance)
- Semicircular canals (contain the receptors for balance).

Drugs applied to the inner ear are localized and they act directly on the affected area.

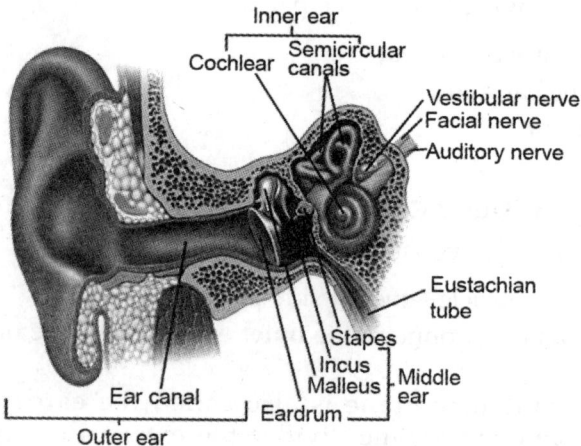

Fig. 8.1: Anatomy of ear

Principle of Hearing

Hearing starts with the outer ear. When a sound is made outside the outer ear, the sound waves, or vibrations, travel down the external ear canal and strike the eardrum (tympanic membrane). The eardrum vibrates. The vibrations are then passed to the three tiny bones in the middle ear called the ossicles. The ossicles amplify the sound and send the sound waves to the inner ear and into the fluid-filled hearing organ (cochlea).

Once the sound waves reach the inner ear, they are converted into electrical impulses that the auditory nerve sends to the brain. The brain then translates these electrical impulses into the perception of sound.

Problems involved in the delivery of drugs to inner ear:

• It is difficult to predict the availability of drug dose in inner ear as no accurate pharmacokinetic studies available and also due to the difference in drug availability due to drainage from the Eustachian tube.

Lack of accurate pharmacokinetic profiles is due to:

• Complexity and tiny size of inner ear that cause difficulty in sampling
• Low quantity of perilymph (about 160 µl) fluid available for sampling
• The perilymph volume of drug distribution is different between animal and human models
• Rapid replacement of ear fluid by CSF shows poor sampling reliability.

Factors to be considered in designing the dosage form:

1. *pH:* The pH range of the formulation should be 3.5–7.5 is acceptable. If out of this range they are unstable and cause local irritation. Buffers are added to maintain the pH of the formulation.
2. *Viscosity:* The viscosity of the ear drops can be increased in order to increase the residence time of the product. The drug when administered to the middle ear may drain into the nasopharynx. Hence, viscosity of the formulation is increased to decrease drug drainage. Inorder to increase the viscosity solvents and polymers are used.

- *Solvents:* Propylene glycol, glycerine
- *Polymers:* Sodium hyaluronate, gelatin, polypropylene fumerate
3. *Tonicity:* Isotonic solutions are more preferred to hypertonic and hypotonic solutions as they cause irritation to the ear.
4. *Sterility:* Sterility of the formulation is to be maintained as it comes in contact with the tympanic membrane and the ear canal. If not sterilized it may spread pathogens to the ear. Preservatives are added in case of multiple dose units to protect the formulation from microbial contamination.

Different dosage forms:

1. *Ear drops:*
   - These are most convenient dosage forms of ear
   - But shows decrease in residence time and increased drainage
   - Physical properties like pH, viscosity and tonicity are to be adjusted in ear drops formulation
2. *Ear ointments and powders:* These are not commonly used as they cause irritation, discomfort, conductive hearing loss. But they increase the retention time of the drug when compared to ear drops

   Systemic therapy: In this drug is delivered through oral or IV or IM route. Examples include:
   - Systemic steroids for Sensorineural hearing loss (SSNHL)
   - Systemic streptomycin for vertigo control. But streptomycin is found to be ototoxic. Now streptomycin is used to treat bilateral Meniere's disease by administering though intramuscular route.
   - Systemic bisphosphonates are used as therapeutic option for otosclerosis.

Limitations and Drawbacks of Systemic Therapy of Otic Disorders

Potential side effects that are life-threatening effects that cause organ damage and may lead to death of patient if given over a sustained period of time, e.g. systemic steroid therapy leads to hyperglycemia, hypertension, hypokalemia, peptic ulcer disease, osteoporosis, immunosupression, adrenal suppression.

Drug Delivery to Middle Ear

The drug delivery to middle ear can be achieved through the following devices:

1. *Injections:* In order to deliver drug to middle ear injections are preferred as the drug is not accessible directly to the middle ear due to tympanic membrane, e.g. administration of antibiotics and anti-inflammatory agents in chronic otitis media.
2. *Fixed catheters or wicks:* These are used for the repeated administration of drug at regular intervals to the middle ear.
3. *Electronically or manually controlled dose device pumps:* These are used to deliver the drugs like local anaesthetics, steroids, antibiotics, neurotransmitters, neurotransmitter agonists and other drugs to middle ear which is transported to the inner ear.

Drug Delivery to the Inner Ear

The drugs which are administered to inner ear have no acceptability to the systemic circulation because of the presence of blood-inner ear barrier similar to that of blood brain barrier. This reduces the systemic side effects. The methods used for drug delivery to inner ear include:

- Transtympanic injection or myringotomy
- The silverstein microwick
- Microcatheter implantation
- Hydrogels
- Nanoparticles

Transtympanic Injection

In this the medication is delivered via injection into the middle ear with a needle or using a myringotomy with or without a tympanostomy tube.

Advantages

Quick delivery of drug to inner ear

Silverstein microinjection: The silverstein microwick is 1–9 mm which is composed of polyvinyl acetate. It is applied though a ventilation tube placed in a myringotomy in the tympanic membrane. It is used for sustain release of medication in the

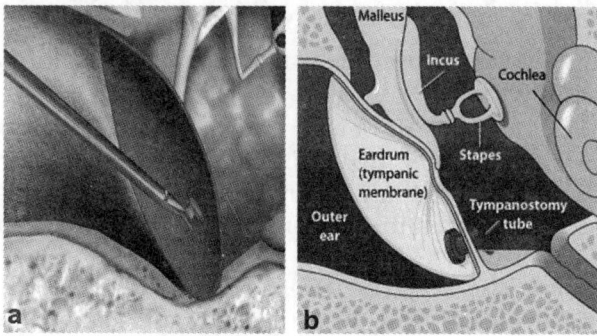

Figs 8.2a and b: (a) Tympanostomy tube insertion to middle ear, (b) Tympanostomy tube in tympanic membrane

inner ear. The patient instills the medication into the external auditory canal, usually several times a day for several weeks that travels through the microwick to the round window membrane.

Applications

- It successfully manages the vertigo attacks in Meniere's disease by delivery of gentamicin.
- Delivery of methylprednisolone in the setting of SSNHL that shows improvement in hearing.

Drawbacks

- It includes development of persistent perfusion of the tympanic membrane
- Infection of the middle ear or external ear
- Fibrosis— a condition in which there is tissue in growth in the middle ear
- Cholesteatoma— a condition in which there is abnormal in growth of epithelial tissue.

Microcatheter Injection

In this system, a microcatheter is placed in the round window niche, traverses a tunnel developed at the tympanic annulus and then through a well in the posterior external auditory canal, and emerges at the external auditory meatus.

Advantage

It delivers medication to the middle ear continuously for several weeks which transports drug to inner ear.

Application

Delivery of steroid medications to treat SSNHL after failed systemic therapy.

Complications

- Development of minor granulation tissue within the middle ear
- Occurrence of catheter dislocation due to partial implantable nature of the device. This is eliminated by placing a thin transparent adhesive over the external portion of the microcatheter.

Hydrogels

- Hydrogels are the medications that are designed for the consistent delivery of medicines to the inner ear. Hydrogels have yet to be used as drug carriers for treating inner ear diseases.
- The formulation consists of a dissolvable matrix which is mixed with the medications before instillation in the middle ear.
- It releases the medication by the hydrolysis of the matrix or by the diffusion of the drug through the matrix in a controlled fashion.
- Polymers used in this formulation include siloxane based polymers, polylactic glycolic acid (PLGA) polymers, gelatin and chitosan glycerophosphate.

Applications

- Delivery of brain derived neurotropic factor (BDNF) to the inner ear by the application of hydrogel containing BDNF was studied in guinea pigs.
- Delivery of insulin-like growth factor-1 and dexamethasone.

Drawbacks

- Accurate placing of the hydrogel over the round window to permit transfer of drug to inner ear is difficult.

- Hearing loss may occur if the middle ear is overfilled with hydrogel.
- Release profile of drug from hydrogel may not be ideal for chronic conditions.

Nanoparticles

This is another methodology of delivery of drug to the inner ear and shows considerable interest in the past several years. These are the colloidal particles whose size ranges from 200 to 1000 nm.

Nanoparticles formed with PLGA are shown to present within the cochlea when delivered either systemically or when applied topically to the round window membrane. These are used for *non viral gene therapy*. This type of delivery system is still in budding stage and many factors are to be considered.

Factors to be considered in designing of nanoparticle drug delivery to ear:
- Biocompatibility
- Drug release profile
- Biosafety

Recent Developments of Drug Delivery to Inner Ear

New strategies are being developed for direct delivery of the medication to the inner ear (intracochlear delivery). It includes:
1. Cochlear implant technologies
2. Osmotic pumps
3. Reciprocating perfusion systems.

Cochlear Implantation

In this the implant is directly placed in the inner ear and the medication is delivered along with the implant. Efforts are also being made to study the potential for coating cochlear implant electrodes with a biorelease polymer which permits diffusion of medication into the inner ear.

Potential Drawbacks

Greater risk of infection and poorer implant performance.

Applications

Research is going on in the development of cochlear implant to deliver neurotrophins and steroids, e.g. application of triamcinolone to the site cochleostomy can be used from the surgical trauma of cochleostomy, application of dexamethasone to the round window shows decrease in traumatic threshold in case of traumatized cochlea.

Osmotic Pump

This is one of the novel drug delivery system intended to deliver drug to inner ear. Recently the micro-cannula portion of the device has been modified to permit longer drug infusion times as well as bolus dosing.

Drawbacks

- Inability to deliver varying dosages or dosing intervals of drug
- It is difficult to start and stop drug delivery externally, without removing the system.

Reciprocating Perfusion System

Novel approaches like microsystems and microfluidics have been developed during the past decade. Entire drug-delivery system including power, electronic control, drug reservoirs, release mechanisms, and sensors can now be packed and implanted in small area within the body.

Advantages

- Greater control and accuracy over delivery profiles
- Enhanced preservation of potentially unstable drug for long periods before release
- Availability of timed-sequence of multiple agents in case of complex dosing of numerous compounds
- Précised drug delivery can be achieved at extremely low volume and flow rates through the system's micropumping elements for hearing damage.

Drawback

Surgical implantation is needed.

EVALUATION OF OTIC PRODUCTS

Particle Size Determination

The desired particle size of the otic suspension is 5–10 µm or less. The particle size of the otic suspension is to be determined as it affects the drug absorption and larger size of the particles cause irritation.

Optical microscopy: Particle size can be measured microscopically by sizing against a graticule and counting, but for a statistically valid analysis, millions of particles must be measured. This is impossibly arduous when done manually, but automated analysis of electron micrographs is now commercially available. Instruments such as the retsch Camsizer can perform this analysis on the run using standard camera technology.

Coulter Counter Method (Electroresistance Counting Methods)

In this the momentary changes in the conductivity of a liquid passing through an orifice is measured when individual nonconducting particles pass through. The particle count is obtained by counting pulses, and the size is dependent on the size of each pulse.

Technique advantages: Very small sample aliquots can be examined.

Technique disadvantages: Sample must be dispersed in a liquid medium as some particles may (partially or fully) dissolve in the medium altering the size distribution. The results are only related to the projected cross-sectional area that a particle displaces as it passes through an orifice. This is a physical diameter, not really related to mathematical descriptions of particles (e.g. terminal settling velocity).

Acoustic Spectroscopy or Ultrasound Attenuation Spectroscopy

In this method ultrasound is employed for collecting information on the particles that are dispersed in fluid. Dispersed particles absorb and scatter ultrasound similarly to light. It turns out that instead of measuring *scattered energy versus angle*, as with light, in the case of ultrasound, measuring the *transmitted energy versus frequency* is a better choice. The resulting ultrasound attenuation frequency spectra are the raw data for calculating particle size distribution. It can be measured for any fluid system with no dilution or other sample preparation. Calculation of particle size distribution is based on theoretical models that are well-verified for up to 50% by volume of dispersed particles.

Laser diffraction methods: These depend upon analysis of the "halo (dark portion)" of diffracted light produced when a laser beam passes through a dispersion of particles in air or in a liquid. The angle of diffraction increases as particle size decreases. This method is particularly good for measuring sizes between 0.1 and 3,000 μm. A particular advantage is that the technique can generate a continuous measurement for analyzing process streams.

Tests for Otic Solutions

Clarity of the solution: Retention of clarity of solution is a main concern regarding stability of solution. In this a microscopic light is projected though a diaphragm into the solution. The solution will remain clear if there are no undissolved particles. If not the solution appears hazy due to the scattering of light by undissolved particles. Light scattering instruments are most widely used to test the clarity of the solution.

Test for Particulate Matter in Otic Solutions

Otic solutions should be essentially free from particulate matter which can be observed on visual inspection. This test describes the physical tests performed to enumerate extraneous particles with specific size ranges. Particulate matter includes mobile, randomly sourced, extraneous substances, other than gas bubbles that cannot quantified by chemical analysis due to less amount and of their heterogeneous compositions.

Methods

- Light obscuration method
- Microscopic method

Light Obscuration Method

This method applies for otic solutions, including solutions constituting from sterile solids, for which the test for particulate matter is specified in the individual monograph.

The otic product meets the requirements of the test if the average numbers of particles present in the units tested does not exceed the appropriate value listed in the following (Table 8.1).

Table 8.1: Light obscuration particle count test		
	Diameter	
	≥10 µm	≥25 µm
Number of particles	50 per ml	5 per ml

If the average number of particles exceeds this limit, the test article is subjected to microscopic method.

Microscopic Method

This method is performed when some particles are not exactly detected by the light obscuration method. This test enumerates the sub-visible particles essentially solid, particulate matter present in the ophthalmic solutions. The test sample is collected on a micro-porous membrane filter.

The otic product meets the requirements of the test if the average number of particles present in the units tested does not exceed the appropriate value listed in Table 8.2.

Table 8.2: Microscopic method particle count test			
	Diameter		
	≥ 10	≥ 25	≥ 50
Number of particles	50 per ml	5 per ml	2 per ml

Test for Sterility

This is used to test the presence of microorganisms in the test solution. It is done by two methods.
• Membrane filtration method
• Direct inoculation (immersion) method.

Membrane filtration method: In this the test solution is first passed through a size exclusion membrane capable of retaining the micro-organisms. The concept is that the microorganisms will collect on the surface of a 0.45 micron pore size filter. The filter is rinsed and then the membrane is transferred to appropriate test medium as specified in the monograph.

Direct inoculation (immersion) method: In this the test article is directly inoculated into the test medium and then the medium is incubated for the growth of microorganisms, if present.

Test media: The test media are fluid thioglycolate medium (FTM) and soybean casein digest medium (SCDM). FTM is selected based upon its ability to support the growth of anaerobic and aerobic microorganisms. SCDM is selected based upon its ability to support a wide range of aerobic bacteria and fungi (i.e. yeasts and molds).

Incubation time: In both the methods the test medium after the transferring of the test solution is to be incubated for 3 days in case of bacteria and 5 days in case of fungi and then the growth is compared with that of standard. If no growth is observed then the sample passes the test and it meets the GMP requirements.

Table 8.3 outlines the requirement for sterility testing as per USP.

Table 8.3: Sterility testing as per USP

Volume/container	Minimum quantity to test in each media
< 1 ml	The entire contents of each container
1–40 ml	Half the contents of each container but not < 1 ml
41–100 ml	20 ml
> 100 ml	10% of the contents of the container, but not < 20 ml

Test for Pyrogens

It is used to check for the presence of pyrogens in the ophthalmic formulation. Two general tests are performed.
- Rabbit test and
- LALs test

Rabbit Test

The pyrogen test is designed to limit to an acceptable level the risks of febrile reaction in the patient to the administration, by injection, of the product concerned. Unless otherwise specified in the individual monograph, inject into an ear vein of each of three rabbits 10 ml of the test solution per kg of body weight, completing each injection within 10 minutes after start of administration. The test solution is *either* the product, constituted if necessary as directed in the labeling, *or* the material under test treated as directed in the individual monograph and injected in the dose specified therein. Assure that all test solutions are protected from contamination. Perform the injection after warming the test solution to a temperature of 37 ± 2°C. Record the temperature at 30 minute intervals between 1 and 3 hours subsequent to the injection.

Test Interpretation

Consider any temperature decreases as zero rise. If no rabbit shows an individual rise in temperature of 0.5°C or more above its respective control temperature, the product meets the requirements for the absence of pyrogens. If any rabbit shows an individual temperature rise of 0.5°C or more, continue the test using five other rabbits. If not more than three of the eight rabbits show individual rises in temperature of 0.5°C or more and if the sum of the eight individual maximum temperature rises does not exceed 3.3°C, the material under examination meets the requirements for the absence of pyrogens.

LAL test: Limulus amoebocyte lysate (LAL) is an aqueous extract of blood cells (amoebocytes) from the horseshoe crab, *Limulus polyphemus.* LAL reacts with bacterial endotoxin or lipopolysaccharide (LPS), which is a membrane component of gram-negative bacteria. This reaction is the basis of the LAL test.

Method: Blood is removed from the horseshoe crab's pericardium and the blood cells are separated from the serum using centrifugation and are then placed in distilled water, which causes them to swell up and burst ("lyse"). This releases the chemicals from the inside of the cell (the "lysate"), which is then purified and freeze-dried. To test a sample for endotoxins, it is mixed with lysate and water; endotoxins are present if coagulation occurs.

Test for Otic Gels, Suspensions and Ointments

- *Viscosity measurement:* Brook-field viscometer, cone and plate viscometer. The flow of fluids through the dropper or tube is influenced by viscosity of the product. In order to have a better flow and to maintain residence time in the ear, the viscosity of the formulation should be checked under controlled temperature.

- *Brook-field viscometer:* It measures the shearing stress on a spindle rotating at a definite, constant speed while immersed in the sample. The degree of spindle lag is indicated on a rotating dial. This reading multiplied by a conversion factor based on spindle size and rotational speed, gives a value for viscosity in centipoise.

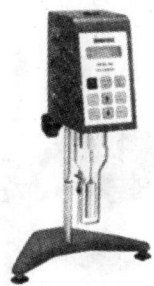

Fig. 8.3: Brook-field viscometer

- *Cone and plate viscometer:* It used a cone of very shallow angle in bare contact with a flat plate. With this system the shear rate beneath the plate is constant to a modest degree of precision and deconvolution of a flow curve; a graph of shear stress (torque) against shear rate (angular velocity) yields the viscosity in a straight forward manner.

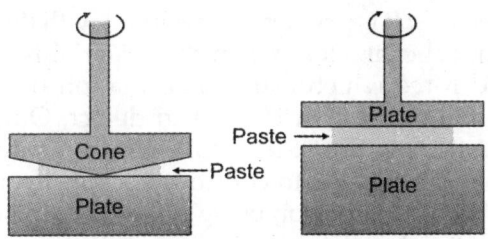

Fig. 8.4: Cone and plate viscometer

- *Consistency measurement*: Penetrometer. It is the measure of penetration of an object into the product to be examined in a container with a specified shape and size. In this the test sample is placed on the base of the penetrometer such that its surface is perpendicular to the vertical axis of penetrating object. The temperature of the penetrating object is maintained at 25 + / – 0.5°C and then its tip is adjusted such that it just touches the surface of the sample. The penetrating object if released and hold it for 5 sec then the penetrating object is clamped and the depth of penetration is measured. The test is repeated for 2 remaining containers (Fig. 8.5).

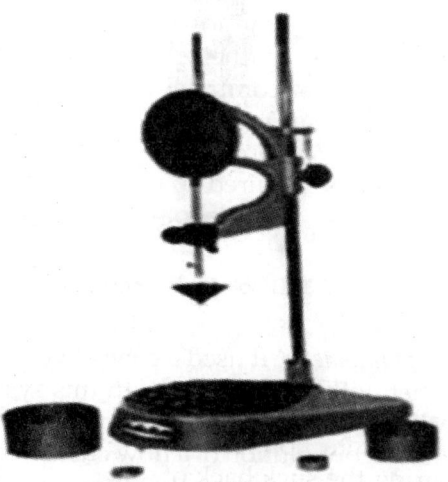

Fig. 8.5: Penetrometer

- *Texture analysis:* It is primarily concerned with the evaluation of mechanical characters when the material is subjected to controlled force which cause deformation of the sample. Texture analyzer which is used to detect. Ointment flow characteristic, e.g. Brook-field CT_3 texture analyser. In this the sample is subjected to controlled forces in compression using a probe or in tension using grips. The resistance of the sample material to these forces is measured by a calibrated load cell and is expressed in either gram or newton. These forces are a function of the properties of the sample and the parameters of the test method.
- *Gel strength:* Gels have gained wide acceptance as semisolid dosage forms. It has been postulated that the strength rather than the viscosity of a gel layer plays a major role in

determining the amount of drug release from hydrophilic matrices. Recent advances have occurred in the development of an optimal apparatus to characterize gel strength. The apparatus consists of a sample holder placed on an electronic microbalance connected to a computer. A probe is lowered into the sample by means of a motor equipped with a speed transformer, and the force required to penetrate the gel is measured. The increase in force with time is a function of the mechanical resistance of the sample to the penetration of the probe. Because the lowering speed is known, the displacement covered by the probe as a function of time is calculated and used to compute the gel-strength parameter or mechanical resistance of the gel system.

- *Sachet or tube extrusion force measurement:* In this the device quantifies the force required to extrude the contents from either tube or sachet style packaging that allows the manufacturers to tests the force required to extrude the content of a sachet or tube at regular intervals over a long period of time, throughout its shelf-life.

Test for Antimicrobial Effectiveness

Generally an antimicrobial agent is used in multiple dose units of otic drops for protection from microbial contamination that may occur during the suck back of an unreleased drop, when the pressure is released after withdrawal of the product. So there is need to check the efficacy of the antimicrobial agent against these microorganisms.

In this cultures of *Candida albicans, Aspergillus niger, Escherichia coli, Pseudomonas aeuroginosa, Staphylococcus aureus* are used. In this a standardized inocula of microorganisms is prepared with a count of 10^5–10^6 per ml. This is used to test the preserved formula. They are incubated for 28 days at 20–25°C and observed for the preservative action at 7, 14, 21 and 28 days.

The products preservative action is found to be effective if it satisfies the following:

- There should be reduction of no more than 0.1% of viable bacteria with that of initial concentrations by day 14th.
- There should be decrease in concentration of viable yeasts and molds when compared to initial by day 14th.

- The concentration of remaining viable organisms should be lower as designated at the end of 28th day.

Cidal test: This is another test employed to determine antimicrobial agent efficacy.

- In this the formulation is tested against 5–14 species of microorganisms including gram –ve, gram +ve, yeast, and fungi in previously standardized inoculums. Cidal times (growth of microorganisms) are measured within 24, 48 and 72 hours of contact.

Conclusion

Administration of drugs to ear is intended mainly for local effect and not for systemic effect. Systemic delivery of drugs to treat otic disorders is avoided as far as possible as they may cause systemic side effects. Research is going on in the development of new drug delivery methods to deliver drug to middle and inner ear.

ISOLATED KEY POINTS

- Drug delivery to ear is intended for local effect to treat ear discorders and not for systemic effects.
- Systemic delivery of drugs to treat otic disorders is avoided as they may cause systemic side effects.
- Various disorders of the ear include Meniere's disease, vertigo, tinnitus, inflammatory diseases.
- Different dosage forms available include ear drops, ear ointment and ear powders among which ear drops are commonly used.
- Delivery devices include fixed catheters or wicks, implants.
- Evaluation parameters are performed to meet the requirements of the dosage form that includes particle size determination, clarity of the solution, test for particulate matter, sterility test, test for antimicrobial agent efficacy, viscosity measurement of otic gels and suspensions, test for consistency of ointments and gels.
- Research is going on in the development of new delivery methods to deliver drug to middle and inner ear.

PRACTICE QUESTIONS

1. Define the term otic products. What are the various factors, which is to be kept in mind in designing the otic dosage form.
2. Explain the anatomy of ear with the help of neat and labeled diagram.
3. What are the different types of otic dosage form? Give their merits and demerits.
4. What are the various evaluation test used for otic formulation?

9

Parenteral Products

Definition

Parenteral (derived from Greek word, *para enteron*, beside the intestine) dosage forms of drugs are injected directly into body tissue through one or more layer of skin and mucous.

Parenteral preparation are introduced directly into body fluid system composing:

- The intra and extra-cellular fluid compartment
- The lymphatic system
- The blood circulatory system.

As highly protective barriers get avoided so introduction of microorganism and toxic agents is very dangerous. Considering this parenteral formulation should be as perfect as possible with respect to:

- Purity
- Freedom for toxicity
- Freedom from contamination.

Advantages

- *Quick onset of action:* 15–30 seconds for IV, 3–5 minutes for IM and subcutaneous (subcut)
- 100% bioavailability for IV injection
- Suitable for drugs not absorbed by the gut or those that are too irritant (anti-cancer)
- One injection can be formulated to last days or even months, e.g. depo provera, a birth control shot that works for three months

- IV can deliver continuous medication, e.g. morphine for patients in continuous pain, or saline drip and glucose for people needing fluids and nutrients.
- Useful for unconscious and vomiting patient
- Suitable for drugs, which are inactivated by GIT fluid or enzymes.

Disadvantages

- Onset of action is quick, hence more risk of addiction when it comes to injecting drugs of abuse.
- Patients are not typically able to self-administer, need trained person.
- Belonephobia, the fear of needles and injection.
- If needles are shared, there is risk of HIV and other infectious diseases.
- It is the most dangerous route of administration because it bypasses most of the body's natural defenses, exposing the user to health problems such as hepatitis, abscesses, infections.
- If not done properly, potentially fatal air boluses (bubbles) can occur.
- Need for strict asepsis.

Classifications

Parenteral dosage forms can be categorized into six categories:

- Solutions ready for injection.
- Dry, soluble products ready to be combined with a solvent just prior to use.
- Suspensions ready for injection.
- Dry insoluble products ready to be combined with a vehicle just prior to use.
- Emulsions.
- Liquid concentrates ready for dilution prior to administration.

Routes of drug Administration

Organs	Injection type
Skin	Intradermal
	Subcutaneous
Organs	Intracavernous
	Intravitreal
	Transscleral
Central nervous system	Intracerebral
	Intrathecal/intraspinal
	Epidural
	Intracisternal
Circulatory/musculoskeletal	Intravenous
	Intracardiac
	Intramuscular
	Intraosseous
	Intra-articular
	Intraperitoneal
	Intra-arterial

Intradermal (In or into the skin): An intradermal injection is given into the skin. It is used for skin testing some allergens, and also for Mantoux test for tuberculosis.

Subcutaneous: Under the skin. "Subcutaneous" implies just under the skin. With a subcutaneous injection, a needle is inserted just under the skin. A drug (for example, insulin) can then be delivered into the subcutaneous tissues. After the injection, the drug moves into small blood vessels and the bloodstream. The subcutaneous route is used with many protein and polypeptide drugs such as insulin which, if given by mouth, would be broken down and digested in the intestinal tract. The amount of medication is around 1 ml, given by holding the needle at 45 degree angle while piercing the skin, skin is pinched tight, insert needle so that hub of needle shaft touches the skin, aspirate to check the location of needle. If blood is aspirated, withdraw the needle and try at other site, if not gently push the medication into subcutaneous tissue, withdraw needle and gently massage the area to help in absorption, never massage insulin or other drug which stains the skin.

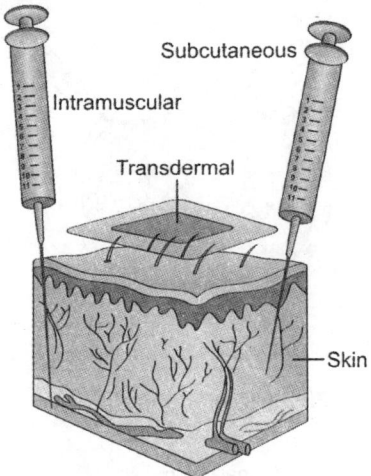

Fig. 9.1: Types of injections

Intracavernous: An intracavernous (or intracavernosal) injection is an injection into the base of the penis. This injection site is often used to administer medications to check for or treat erectile dysfunction in adult men.

Intravitreal: Intravitreal (Intravitreal is a route of administration of a drug, or other substance, in which the substance is delivered via an eye. "Intravitreal" literally means "inside an eye") (Fig. 9.2).

Trans-scleral (trans- + sclera + -al): Injected into sclera (sclera- the white of the eye. It is the tough outer coat of the eye that covers the eyeball except for the cornea).

Intracerebral (L, intra + cerebrum, brain, pertaining to the area or substance within the cerebrum): Injected in cerebrum.

Intrathecal: Intrathecal (Latin intra – "inside", Greek theka "capsule", "hull" is an adjective that refers to something introduced into or occurring in the space under the arachnoid membrane of the spinal cord) injection of a substance through the theca of the spinal cord into the subarachnoid space.

Epidural: Injection of an anesthetic substance into the epidural space of the spinal cord in order to produce epidural anesthesia (Fig. 9.3).

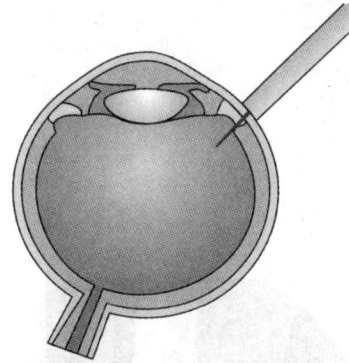

Fig. 9.2: Intravitreal injection

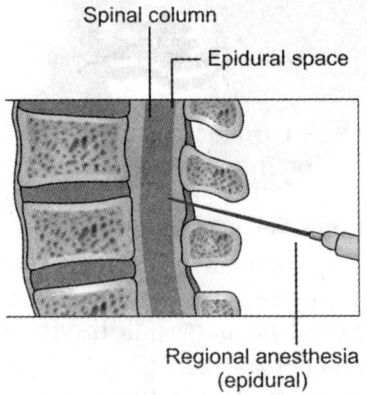

Fig. 9.3: Epidural injection

Intraosseous infusion: (Into the bone marrow) is, in effect, an indirect intravenous access because the bone marrow drains directly into the venous system. This route is occasionally used for drugs and fluids in emergency medicine and pediatrics when intravenous access is difficult.

Intracisternal: It is given between the first and second cervical vertebrae—used to withdraw cerebrospinal fluid for diagnostic purposes.

Intravenous: Intravenous therapy or IV therapy is the giving of substances directly into a vein. The word intravenous simply means "within a vein".

Intracardiac: Intracardiac (into the heart), injection given into the heart, e.g. adrenaline during cardiopulmonary resuscitation, nowadays not commonly performed.

Intramuscular: Intramuscular injection into a muscle, e.g. many vaccines, antibiotics, and long-term psychoactive agents.

Intra-articular (Origin: intra- + L. articulus, joint), drug injected with in joints.

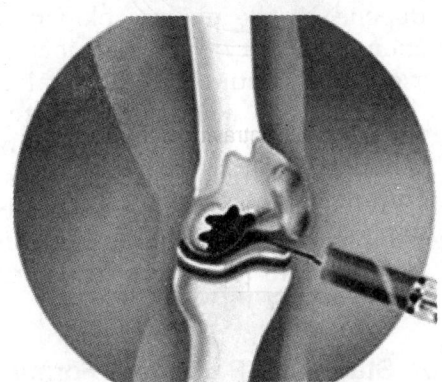

Fig. 9.4: Intra-articular injection

Intraperitoneal (infusion or injection into the peritoneum): Intraperitoneal injection or IP injection is the injection of a substance into the peritoneum (body cavity). IP injection is more often applied to animals than humans, e.g. peritoneal dialysis

Intra-arterial (arterial-arteries): Injected into arteries, e.g. vasodilator drugs in the treatment of vasospasm and thrombolytic drugs for treatment of embolism.

The most common routes of parenteral administration are intravenous (IV), subcutaneous (SC), and intramuscular (IM).

Classification of Injections on the Basis of Injection Volumes

Pharmacopoeias classify injectables into two, on the basis of injection volumes:

- Small-volume parenterals (SVPs)
- Large-volume parenterals (LVPs).

Small-volume parenterals (SVPs): The US pharmacopoeia (USP) defines SVPs as containing less than 100 ml.

Large-volume parenterals (LVPs): The US pharmacopoeia (USP) defines LVPs as containing more than 100 ml.

SVPs given rapidly in a small volume are known as a bolus. SVPs may also be added to LVPs, such as 5% dextrose and 0.9% sodium chloride infusion/injection, for administration by intravenous infusion. The selection of bolus or infusion will depend on the pharmacokinetics of the drug, and the distinction is not very clear. Infusions can be as brief as 15 minutes or may continue for several days. Usually infusions are formulated as a concentrate, which will subsequently be diluted by the practitioner or pharmacist prior to administration. Intramuscular or subcutaneous injections are almost always administered as a bolus. Usually volume of injection administered through subcutaneous route is less than 1 to 1.5 ml and for intramuscular route not more than 2 ml.

Preformulation Studies of Parenteral Formulation

Characterization of Drug Substance

The drug substance attributes that were considered during product development are:

- The drug substance solubility.
- The drug substance stability.
- The particle size of the drug substance.
- The compatibility between the excipients and the drug substance.
- The partition and distribution coefficients.

The Drug Substance Solubility

Solubility is one of the most important physicochemical properties studied during pharmaceutical preformulation. Solubility is the maximum concentration that can be attained by a solute in a specific solvent. pH effects on solubility also can be of particular utility in the preparation of parenteral solutions (i.e. intravenous). The US pharmacopoeia (USP) gives following definitions of solubility:

Table 9.1: Pharmacopoeia (USP)—definitions of solubility

Descriptive term	Parts of solvent required for 1 part of solute
Very soluble	Less than 1
Freely soluble	From 1 to 10
Soluble	From 10 to 30
Sparingly soluble	From 30 to 100
Slightly soluble	From 100 to 1,000
Very slightly soluble	From 1,000 to 10,000
Practically insoluble	10,000 and over

Factors that can affect solubility:
- Nature of the drug substance
- Particle size
- Solvent system
- pH of solution
- Temperature
- Solubilizing agents
- Complexing agents

The Drug Substance Stability

Drug substance stability has big commercial and safety related impact on the product. A highly unstable protein drug cannot be placed in anything but needs preserved and protected parenteral form.

The Particle Size of the Drug Substance

The particle size of a new drug substance is a critical parameter. Appropriate particle size is required to achieve control sedimentation and flocculation in parenteral suspensions and it effects solubility for parenteral solution.

The Compatibility Between the Excipient and the Drug Substance

The drug excipients shall be evaluated by forced degradation and stability studies at various temperature/humidity conditions. After force degradation studies, we can trace out whether drug substance undergo oxidation/reduction/

hydrolytic or thermal degradation. Whereas the choice of excipients starts with the stages of formulation, some excipients are historically used in specific drug formulations; for example, if the newly discovered drug is a cephalosporin for use as an intravenous product, compatibility with arginine or sodium carbonate would be advised as these are the most commonly used active excipients for solubilization.

Components of Parenteral Formulation

The components of the product to be accumulated and selected include:

- Vehicles
- Solute
- Container and
- Closure

Vehicles

Majority of the injections are diluted so vehicle makes highest portion of the injection. Vehicles are categories into following headings:

- Aqueous vehicles
- Water-miscible vehicles
- Nonaqueous vehicles

Aqueous vehicles: The vehicle of greatest importance is water, i.e. water for injection (WFI) usually aqueous vehicles are isotonic vehicles to which a drug may be added at the time of administration. For example, sodium chloride injection, ringer's injection, dextrose injection, dextrose and sodium chloride injection, and lactated ringer's injection.

Water for Injection

The USP monograph states: "Water for injection (WFI) is water purified by distillation or reverse osmosis."

WFI is produced by either distillation or 2-stage RO. It is usually stored and distributed hot (at 80°C) in order to meet microbial quality requirements and should not be used after 24 hours of storage.

Preparation of Water for Injection (WFI)

Conventional still consists of:

- Boiler (evaporator) containing feed water (distilland).
- A source of heat to vaporize the water in the evaporator.
- A headspace above the level of distilland, with condensing surfaces for refluxing the vapor, there by returning nonvolatile impurities to the distilland; a means for removing volatile impurities before the hot water vapor is condensed.
- A condenser for removing the heat of vaporization thereby converting the water vapor to a liquid distillate.

Following factors are considered while selecting the process of purification of water so that purified water meets the specification or criteria of water for injection:

i. *Quality of the water feed:* The quality of the feed water will affect the quality of the distillate. Controlling the quality of the feed water is essential for meeting the required specifications for the distillate.

ii. *Size of the evaporator:* The size of the evaporator will affect the efficiency, i.e. larger the sizes better the efficiency.

iii. *Design of baffles (condensing surfaces):* The baffles (condensing surfaces) determine the effectiveness of refluxing. They should be designed for efficient removal of the entrainment at optimal vapor velocity, collecting and returning the heavier droplets contaminated with the distilland.

iv. Redissolving volatile impurities in the distillate reduces its purity. Therefore, they should be separated efficiently from the hot water vapor and eliminated by aspirating them to the drain or venting them to the atmosphere.

v. Contamination of the vapor and distillate from the metal parts of the still can occur. Present standards for high-purity stills are that all parts contacted by the vapor or distillate should be constructed of metal coated with pure tin, 304 or 316 stainless-steel, or chemically resistant glass.

Common used apparatus designed for the production of high purity water are as follows:

1. Compression distillation
2. Multiple effect distillation
3. Reverse osmosis (RO)

Vapor Compression Distillation

Step 1: In a vapor compression (VC) system, the distillation process begins in the boiling chamber, just as it does in virtually any other distiller. What separates this method from other distillation methods is what comes after the boiling chamber.

Step 2: In a vapor compression system the boiling process begins with both heating elements turned on. As the water in the boiling chamber reaches near boiling temperatures, the compressor turns on.

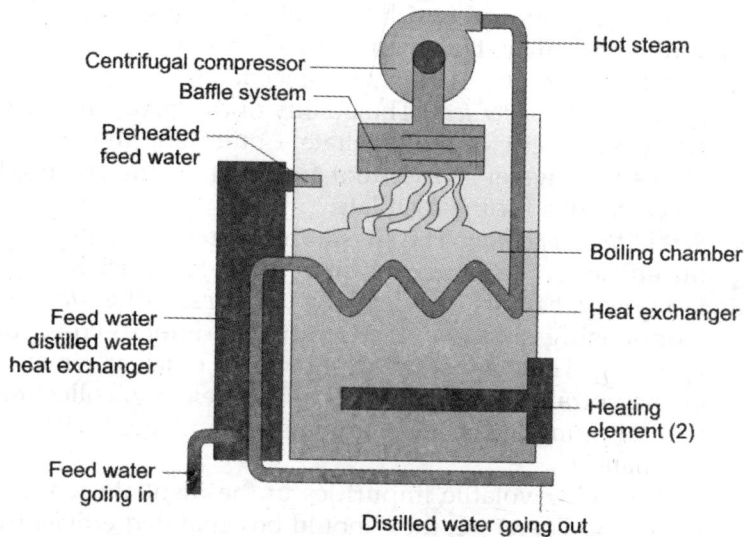

Fig. 9.5: Vapor compression system

When the boiling begins, the heating element turns off and the heating element cycles on and off maintaining the boiling at just the right temperature for maximum efficiency. The steam from the boiling water flows through a baffling system and then into the compressor.

Step 3: In the compressor, the steam is pressurized, which raises the steam's temperature before it is routed through a special heat exchanger located inside the boiling chamber. The steam (under pressure) is at a higher temperature than the feed water inside the boiling chamber.

Step 4: The pressurized steam gives off its heat to the tap water inside the boiling chamber, causing this water to boil, which creates more steam. In technical terms, the steam "gives up its latent heat of vaporization" to the water inside the boiling chamber.

Step 5: While the pressurized steam is giving up its latent heat, the steam will condense. One of the heating elements will cycle on and off periodically as needed to provide any "make-up" heat that is required to keep the system operating at optimum temperature for maximum efficiency.

Step 6: At this stage, the condensed steam is considered distilled water but is still very hot-only slightly cooler than boiling temperature. To get maximum efficiency from the VC systems, the hot distilled water preheats the incoming feed water that will be distilled.

Multiple Effect Distillation

The multiple-effect still is designed to conserve energy and water usage. It is simply a series of single-effect stills running at differing pressures. A series of up to seven effects may be used, with the first effect operated at the highest pressure and the last effect at atmospheric pressure (see a schematic drawing of a multiple-effect still). Steam from an external source is used in the first effect to generate steam under pressure from feed water; it is used as the power source to drive the second effect. The steam used to drive the second effect condenses as it gives up its heat of vaporization and forms a distillate. This process continues until the last effect, when the steam is at atmospheric pressure and must be condensed in a heat exchanger. The capacity of a multiple-effect still can be increased by adding effects. The quantity of the distillate also will be affected by the inlet steam pressure; thus, a 600 gal/hr unit designed to operate at 115 psig steam pressure could be run at approximately 55 psig and would deliver about 400 gal/hr. These stills have no moving parts and operate quietly. They are available in capacities from 50 to 7000 gal/hr (Fig. 9.6).

Reverse Osmosis

As the name suggests, the natural process of selective permeation of molecules through a semipermeable membrane

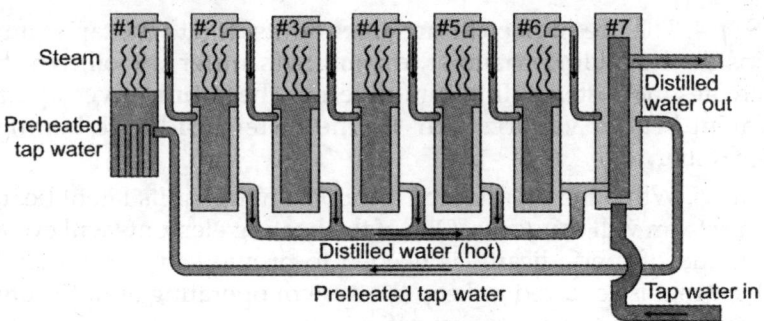

Fig. 9.6: Multiple effect distillation (P1→P2→P3→P4→P5→P6→P7 and P7 is at atmospheric pressure)

separating two aqueous solutions of different concentrations is reversed using pressure (Fig. 9.7). Pressure, usually between 200 and 400 psig, is applied to overcome osmotic pressure and force pure water to permeate through the membrane. Membranes, usually composed of cellulose esters or poly-amides, are selected to provide an efficient rejection of contaminant molecules in raw water. The molecules most difficult to remove are small inorganic ones such as sodium chloride. Passage through two membranes in series is sometimes used to increase the efficiency of removal of these small molecules and to decrease the risk of structural failure of a membrane to remove other contaminants, such as bacteria and pyrogens (Fig. 9.7).

It is important to note that whatsoever purification method is to be used should be validated first.

Microbial Quality

The monograph specifies that WFI should not contain more than 0.25 USP endotoxin units (EU) per mL. Endotoxins are a class of pyrogens that are components of the cell wall of gram-negative bacteria (the most common type of bacteria in water). They are shed during bacterial cell growth and from dead bacteria. Indirectly, the water must be of a very high microbial quality in order to have a low endotoxin concentration. The USP informational section recommends an action limit of 10 cfu/100 ml (CFU-colony forming unit). The

Reverse osmosis

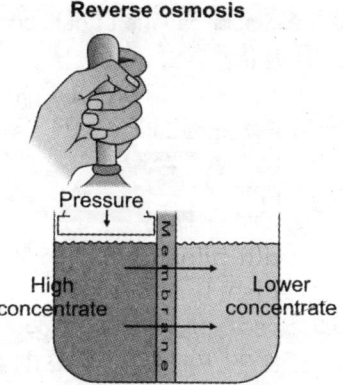

Fig. 9.7: Showing principle of reverse osmosis

recommended method of testing is membrane filtration of a 100 ml sample and plate count agar at an incubation temperature of 30–35 °C for a 48 hour period.

Chemical and Physical Quality

The only physical and chemical tests are:

1. Total organic carbon (TOC), with a limit of 500 ppb.
2. Conductivity test with a limit of 1.3 μS/cm at 25°C or 1.1 μS/cm at 20°C. The TOC is an instrumental method capable of detecting all organic carbon present, and the conductivity is a three-tiered instrumental test measuring the conductivity contributed by ionized particles (in microSiemens (μS) or micromhos) relative to pH. The TOC and conductivity specifications are now considered to be adequate minimal predictors of the chemical and physical purity of WFI (Tables 9.2 and 9.3).

Water-miscible vehicles: A number of solvents that are miscible with water is used in the formulation of parenterals as cosolvent. These solvents are used primarily to affect the solubility of certain drugs and to reduce hydrolysis. Cosolvents are reportedly used in 10% of FDA-approved parenteral products, although the range is limited to glycerin, ethanol, propylene glycol, polyethylene glycol, and N, N-dimethylacetamide.

Table 9.2: Specifications of purified water

Parameter	Unit	USP 24	Ph. Eur.
TOC	ppbC	500	500
Conductivity	µS/cm @ 20°C	–	<4.3
Conductivity	µS/cm @ 25°C	<1.3	–
Nitrate (NO_3)	ppm	–	<0.2
Heavy metals	ppm as Pb	–	< 0.1
Aerobic bacteria	CFU/ml	<100	<100

Table 9.3: Specifications of water for injection

Parameter	Unit	USP 24	Ph. Eur.
TOC	ppbC	500	500
Conductivity	µS/cm @ 20°C	–	<1.1
Conductivity	µS/cm @ 25°C	<1.3	–
Dry residue	%	–	<0.001
Nitrate (NO_3)	ppm	–	<0.2
Heavy metals	ppm as Pb	–	<0.1
Aerobic bacteria	CFU/100 ml	<10	<10
Bacterial endotoxins	EU/ml	<0.25	<0.25

Marketed Products Containing Cosolvent (Table 9.4)

Table 9.4

Active ingredient	Route	Vehicle composition	Special instructions
Diazepam	IM/IV	40% propylene glycol 10% benzoate butter 1.5% benzyl alcohol	Inject slowly (at least 1 min/mL) if giving IV Do not use small veins
Co-trimoxazole	IV	40% propylene glycol 10% ethyl alcohol 0.3% diethanolamine 1% benzyl alcolol 0.1% sodium meta-bisulfite	Must be diluted with 5% dextrose infusion Discard if cloudy or if there is evidence of crystallization

Contd.

Table 9.4 (Contd.)

Active ingredient	Route	Vehicle composition	Special instructions
Etoposide	IV	65% w/v PEG 300 30.50% w/v 8% w/v polysorbate 80 3% w/v benzyle alcohol 0.2% w/v citric acid	Must be diluted. At concentrations >0.4 mg/alcohol ml, precipitation may occur.
Loxapine	IM	70% propylene glycol 5% polysorbate 80	
Lorazepam	IV/IM	80% propylene glycol 18% ethanol 2% benzyl alcohol	Dilute two-fold for IV injection.

Nonaqueous vehicles: The most important group of nonaqueous vehicles are the fixed oils. The fixed oils used inparenteral must be of vegetable origin because of following characteristics:

- They will be metabolized and
- Remain liquid at room temperature, and
- Will not become rancid readily.

The USP also specifies limits for the degree of unsaturation. and free fatty acid content. Examples of fixed oils are corn oil, cottonseed oil, peanut oil, and sesame oil. Fixed oils are used particularly as vehicles for certain hormone preparations and poorly soluble drugs for intramuscular administration can be formulated in a nonaqueous vehicle; this can have the additional benefit of providing a slow release of the active moiety. The label must state the name of the vehicle so that the user may beware in case of known sensitivity or other reactions to it.

Solutes

The requirement of purity of medical compound used in an injection often makes it necessary to take special purification of chemical grade used. The best chemical grade to be used

but further purification may be necessary. Factors to be consider for the quality of solute:
- Purity.
- Freedom for toxicity.
- Freedom from contamination (microbial and pyrogen contamination).
- Solubility of compound.
- Freedom from gross dirt.

Added Substances

The USP includes in this category all substances added to a parenteral preparation to improve or safeguard its quality. An added substance may:
- Effect solubility, as does sodium benzoate in caffeine and sodium benzoate injection.
- Provide patient comfort, as do substances added to make a solution isotonic or near physiological pH.
- Enhance the chemical stability of a solution, as do antioxidants, inert gases, chelating agents and buffers.
- They may preserve the preparation against microbial growth.

Antimicrobial agents:
- The USP states that antimicrobial agents in bacteriostatic or fungistatic concentrations must be added to preparations contained in multiple-dose containers.
- They must be present in adequate concentration at the time of use to prevent the multiplication of microorganisms inadvertently introduced into the preparation while withdrawing a portion of the contents with a hypodermic needle and syringe.
- The USP provides a test for antimicrobial preservative effectiveness to determine that an antimicrobial substance or combination adequately inhibits the growth of microorganisms in a parenteral product (Table 9.5).
Compatability studies of the microbial agents should be performed before using them into the formulation.

Buffers

Buffers are used primarily to stabilize a solution against pH, which result into reduction in the chemical degradation that

Table 9.5: Preservative used and their concentration

Preservative	Typical concentration (%)
Benzyl alcohol	1–2
Chlorbutanol	0.5
Methylparaben	0.1–0.18
Propylparaben	0.01–0.02
Phenol	0.2–0.5
Thiomersal	<0.01

might occur if the pH changes. Buffer systems employed should normally have low buffering capacity as if buffering capacity of product is high it may disturb significantly the body's buffering systems when injected. In addition, the buffer range and effect on the activity of the product must be evaluated carefully (Table 9.6).

Table 9.6: Buffers used in parenteral products

Buffer	pH range
Acetate	3.8–5.8
Ammonium	8.25–10.25
Ascorbate	3.0–5.0
Benzoate	6.0–7.0
Bicarbonate	4.0–11.0
Citrate	2.1–6.2
Diethanolamine	8.0–10.0
Glycine	8.8–10.8
Lactate	2.0–4.1
Phosphate	3.0–8.0
Succinate	3.2–6.6
Tartrate	2.0–5.3
Tromethamine (TRIS. THAM)	7.1–9.1

A parenteral product should be formulated with a pH close to physiological, unless stability or solubility considerations preclude this. Often, the pH selected for the product is a compromise between the pH of maximum stability, solubility, and physiological acceptability.

Antioxidants

Antioxidants are required to preserve products because of the ease with which many drugs are oxidized. Antioxidants are included in parenteral formulations, although their use is now in decline, and EU guidelines discourage their use unless no other alternative exists. A preferred method of preventing oxidation is simply to exclude oxygen; this is usually achieved by purging the product with nitrogen and creating a nitrogen headspace within the container. Where this process is insufficient:

- A metal chelator, such as disodium edentate (0.05%)
- An antioxidant compound, such as ascorbic acid or sodium metabisulfite (1%, and 0.3%, respectively).

Tonicity agents are used in many parenteral and ophthalmic products to adjust the tonicity. However, not all preparations need to be isotonic. The agents most commonly used are electrolytes and mono-or disaccharides.

CONTAINER TYPES

The container closure system is an intrinsic part of the parenteral product and is essential to delivery and handle the pharmaceutical product. It defines the closure, protection, and functionality of a container while it ensures the safety and quality of the drug product over the product shelf-life. Changes to components and materials, suppliers, and processing flow are also part of product life cycle.

The selection of container is based on:

- Composition of container
- Composition of solution
- Treatment to which it is to be subjected

Container types:

- Plastic
- Glass

PLASTIC

Thermoplastic polymers have been established as packaging materials for sterile preparations such as large-volume parenterals, ophthalmic solutions, and, increasingly, small volume parenterals.

Advantages

- Not breakable
- Less weight
- Flexible
  Sterlization technique used for plastic containers: Ethylene oxide or radiation sterilization may be employed for the empty container with subsequent aseptic filling.

Disadvantages

- Permeation of vapors and other molecules in either direction through the wall of the plastic container, e.g. permeation of volatile constituent and water.
- Leaching of constituents from the plastic into the product, e.g. constituent of plastic like plasticizer and antioxidant migrate into the product.
- Sorption (absorption and/or adsorption) of drug molecules or ions on the plastic material, e.g. sorption of insulin, vitamin A acetate, and warfarin sodium has been shown to occur on PVC bags.
- Not as clear as glass, therefore, inspection of contents is difficult.

GLASS

Types I, Type II, and Type III glass containers are all suitable for parenteral (injection or intravenous) preparations as specified by the US pharmacopoeia on the basis of chemical durability tests.

Type I Glass

Type I glass bottles are made from borosilicate, which have has a highly resistant composition and releases the least amount of alkali. It is commonly used for pharmaceutical or fine chemical products that are sensitive to pH changes.

Type II Glass

Type II glass containers are made from commercial soda lime glass that has been de-alkalized to obtain a great improvement in chemical resistance by treating the interior surfaces at a high temperature to eat away the alkali on or near the glass surfaces.

The undesirable characteristic of type II glass is that the treating etches the surface, causing a frosted (snowy) appearance.

Type III Glass

Type III glass bottles and containers are made of untreated commercial soda-lime glass and has average or somewhat above average chemical resistance.

Type NP Glass

Untreated glass containers made of ordinary soda-lime glass. This glass cannot be used for parenteral preparations.

USP tests for determining glass type:

- The powdered glass test.
- The water attack test.

The water attack test is used only for type II glass and is performed on the whole container, because of the dealkalized surface.

The powdered glass test is performed on powdered glass, which exposes internal surfaces of the glass compound. The results are based upon the amount of alkali titrated by 0.02 N sulfuric acid after an autoclaving cycle with the glass sample in contact with a high purity distilled water. Thus, the powdered glass test challenges the leaching potential of the interior structure of the glass while the water attack test challenges only the intact surface of the container.

Uses

- Type I glass will be suitable for all products.
- Type II glass may be suitable, for example, for buffered solution, has a pH below 7, or is not reactive with the glass.
- Type III glass usually will be suitable principally for anhydrous liquids or dry substances.

Physical Shapes

Ampuls and vials sizes are up to 100 ml and bottles can be of larger size (up to 1000 ml). The physical shapes of glass container can be:

- Ampoules
- vials
- Glass bottles

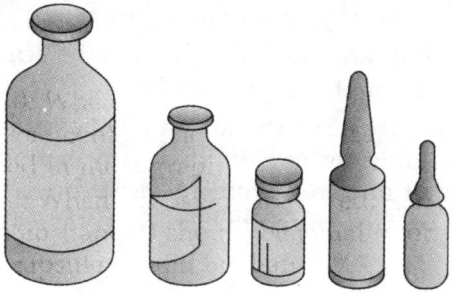

Fig. 9.8: Ampoules and vials

Desired characterstics of glass container:

- Glass containers should be strong enough to withstand the physical shocks of handling and shipping and the pressure differentials that develop, particularly during the autoclave sterilization cycle.

- The container also must be transparent to permit inspection of the contents.

- Preparations that are light-sensitive must be protected by placing them in amber glass containers or by enclosing flint glass containers in opaque cartons labeled to remain on the container during the period of use. As amber color bottles can have impeachable iron, which can leach to parenteral preparation. To avoid leaching of iron silicon coating can be given over amber color glass.

CLOSURE

Rubber Closure

Rubber closures for containers for aqueous parenteral preparations for powders and for freeze-dried powders. They are made of materials obtained by vulcanisation (cross-linking) of macromolecular organic substances (elastomers), with appropriate additives. The elastomers are produced from natural or synthetic substances by polymerisation, polyaddition or polycondensation. The nature of the principal components and of the various additives (for example, vulcanisers, accelerators, stabilisers, pigments) depends on the properties required for the finished article.

Rubber closures may be classified in 2 types:

Type I: Closures are those which meet the strictest requirements and which are to be preferred;

Type II: Closures are those which, having mechanical properties suitable for special uses (for example, multiple piercing), cannot meet requirements as severe as those for the first category because of their chemical composition.

Table 9.7: Components of rubber

Ingredient	*Examples*
Elastomer	Natural rubber (latex) butyl rubber neopene
Vulcanizing (curing) agent	Sulfur, peroxides
Accelerator	Zinc dibutyldithicarbamate
Activator	Zinc oxide, stearic acid
Antioxidant	Diaryl thiodipropionate
Plasticizer, lubricant	Paraffinic oil, silicon oil
Fillers	Carbon black, clay, barium sulfate
Pigments	Inorganic oxides, carbon black

Criteria for Selecting Closure

The closures chosen for use with a particular preparation are such that:

- The components of the preparation in contact with the closure are not adsorbed onto the surface of the closure and do not migrate into or through the closure to an extent sufficient to affect the preparation adversely.
- The closure does not yield to the preparation substances in quantities sufficient to affect its stability or to present a risk of toxicity.
- The closures are compatible with the preparation for which they are used throughout its period of validity.
- The manufacturer of the preparation must obtain from the supplier an assurance that the composition of the closure does not vary and that it is identical to that of the closure

used during compatibility testing. When the supplier informs the manufacturer of the preparation of changes in the composition, compatibility testing must be repeated, totally or partly, depending on the nature of the changes.
* The closures are washed and may be sterilised before use.

Rubber Closures Compendial Test Series

Depending on a drug product's targeted global market, the primary elastomeric closure component(s) used to package the drug must be tested for and comply with respective compendial standards. The major compendial standards are the United States Pharmacopoeia (USP) <381> "Elastomeric Closures for Injections," European Pharmacopoeia (Ph. Eur.) 3.2.9, "Rubber closures for containers for aqueous parenteral preparations, for powders, and for freeze dried powders," pharmacopoeia of Japan (JP), section 7.03, "test for rubber closure for aqueous infusions," and international organization for standardization (ISO). These tests are applied to address anticipated regulatory concerns and for quality control. Compendial tests are performed to determine if the material's specifications are met and/or to address anticipated regulatory concerns. These test series can also be applied to determine general drug compatibility or for routine quality control.

Analyses
USP <381> Physicochemical and functional test series
Ph. Eur. 3.2.9 Rubber closures—Physicochemical and functional test series
JP 7.03 Rubber closures
ISO 8362–2 : 1988 Closures for injection vials
ISO 8871 : 1990 Elastomeric parts for aqueous parenteral preparations

Elastomeric Closure/Plunger Test Series

A variety of base formulations, treatments and post-manufacturing processes are used to manufacture elastomeric closures and medical device components. Package testing represents a critical element in determining product qualification and product compatibility, and in evaluating performance characteristics of components before and after they are processed.

Methods such as total ash and specific gravity can be used for quality control identification tests. Additionally, other methods are:

* Validation of drying cycles for lyophilization closures
* Validation of washing cycles for particulate levels on components
* Validation of component siliconization
* Determining closure reseal
* Evaluating affects of sterilization on component functionality
* Evaluating the functionality of prefilled cartridges or syringe units.

General

Analyses
Determination of% ash
Determination of volume swell in solvents
Proved clean index (PCI)
Quantification of silicone oil (rubber closures)
Quantification of surface silicone on cotton swabs
Quantification of silicone oil in aqueous solutions
Karl fischer moisture quantification
Determination of specific gravity

Functional

Analyses
Determination of fragmentation (Ph. Eur. 3.2.9)
Determination of penetrability (Ph. Eur. 3.2.9)

COMPENDIAL DRUG PRODUCT TESTING

Packaging components can produce particulate matter in injectable drugs. Injectable solutions, including solutions constituted from sterile solids intended for parenteral use, should be free from visible particles. The USP provides a standard for particulate matter testing that includes a light obstruction and a microscopic procedure. Depending on the drug product form and the clarity and viscosity of the injectable solution.

For drug product testing requirements, various compendial methods are applied. Some common methods that are used for routine analysis or during stability shelf-life studies are presented.

Analyses
USP <788> Particle count—Microscopic count
USP <788> Particle Test—Light obscuration
USP <791> pH measurement
USP <643> Total organic carbon

Plastics Test Series

Pharmaceutical containers constructed of plastic materials such as but not limited to polyethylene and polypropylene must be qualified and meet USP <661> standards for testing. If the container is intended to provide protection from light (light resistant), it must meet the requirements for light transmission. Additionally the containers must meet the requirements for physicochemical tests to determine physical and chemical properties. These standards are applied and used routinely to test pharmaceutical products.

Pharmaceutical Container Testing

Pharmaceutical containers constructed of materials such as plastic and glass must be qualified and meet USP <661> containers and <671> containers-permeation standards. For example, if the container is intended to provide protection from light (light resistant), it must meet requirements for light transmission. Additionally the containers must meet the requirements for physicochemical tests to determine physical and chemical properties. The following tests are routinely offered.

Analyses
USP <671> Light transmission
USP <660> Chemical resistance—Glass containers
USP <661> Physicochemical tests—Plastics
USP <661> Polyethylene containers
USP <661> Polyethylene terephthalate and polyethylene terephthalate
     G bottles
USP <671> Multiple—Unit container
USP <671> Single—Unit container

Container Closure Integrity Testing Methodologies

Container closure integrity is defined as the ability and quality of a container closure system to provide protection and maintain efficacy and sterility during the shelf-life of a sterile drug product. The ability of rubber components to prevent microbial ingress of parenteral containers can be measured by seal integrity. To determine container closure integrity various testing methodologies are used. Some are for research and development purposes and help to characterize immediate container systems. Others are part of a sound control strategy and verify the constant performance of the manufacturing line during operation.

The most frequently used ones are:

- Helium integrity
- Determination of sealability (methylene blue dye filled vials).

In practice, there are numerous types of container closure integrity test methods that are available with varying sensitivities. A helium leak test method is state of the art and there are conventional methods used by the industry for many years.

Helium Leak Testing

The most sensitive seal integrity testing technique uses helium leak detection. This technique offers advantages over conventional seal integrity methods. The system is based on a helium mass spectrometer leak detector equipped with custom fixtures for the particular vial or parenteral container to be tested. Such instruments can be calibrated against traceable standard leaks and measure the rate of helium leak from the container, as well as the actual percent of helium that is filled within the container.

Various types of containers including vials, syringe systems, cartridges and blister packs can be evaluated. By using the tracer helium gas technique,the leakages could be determined quantitatively. Helium leak rate greater than 10^{-6} cm^3/sec can be considered a failure for closure integrity. Helium leak rates lower than 10^{-6} cm^3/sec has been associated with acceptable microbial challenge results. For sensitivity comparison, conventional seal integrity methods (i.e. dye leakage) have leak rates of 10^{-3} cm^3/sec.

Recommended applications of this technology include:

   i. General container closure integrity testing
   ii. Seal integrity monitoring during stability studies
  iii. Closure formulation/configuration selection
  iv. Sealing machinery optimization/validation
   v. Prediction of shelf-life seal integrity
  vi. Identifying the source of leaks.

Conventional Methods

Conventional seal integrity test methods are widely accepted by the industry and regulators and are routinely used for research and development studies, problem solving and to generate baseline data. Basic testing methods include but are not limited to:

- Determination of sealability of rubber closures by methylene blue ingress
- Determination of the amount of vacuum within a sealed vial
- Residual seal force.

The most common testing method uses methylene blue dye which after being filtered is placed into a vacuum vessel. Test samples filled with a suitable medium are then inserted into the vessel so that the samples are completely immersed in the dye. The vacuum vessel is then sealed and air is removed slowly. After a predefined length of time, the vacuum is slowly released. Samples then are removed from the vessel and cleaned to remove the dye. Samples are analyzed using either visual analysis or ultraviolet spectrophotometers. An aliquot from an untested sample is placed into a test tube. The detection limit is determined by adding a specific amount of dye to the untested sample until the dye is detectable visually or by the used instrumentation. Another aliquot is taken from an untested sample and transferred to a test tube to be used as the negative control. Aliquots from the contents of each sample are taken and place into a test tube, including a positive control. The negative control is compared to the test samples and the test tube used to determine the detection limit. Evidence of blue dye ingress is considered a failure.

Cleaning and Sterilization of Containers/Closures

Containers and closures should be rendered sterile and, for parenteral pharmaceutical drug products, nonpyrogenic. The process depend primarily on the nature of the container and/or closure materials. The process should be adequate to demonstrate its ability to render materials sterile and non-pyrogenic and should be validated. Pre-sterilization of glass containers usually involves a series of wash and rinse cycles. These cycles serve an important role in removing foreign matter. We recommend use of rinse water of high purity so as not to contaminate containers for parenteral products, final rinse water should meet the specifications of WFI, USP. The adequacy of the depyrogenation process can be assessed by spiking containers and closures with known quantities of endotoxin, followed by measuring endotoxin content after depyrogenation. The challenge studies can generally be performed by directly applying a reconstituted endotoxin solution onto the surfaces being tested. The endotoxin solution should then be allowed to air dry. Positive controls should be used to measure the percentage of endotoxin recovery by the test method. Validation study data should demonstrate that the process reduces the endotoxin content by at least 99.9 percent.

Subjecting glass containers to dry heat generally accomplishes both sterilization and depyrogenation. Validation of dry heat sterilization and depyrogenation should include appropriate heat distribution and penetration studies as well as the use of worst-case process cycles, container characteristics (e.g. mass), and specific loading configurations to represent actual production runs. Plastic containers used for parenteral products also should be non-pyrogenic. Where applicable, multiple WFI rinses can be effective in removing pyrogens from these containers. Plastic containers can be sterilized with an appropriate gas, irradiation, or other suitable means. For gases such as ethylene oxide (EtO), certain issues should receive attention. For example, the parameters and limits of the EtO sterilization cycle (e.g. temperature, pressure, humidity, gas concentration, exposure time, degassing, aeration, and determination of residuals) should be specified and monitored closely. EtO is an effective surface sterilant and is also used to penetrate certain packages with porous overwrapping. Biological indicators are of special importance in demonstrating the effectiveness of EtO and other gas sterilization processes. We recommend that these methods be carefully controlled and validated to evaluate whether consistent penetration of the sterilant can be achieved and to minimize residuals. Residuals from EtO processes typically include ethylene oxide as well as its byproducts. and should be within specified limits.

Rubber closures (e.g. stoppers and syringe plungers) can be cleaned by multiple cycles of washing and rinsing prior to final steam or irradiation sterilization. At minimum, the initial rinses for the washing process should employ at least purified water, USP, of minimal endotoxin content, followed by final rinse (s) with WFI for parenteral products. Normally, depyrogenation can be achieved by multiple rinses of hot WFI The time between washing, drying (where appropriate), and sterilizing should be minimized because residual moisture on the stoppers can support microbial growth and the generation of endotoxins. Because rubber is a poor conductor of heat, extra attention is indicated in the validation of processes that use heat with respect to its penetration into the rubber stopper load. Validation data from the washing procedure should demonstrate successful endotoxin removal from rubber materials. A potential source of contamination is the siliconization of rubber stoppers. Silicone used in the preparation of rubber stoppers should meet appropriate quality control criteria and not have an adverse effect on the safety, quality, or purity of the drug product. Contract facilities that perform sterilization and/or depyrogenation of containers and closures are subject to the same CGMP requirements as those established for in-house processing. The finished dosage form manufacturer should review and assess the contractor's validation protocol and final validation report.

Inspection of Container Closure System

A container closure system that permits penetration of microorganisms is unsuitable for a sterile pharmaceutical product. Any damaged or defective units should be detected, and removed, during inspection of the final sealed product. Safeguards should be implemented to strictly preclude shipment of product that may lack container closure integrity and lead to nonsterility. Equipment suitability problems or incoming container or closure deficiencies can cause loss of container closure system integrity. For example, failure to detect vials fractured by faulty machinery as well as by mishandling of bulk finished stock has led to drug recalls. If damage that is not readily detected leads to loss of container closure integrity, improved procedures should be rapidly implemented to prevent and detect such defects. Functional defects in delivery devices (e.g. syringe device defects, delivery volume) can also result in product quality problems and should be monitored by appropriate in-process testing. Any defects or results outside the specifications established for in-process and final inspection are to be investigated.

Pyrogen

"Microbial pyrogen" as opposed to "gram-negative bacterial endotoxin" has become a general descriptive term for many substances. However, some gram-negative bacteria, myco-bacteria fungi and also some viruses can produce pyrogenic substances, but the pyrogens produced by gram- negative bacteria, i.e. the endotoxins, are of significance to the pharmaceutical industry.

Bacterial endotoxins, found in the outer membrane of gram-negative bacteria are members of a class of phospholipids called lipopolysaccharides (LPS). LPS are not exogenous products of gram-negative bacteria. The release of LPS from bacteria takes place after death and lysis of the cell. Good examples of pyrogen producing gram-negative bacteria are *Escherichia coli, Proteus, Pseudomonas, Enterobacter* and *Klebsiella.*

Sources: There are several sources of pyrogens in parenteral and medical device products. Usual sources are: the water used as the solvent or in the processing; packaging components; the chemicals, raw materials or equipment used in the preparation of the product. Good practices include the control of microbiological contamination and endotoxin levels of contamination in the potential sources mentioned above. Additionally, if the drug substance is biological, the incomplete process of removal of the microorganism during purification can result in high endotoxin levels.

Control: General processing procedures for physical components of parenteral products such as stoppers and vials provide fore washing these components with pyrogen-free water prior to sterilization. Another source of endotoxin is WFI Generally ambient temperature WFI systems present the greatest problems. Remember—endotoxins result from high levels of microorganisms and are not removed by sterilizing or filtration. It is difficult to remove endotoxins from products once present. It is better to keep products and components relatively endotoxin-free than to have to remove them once present. The most common depyrogenation procedures for physical components include incineration and removal by washing (also called dilution). Distillation has been shown to be effective and the most reliable method in removing endotoxin from contaminated water samples. For physical components, such as stoppers and tubing, rinsing or dilution with pyrogen-free water systems is most common. Historically, glass components are rinsed with pyrogen-free water and dry heat sterilized at high temperatures. There are other methods used for chemical components and manufacturing equipment. Pyrogen testing is discussed latter in this chapter.

METHOD OF PREPARING PARENTERAL SUSPENSION AND SOLUTION

Two basic methods are used to prepare parenteral suspension or solution.

Method 1

Step 1: Aseptically combining sterile powder and vehicle.

Step 2: This method involves dispersing or dissolving sterile milled active ingredients into sterile vehicle system (Solvents + necessary excipients).

Step 3: Aseptically milling the resulting suspension as required.

Step 4: Aseptically filling the milled suspension or solution in to suitable containers.

For example, this process is used to prepare penicillin G suspension. As shown in the (Fig. 9.9).

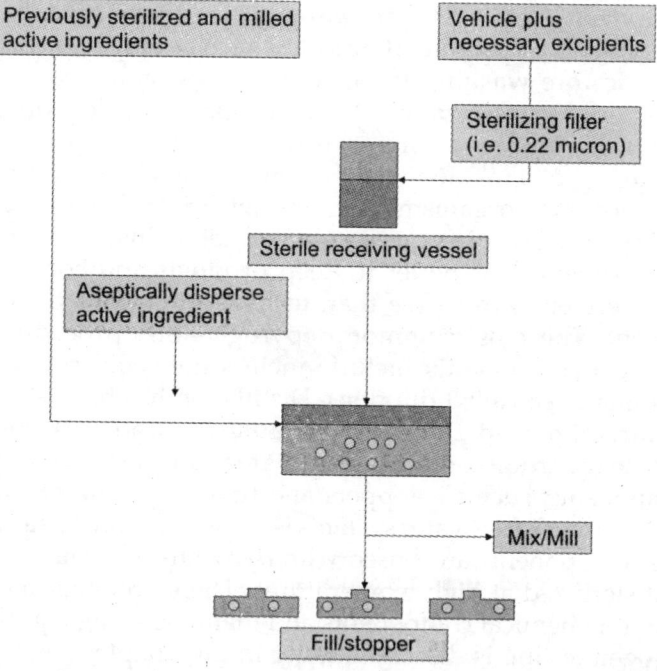

Fig. 9.9: Method 1 of preparing parenteral suspension and solution

Method 2

In situ formation of parenteral suspension:

Step 1: In situ crystal formation by combining sterile solutions (Fig. 9.10).

Step 2: In this method active ingredients are dissolved in suitable solvent system.

Step 3: A sterile vehicle system or counter solvent is added to step 2 solution that causes active ingredient to crystallize.

Step 4: The organic solvent is aseptically removed the resulting suspension is aseptically milled as necessary and then filled in suitable container.

For example, testosterone in parenteral insulin suspension.

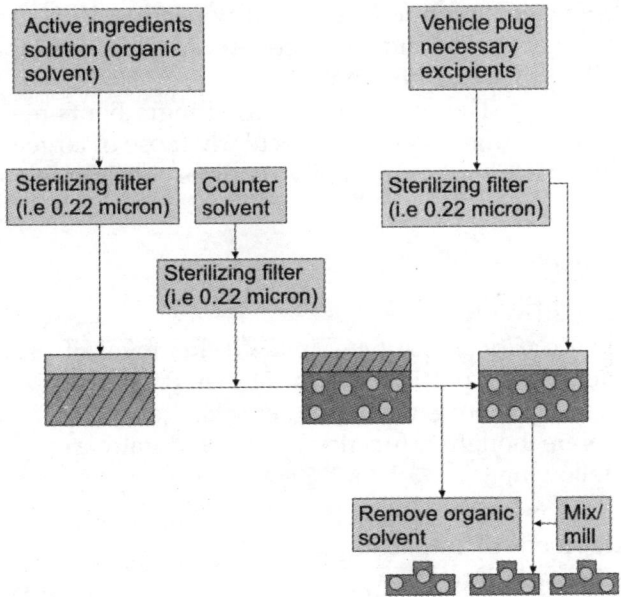

Fig. 9.10: Method 2 of preparing parenteral suspension

Important Unit Operations Involved during Parenteral Preparation

There are five critical steps involved in preparation of parenteral products:

1. Compounding of product
2. Filtration
3. Filling

4. Sealing-ampoules and vials
5. Sterilization.

1. Compounding

In general following steps are involved:

1. Preparation of master formula (MF).
2. All the excipients and active substance should be weighed accurately.
3. Dispensing must be done by weight as weight can be taken more accurately than volume.
4. During calculation for the amount of active drug substance to be taken, assay and water content of drug substance is to be taken into consideration.
5. *Mixing time:* The order of mixing of ingredients may affect the product significantly, particularly those of large volume, where attaining homogeneity requires considerable mixing time.

2. Filtration

Purpose of filtration:

1. *Getting clarity of parenteral solution:* Removal of particulate matter having particle size more than 0.2 µm in size.
2. Remove microorganism (cold sterilization).
   Filters are thought to function by one or, usually, a combination of the following:

• Sieving or screening.
• Entrapment or impaction.
• Electrostatic attraction.

Sieving or screening: When a filter retains particles by sieving, they are retained on the surface of the filter.

Entrapment or impaction: Entrapment occurs when a particle smaller than the dimensions of the passageway (pore) becomes lodged in a turn or impacted on the surface of the passageway.

Electrostatic attraction: Electrostatic attraction causes particles opposite in charge to that of the surface of the filter pore to be held or adsorbed to the surface.

Membrane filters used for parenteral preparation should be nonshedding and nonreactive to components of parenteral preparation. The most common membranes are composed of cellulose esters, nylon, polysulfone, polycarbonate, polyvinylidene difluoride, or polytetrafluoroethylene (teflon).

Each filter in its holder should be tested for integrity before and after use, particularly if it is being used to eliminate microorganisms. This integrity test usually is performed as the bubble point test.

A bubble point test is a test designed to determine the pressure at which a continuous stream of bubbles is initially seen downstream of a wetted filter under gas pressure. To perform a bubble point test, gas is applied to one side of a wetted filter, with the tubing downstream of the filter submerged in a bucket of water. The filter must be wetted uniformly such that water fills all the voids within the filter media. When gas pressure is applied to one side of the membrane, the test gas will dissolve into the water, to an extent determined by the solubility of the gas in water. Downstream of the filter, the pressure is lower. Therefore, the gas in the water on the downstream side is driven out of solution. As the applied upstream gas pressure is increased, the diffusive flow downstream increases proportionally. At some point, the pressure becomes great enough to expel the water from one or more passageways establishing a path for the bulk flow of air. As a result, a steady stream of bubbles should be seen exiting the submerged tubing. The pressure at which this steady stream is noticed is referred to as the bubble point.

Test Method

1. Record the filter part number(s), lot number, and product information. Also include physical observations.
2. Wet the filter to be tested with the appropriate solvent (water for hydrophilic filters, alcohol for hydrophobic filters).
3. Place the wetted filter in the appropriate housing.
4. Connect the outlet fitting from the compressed air pressure regulator to the upstream side of the test filter. Check that the gauge which is connected to the pressure regulator has subdivisions of at least 0.5 psig, and has the capacity to measure up to 100 psig. A digital pressure gauge can also be used.
5. Connect the outlet fitting from the compressed air pressure regulator to the upstream side of the test filter.

6. Connect a piece of flexible tubing from the downstream port of the test filter into a beaker filled with water.

7. Starting from zero pressure, gradually increase the pressure to the test filter using the pressure regulator.

8. Observe the submerged end of the tubing for the production of bubbles as the upstream pressure is slowly increased in 0.5 psig increments. Note the rate that the bubbles appear for the end of the submerged tube.

9. The bubble point of the test filter is reached wher. bubbles are produced from the tube at a steady rate. Record the pressure to the nearest 0.5 psig as indicated on the pressure gauge.

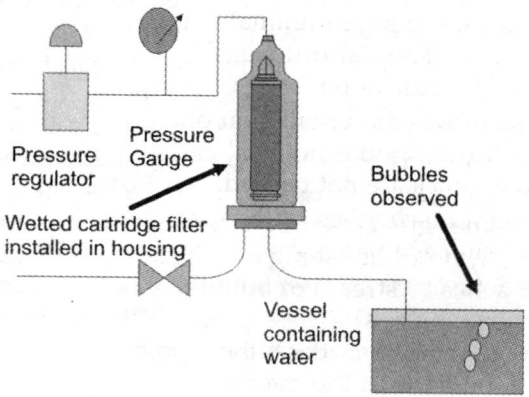

Fig. 9.11: Bubble point test

Filling

Aseptic filling must be exercised to prevent contamination, particularly when there is no terminal sterilization. This unit operation is carried out under blanket of HEPA filtered laminar flow in an aseptic area. Filling machine is provided for repetitively forcing a measured volume of the liquid through the orifice of a delivery tube that is introduced into the container. For large volumes the quantity delivered usually is measured in the container by the level of fill in the container and the force required to transfer the liquid being provided either by gravity or by pump (like pressure and a vacuum pump) or both.

AMPOULE FILLING

The narrow neck of an ampoule limits the clearance possible between the delivery tube and the inside of the neck. Since a drop of liquid normally hangs at the tip of the delivery tube after a delivery, the neck of an ampoule will be wet as the delivery tube is withdrawn, unless the drop is retracted. Therefore, filling machines should have a mechanism by which this drop can be drawn back into the lumen of the tube.

Features of Ampoule Filling Machines

- Most ampoule fillers are characterised with fast changeover time to accommodate a variety of ampoules in terms of shapes and size.
- These machines require minimal maintenance and are very easy to clean. They should easily be demountable for cleaning and sterilization.
- Another feature is the installation of speed adjusting equipment and 'no ampoule no fills' capability to ensure that unfilled ampoules are not packed.
- Check weight mechanism of the machine helps to maintain consistency in each batch.
- Sealing is done either by laser sealing system or conventional gas flame.

Material of construction: Since, the liquid will be in intimate contact with the parts of the machine through which it flows, these must be constructed of non-reactive materials such as borosilicate glass or stainless-steel. Stainless-steel syringes are required with viscous liquids because glass syringes are not strong enough to withstand the high pressures developed during delivery.

Solid filling: Sterile solids, like antibiotics, are more difficult to subdivide evenly into containers than are liquids as the rate of flow of solid material is slow and often irregular. Some sterile solids are subdivided into containers by individual weighing using filling machines.

Sealing

Ampoules: Filled containers should be sealed as soon as possible to prevent the contents from being contaminated by the environment. Ampoules are sealed by melting a portion of the glass neck.

Two types of seals are employed normally:

- Tip-seals (bead-seals).
- Pull-seals.
    1. *Tip-seals:* Those made by melting sufficient glass at the tip of the ampule neck to form a bead of glass and close the opening.
    2. *Pull-seals:* Those made by heating the neck of a rotating ampule below the lip, then pulling away the tip to form a small, twisted capillary just prior to being melted closed.

Manual pull-sealing of ampoules: Using a twin-jet burner (Fig. 9.12), adjust the platform height and flame intensity.

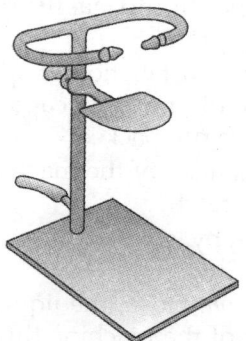

Fig. 9.12: Twin-jet burner

Try an empty ampoule first before sealing your products. Position the ampoule between the flames. Grip the end of the neck with a blunt-nosed forceps and when the glass is soft enough, pull off the top of the ampoule vertically and gently. Leave the tip in the flame for a second or two longer and then remove. The tip should now be smoothly and evenly rounded (Figs 9.13a to e) Ampoules should have a reliable seal which can be readily leak tested. A good seal will not deteriorate during the lifetime of the product.

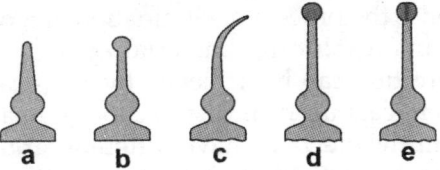

Figs 9.13a to e: (a) Good seal, (b to e) faulty ampoules seal

Sealing of Vials and Bottles

These are sealed by closing the opening with a rubber closure (stopper). This must be accomplished as rapidly as possible after filling and with reasoned care to prevent contamination of the contents. Rubber closures are held in place by means of aluminum caps. The caps cover the closure and are crimped under the lip of the vial or bottle to hold them in place (Fig. 9.14). The closure cannot be removed without destroying the aluminum cap; it is tamperproof. Therefore, an intact aluminum cap is proof that the closure has not been removed intentionally or unintentionally. Such confirmation is necessary to ensure the integrity of the contents as to sterility and other aspects of quality.

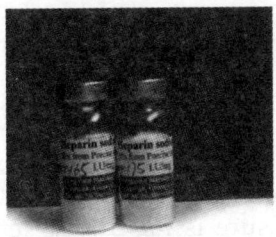

Fig. 9.14: Vials of heparin, where closures was held in place by means of aluminum caps

Sterilization and disinfection: Sterilization can be achieved by means of:
- Physical treatment;
- Chemical treatment; and
- Physiochemical treatment.

Disinfection is the process of elimination of most pathogenic microorganisms (excluding bacterial spores) on inanimate objects. Disinfection can be achieved by physical or chemical methods. Chemicals used in disinfection are called disinfectants. Different disinfectants have different target ranges, not all disinfectants can kill all microorganisms. Some methods of disinfection such as filtration do not kill bacteria, they separate them out. Sterilization is an absolute condition while disinfection is not. These are not same.

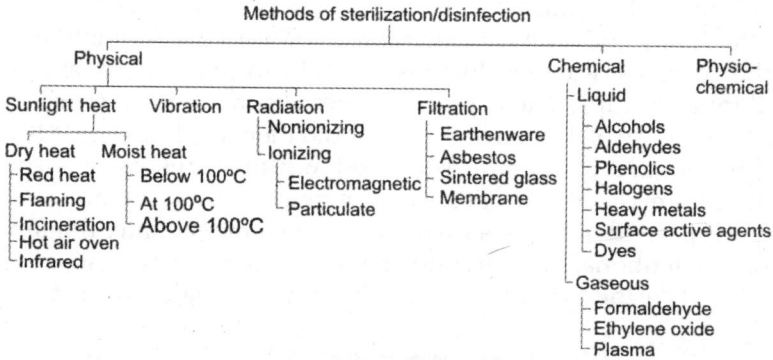

Fig. 9.15: Classification of various methods of sterilization/disinfection

Autoclave

Sterilization can be effectively achieved at a temperature above 100°C using an autoclave. Water boils at 100°C at atmospheric pressure, but if pressure is raised, the temperature at which the water boils also increases. In an autoclave the water is boiled in a closed chamber. As the pressure rises, the boiling point of water also raises. At a pressure of 15 lbs inside the autoclave, the temperature is said to be 121°C. Exposure of articles to this temperature for 15 minutes sterilizes them. To destroy the infective agents associated with spongiform encephalopathies (prions), higher temperatures or longer times are used; 135°C or 121°C for at least one hour are recommended.

Advantages of steam: It has more penetrative power than dry air, it moistens the spores (moisture is essential for coagulation of proteins), condensation of steam on cooler surface releases latent heat, condensation of steam draws in fresh steam.

Different Types of Autoclave

Simple "pressure cooker type" laboratory autoclave, steam jacketed downward displacement laboratory autoclave and high pressure pre-vacuum autoclave.

Construction and Operation of Autoclave

A simple autoclave has vertical or horizontal cylindrical body with a heating element, a perforated try to keep the articles, a lid that can be fastened by screw clamps, a pressure gauge, a safety valve and a discharge tap. The articles to be sterilized must not be tightly packed. The screw caps and cotton plugs must be loosely fitted. The lid is closed but the discharge tap is kept open and the water is heated. As the water starts boiling, the steam drives air out of the discharge tap. When all the air is displaced and steam start appearing through the discharge tap, the tap is closed. The pressure inside is allowed to rise upto 15 lbs per square inch. At this pressure the articles are held for 15 minutes, after which the heating is stopped and the autoclave is allowed to cool. Once the pressure gauge shows the pressure equal to atmospheric pressure, the discharge tap is opened to let the air in. The lid is then opened and articles removed.

Advantage

Very effective way of sterilization, quicker than hot air oven.

Disadvantage

Wetting of articles may occur, trapped air may reduce the efficacy, takes long-time to cool (Fig. 9.16).

Products that will not withstand autoclaving temperatures may withstand marginal thermal methods such as tyndallization or pasteurization, e.g. 10–12 hr at 60°C. These methods may be more effective for some injections by the inclusion of a bacteriostatic agent in the product.

Packaging, Labeling, and Storage of Injections

Containers for injections, including closures, must not interact physically and chemically with the preparation.

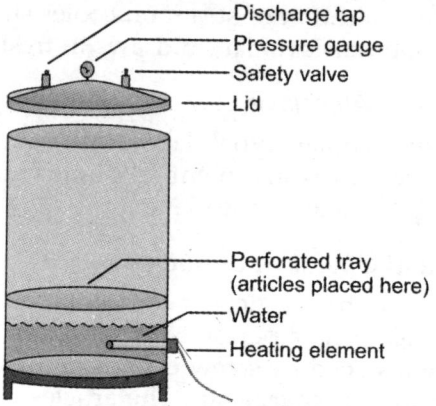

Discharge tap
Pressure gauge
Safety valve
Lid

Perforated tray
(articles placed here)
Water
Heating element

Fig. 9.16: Autoclave

- *Single-dose container:* A single dose container is a hermetic container holding a quantity of sterile drug intended for parenteral administration as a single dose, and which when opened cannot be re-sealed with assurance that sterility has been maintained.
- *Multiple-dose container:* A multiple-dose container is a hermetic container that permits withdrawal of successive portions of the contents without changing the strengths, quality, or purity of the remaining portion.

The labels on containers of parenteral products must state:

1. The name of the preparation.
2. For liquid preparation, the percentage content of the drug or amount of the drug; for dry preparation—the amount of the active ingredient present and the volume of liquid to be added to the dry preparation to prepare a solution or suspensions.
3. The route of administration.
4. Statement of storage conditions and expiration.
5. The name of the manufacturer and distributor.
6. The identifying lot number.

LYOPHILIZATION

Lyophilization (freeze drying) is the removal of water from frozen material. It is an excellent method for preserving microbes and heat-sensitive materials such as proteins, plasma, etc.

Water is removed from frozen samples mainly by sublimation—water is converted from the frozen state into vapor, thus bypassing the liquid phase. The rate of sublimation depends on vapor pressure, which is affected by the system vacuum and sample temperature. The frozen sample absorbs heat, causing water in the sample to enter the vapor phase and migrate into the instrument atmosphere where it is removed by refreezing on the condenser. Drying first occurs at the surface of the sample. As drying proceeds, water is removed from deeper layers of the sample and the drying rate slows.

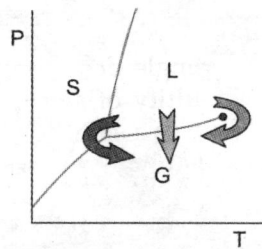

Fig. 9.17: In a typical phase diagram, the boundary between gas and liquid runs from the triple point to the critical point. Freeze-drying brings the system around the triple point, avoiding the direct liquid-gas transition seen in ordinary drying

Three steps in lyophilization:
1. *Freezing:* The sample is placed in a freezing vial/flask. The purpose is to completely freeze the sample.
2. *Primary drying:* Approximately 90% of the total water in the sample (essentially all of the free water and some of the bound water) is removed by sublimation.
3. *Secondary drying:* Bound water is removed by desorption, resulting in a product that has <1–3% residual water. This step requires time about one-third to half the time needed for primary drying.

Methods of Sample Frozen

There are two freezing methods and their use depends on the type of container holding the sample. Small volumes (less than a few milliliters) may be placed in a vial and frozen in a regular freezer. Larger volumes (up to about 100 ml per freezing flask) are shell frozen and dried by the manifold method. In manifold method, flook ampules or vials are in clinidually attached to the part of manifold or dring chamber. Shell freezing involves rotating the flask containing the sample in a freezing bath so the sample freezes on the walls of the flask. This method maximizes the surface area to thickness ratio thereby facilitating water removal from the sample (Fig. 9.18).

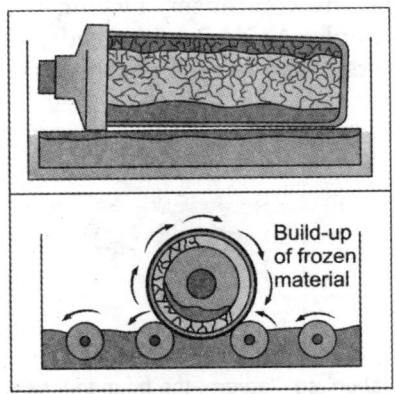

Fig. 9.18: Shell freezing (increase the surface area)

Do not freeze a large block of sample in the bottom of the freezing flask; the sample will be too thick for efficient water removal and may melt during drying.

Rapid freezing results in small ice crystals which reduce drying efficiency (although it is good for preserving structure for microscopic examination). Slower freezing produces larger ice crystals that improve the efficiency of drying.

For freezing purposes, there are two kinds of samples: solutions and suspensions. Solutions usually have water as the solvent. Solutes tend to form eutectics, a combination of solutes that freeze at a lower temperature than water or other solutes. The entire sample must be frozen, including the eutectics, before the sample is ready for drying; otherwise, the unfrozen material will expand and melt when the sample is placed under a vacuum. The freezing temperature of eutectics is known as the *eutectic temperature.*

Suspensions form a glass as they become more viscous during freezing. Eutectics do not form. At the glass transition point the suspension forms a vitreous solid. Each suspension has a unique glass transformation temperature. Suspensions are very difficult to freeze dry.

Three basic formats for freeze drying:

1. Manifold drying is the most commonly used method. Drying flasks or ampules are attached to individual ports on a central manifold. The samples are usually frozen by the shell method, and are quickly attached to the manifold and placed under vacuum to prevent melting. Room temperature provides heat for the sample. This method is useful for relatively small volumes (Figs 9.19 and 9.20).

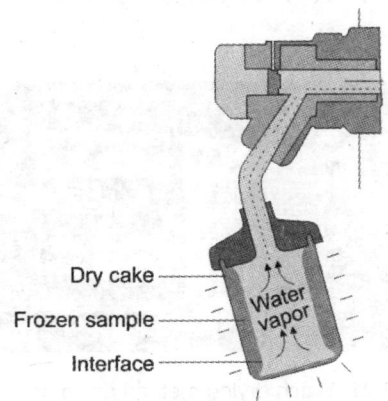

Dry cake

Frozen sample

Interface

Water vapor

Fig. 9.19: Manifold drying-room temperature provides heat for removal of water vapor from frozen samples

2. The batch method is used when large numbers of similar-sized containers are simultaneously freeze dried, e.g. serum vials. A tray system is used instead of a manifold. Heating elements in the trays supply the heat. Most batch systems have a mechanism to seal the vials before they are exposed to air (Fig. 9.21).

3. The bulk method is used for large volumes of a single sample. The sample is poured into special trays, frozen, and then dried in a lyophilizer. Bulk dried samples cannot be sealed

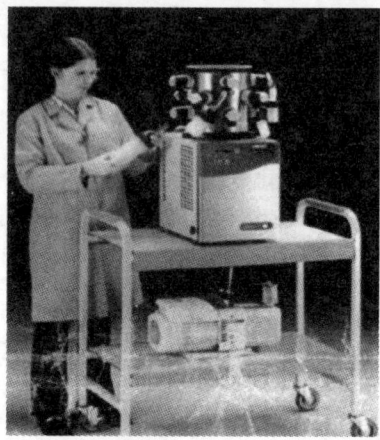

Fig. 9.20: Manifold drying (drying flasks or ampules are attached to individual ports)

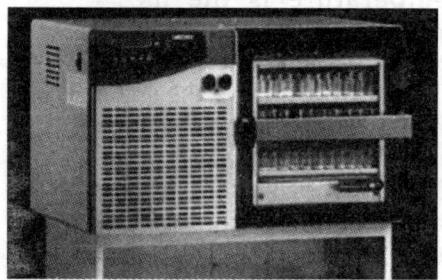

Fig. 9.21: Batch drying method using tray dryer

while in the instrument. Exposure to air before packaging may affect shelf-life (Fig. 9.22).

Factors that affect the efficiency of lyophilization:

- Sample size
- Surface area of the sample
- Thickness of the sample
- Sample characteristics
- Eutectic temperature
- Solute concentration
- Instrument factors

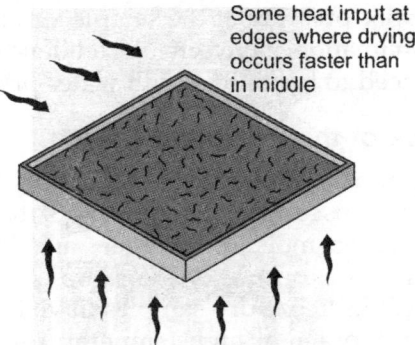

Fig. 9.22: Bulk drying-heat is provided primarily through conduction from shell

- Condenser temperature
- Vacuum

Eutectic temperature is the most important factor determining how much sample can be lyophilized at one time. Vapor pressure decreases as the eutectic temperature lowers, but the rate of heat absorption by the sample remains the same and may cause melting. Diluting the sample with water prior to freezing can prevent melting.

Generally, the larger the surface area of the frozen material, the faster the rate of lyophilization, and, conversely, the thicker the frozen material, the slower the rate of lyophilization. Sample thickness affects the ability of a sample to absorb and transfer heat to the surface undergoing sublimation. Because water vapor must pass through dried material, the rate of lyophilization in thick samples is slower, especially if the dried material collapses onto the surface of the frozen material. Shell freezing minimizes collapsing by increasing the surface area. Generally, the volume of the freeze dry flask should be 2 to 3 times that of the material being frozen. The condenser must be 10–15°C colder than the eutectic temperature of the material being frozen. A vacuum of at least 133×10^{-3} m bar is required for lyophilization. Vapor pressure depends on eutectic temperature and solute concentration. The vapor pressure of water decreases as the concentration of the sample increases, thereby slowing the rate of sublimation. Volatile chemicals increase the vapor pressure at the sample surface and require less heat for sublimation, increasing the tendency to melt. These samples may need to be diluted with water prior to freezing.

Characteristics of the Finished Product

Freeze dried products have from <1–3% residual water content and are very hygroscopic. The stability of the freeze-dried product depends on moisture, oxygen, and temperature. A good seal prevents exposure of the sample to moisture and oxygen. It is best to freeze dry samples in vials and seal them under vacuum. Storage at high temperatures reduces shelf-life. Refrigeration or freezing is best for long-term storage.

Contamination of the Lyophilizer

The main contaminants in a lyophilizer are microorganisms and harmful chemicals. Microorganisms will contaminate any freeze drying instrument unless each vial or flask is fitted with a bacteriological filter. Cross contamination between vials is more likely in the batch method and vials should be decontaminated upon removal from the lyophilizer. The condenser is the most contaminated portion of the instrument and should be decontaminated periodically. Corrosive chemicals and organic solvents can damage lyophilizers. Organic solvents are generally not removed by the condenser and pass into the vacuum pump where they mix with the pump oil, thinning the oil and damaging the pump if the oil is not changed periodically. Corrosive chemicals can damage all portions of a lyophilizer. Wash the system to remove these chemicals after processing samples.

Sample Protocols

The goal is an uncontaminated and stable microbial culture with little or no variation or mutation. Upon reconstitution, the microorganism should exhibit the same growth characteristics it had prior to freezing. Additives are frequently used in suspension fluids to enhance product stability.

Bacteria: Late logarithmic phase cultures are usually best for freeze drying. Collect cultures grown on agar by scraping into a suspension fluid. Cultures grown in broth are harvested by centrifugation, followed by resuspension in a suspension fluid.

Suspension Fluids

1. Meso-inositol 5% in horse serum
2. Inositol broth 2.5% meso-inositol 5% in water.

Note: Inositol serum (#1) is not recommended for enterobacteria.

Fungi: Add equal volumes of a 72 hour shake culture and a solution of 7.5% glucose in serum. Sucrose or inositol (5%) can be substituted for glucose. Refrigerate immediately to prevent further replication.

Add 0.5–1.0 ml of suspension to a 2.0 ml freezing vial. Freeze by placing in a laboratory freezer (–20 degrees or below). Place in lyophilizer and dry using the batch method.

The Basics of Freeze Drying

Freeze drying or lyophilization: This is a process of stabilizing initially wet materials (aqueous solutions or suspensions) by freezing them, then sublime the ice while simultaneously desorbing some of the bound moisture (primary drying). Following the disappearance of the ice, desorption may be prolonged (secondary drying). This process is usually conducted under vacuum.

Desorption: The release of liquids and gas trapped within a substance.

Sublimation: Vaporization or evaporation wholly from a solid phase without melting.

Primary drying: Stage of freeze drying involving the sublimation of ice, although this is usually accompanied by concurrent desorption of bound moisture.

Secondary drying: Prolonged drying stage (when all visible ice is sublimed) for continued desorption until desired product consistency.

Science of Freeze Drying

When to preserve a product without altering it, there is no replacement for freeze-drying. This gentle process removes moisture from aqueous product, without affecting its biological, chemical or structural properties. Because a rigid ice matrix holds the solid components in place, the freeze drying process maintains product integrity. Compare this with conventional drying, which typically causes shrinkage or chemical reactions, damaging cells and rendering an end-product useless for additional chemical analysis, or for final product display. For many years, freeze-drying was as much guess work and intuition as science. But you can now count on precise, repeatable results, time after time. While the chemistry involved in freeze drying may be complex, the process itself can be divided into three basic process steps:

Freezing

In the first step, the product is frozen solid, which converts the water content of the material to ice. The final temperature must be below the product's eutectic, or collapse temperature, so that it maintains its structural soundness. Once the product is frozen solid, the condenser and vacuum systems are energized for the next critical process step.

Primary Drying

In the second step, the objective is to remove the unbound, or easily removed ice from the product. This water is now in the form of free ice, which is removed by converting it directly from a solid to a vapor, in a process called sublimation. To accomplish sublimation, a uniform source of heat energy is applied to the ice crystals, turning them directly into water vapor. The product and condenser chambers are placed under vacuum to encourage the orderly migration of water vapor to the system's ice-collecting condenser, and to ensure that the pressure of the water vapor remains below its "triple point", as required for sublimation to occur.

Secondary Drying

Even after all the free ice is removed by the sublimation process, your product may still contain enough bound water to limit its structural integrity and shelf-life. During secondary drying, the sorbed water, or the water that was bound strongly to the solids in the product, is converted to vapor. This can be a slow process; the remaining bound water has a lower pressure than free liquid at the same temperature, which makes it difficult to remove. Secondary drying actually starts during the primary drying phase, but must be extended after the total removal of the free ice to achieve low enough residual moisture levels. Freeze-drying is complete when all the free and bound water has been removed, resulting in a residual moisture level that guarantees the desired biological and structural characteristics of the final product.

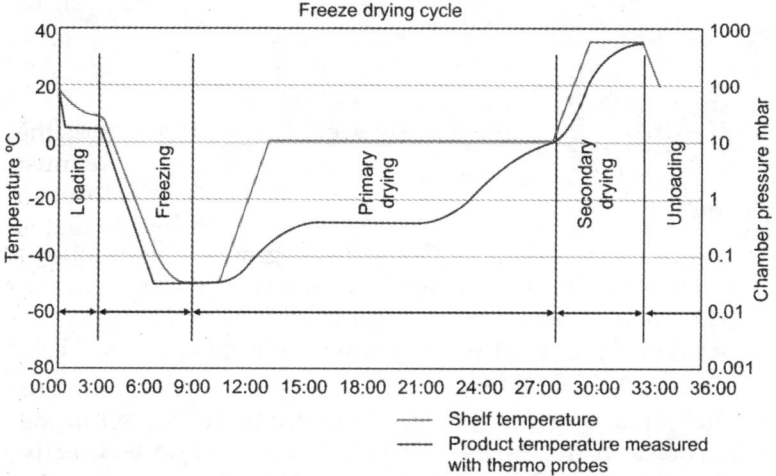

Fig. 9.23: Freeze drying cycle

CLEAN ROOM AREA FOR STERILE PRODUCTS

Clean rooms are classified by the cleanliness of their air. As per federal standard 209 class limits clean area classified in Table. 9.8.

Table 9.8: Federal standard 209 class limits

Measured particle size (micrometers)

Class	0.1	0.2	0.3	0.5	5.0
1	35	7.5	3	1	NA
10	350	75	30	10	NA
100	NA	750	300	100	NA
1,000	NA	NA	NA	1,000	7
10,000	NA	NA	NA	10,000	70
100,000	NA	NA	NA	100,000	700

For the manufacture of sterile medicinal products four grades are given. The airborne particulate classification for these grades is given in Table 9.9.

Table 9.9: Maximum permitted number of particles/ m³.

Grade	At rest (b)		In operation	
	0,5 um	5 um	0,5 um	5,0 um
A	3 500	0	3 500	0
B (a)	3 500	0	350 000	0
C (a)	350 000	2 000	3 500 000	2 000
D (a)	3 500 000	20 000	Not defined (c)	Not defined (c)

Notes

a. In order to reach the B, C and D air grades, the number of air changes should be related to the size of the room and the equipment and personnel present in the room. The air system should be provided with appropriate filters such as HEPA for grades A, B and C.

b. The guidance given for the maximum permitted number of particles in the "at rest" condition corresponds approximately to the US Federal Standard 209 as follows: Grades A and B correspond with class 100. Grade C with class 10, 000 and grade D with class 100,000.

c. The requirement and limit for this area will depend on the nature of the operations carried out.

The particulate conditions given in the table for the "at rest" state should be achieved in the unmanned state after a short "clean up" period of 15–20 minutes, after completion of operations. The particulate conditions for grade A in operation given in the table should be maintained in the zone immediately surrounding the product whenever the product or open container is exposed to the environment. It is accepted that it may not always be possible to demonstrate conformity with particulate standards at the point of fill when filling is in progress, due to the generation of particles or droplets from the product itself. Examples of operations to be carried out in the various grades are given in Table 9.10.

Table 9.10: Operations to be carried out in the various grades

Grade	Examples of operations for terminally sterilized products
A	Filling of products, when unusually at risk.
C	Preparation of solutions, when unusually at risk filling of products.
D	Preparation of solution and components for subsequent filling.

Grade	Examples of operations for terminally sterilized products
A	Aseptic preparation and filling
C	Preparation of solutions to be filtered
D	Handling of components after washing

Additional microbiological monitoring is also required outside production operations, e.g. after validation of systems, cleaning and sanitization (Table. 9.11).

Table 9.11: Recommended limits for microbial contamination

Grade	Air sample cfu/m$_3$	Settle plates (diam. 90 mm), cfu/ 4 hours (b)	Contact plates (diam. 55 mm), cfu/ plate	Glove print, 5 fingures, cfu/ glove
A	<1	<1	<1	<1
B	10	5	5	5
C	100	50	25	.
D	200	100	50	–

Notes

a. These are average values
b. Individual settle plates may be exposed for less than 4 hours.
c. Appropriate alert and action limits should be set for the results of particulate and microbiological monitoring. If these limits are exceeded operating procedures should prescribe corrective action.

Two areas are defined. The 'critical area' is where the sterilized dosage form, containers, and closures are exposed to the environment. The 'controlled area' is where unsterilized product, in-process materials, and container/closures are prepared.

Critical areas: Air in the immediate proximity of exposed sterilized containers/closures and filling/closing operations is of acceptable particulate quality when it has a per-cubic foot particle count of no more than 100 in a size range of 0.5 micron and larger (class 100) when measured not more than one foot away from the work site, and upstream of the airflow, during filling/closing operations. The agency recognizes that some powder filling operations may generate high levels of powder particulates, which by their nature do not pose a risk of product contamination. It may not, in these cases, be feasible to measure air quality within the one-foot distance and still differentiate "background noise" levels of powder particles from air contaminants, which can impeach product quality. In these instances, it is nonetheless important to sample the air in a manner, which to the extent possible characterizes the true level of extrinsic particulate contamination to which the product is exposed.

Air in critical areas should be supplied at the point of use as HEPA filtered laminar flow air, having a velocity sufficient to sweep particulate matter away from the filling/closing area. Normally, a velocity of 90 feet per minute, plus or minus 20%, is adequate, although higher velocities may be needed where the operations generate high levels of particulates or where equipment configuration disrupts laminar flow.

Air should also be of a high microbial quality. An incidence of no more than one colony forming unit per 10 cubic feet is considered as attainable and desirable.

Critical areas should have a positive pressure differential relative to adjacent less clean areas; a pressure differential of 0.05 inch of water is acceptable.

Controlled areas: Air in controlled areas is generally of acceptable particulate quality if it has a per-cubic-foot particle count of not more than 100,000 in a size range of 0.5 micron and larger (class 100,000) when measured in the vicinity of the exposed articles during periods of activity. With regard to microbial quality, an incidence of no more than 25 colony forming units per 10 cubic feet is acceptable.

In order to maintain air quality in controlled areas, it is important to achieve a sufficient airflow and a positive pressure differential relative to adjacent uncontrolled areas. In this regard, airflow sufficient to achieve at least 20 air changes per hour and, in general, a pressure differential of at least 0.05 inch of water (with all doors closed), are acceptable. When doors are open, outward airflow should be sufficient to minimize ingress of contamination'.

Evaluation tests for parenteral preparations:
- Pyrogen test
- Test for particulate matter
  - Light obstruction particle count test
  - Microscopic particle count test
- Test for sterility of parenteral products
- Leak test (already discussed).

Test for Pyrogens

It is used to check for the presence of pyrogens in the parenteral formulation. Two general tests are performed.
- Rabbit test and
- LALs test

Rabbit Test

The pyrogen test is designed to limit to an acceptable level the risks of febrile reaction in the patient to the administration, by injection, of the product concerned. Unless otherwise specified in the individual monograph, inject into an ear vein of each of three rabbits 10 ml of the test solution per kg of body weight, completing each injection within 10 minutes after start of administration. The test solution is either the product, constituted if necessary as directed in the labeling, or the material under test treated as directed in the individual monograph and injected in the dose specified therein. Assure that all test solutions are protected from contamination. Perform the injection after warming the test solution to a temperature of 37 ± 2°. Record the temperature at 30 minute intervals between 1 and 3 hours subsequent to the injection.

Test Interpretation

Consider any temperature decreases as zero rise. If no rabbit shows an individual rise in temperature of 0.5° or more above its respective control temperature, the product meets the requirements for the absence of pyrogens. If any rabbit shows an individual temperature rise of 0.5° or more, continue the test using five other rabbits. If not more than three of the eight rabbits show individual rises in temperature of 0.5° or more and if the sum of the eight individual maximum temperature rises does not exceed 3.3°, the material under examination meets the requirements for the absence of pyrogens.

LALs test: Limulus amebocyte lysate (LAL) is an aqueous extract of blood cells (amoebocytes) from the horseshoe crab, Limulus polyphemus. LAL reacts with bacterial endotoxin or lipopolysaccharide (LPS), which is a membrane component of Gram-negative bacteria. This reaction is the basis of the LAL test.

Method: Blood is removed from the horseshoe crab's pericardium and the blood cells are separated from the serum using centrifugation and are then placed in distilled water, which causes them to swell up and burst ("lyse"). This releases the chemicals from the inside of the cell (the "lysate"), which is then purified and freeze-dried. To test a sample for endotoxins, it is mixed with lysate and water; endotoxins are present if coagulation occurs.

Particulate Evaluation

Parenteral solutions should be essentially free from particulate matter which can be observed on visual inspection. This test describes the physical tests performed to enumerate extraneous particles with specific size ranges. Particulate matter includes mobile, randomly sourced, extraneous substances, other than gas bubbles that cannot quantified by chemical analysis due to less amount and of their heterogeneous compositions.

Methods

* Light obscuration method
* Microscopic method

Light Obscuration Method

This method applies for parenteral product including solutions constituting form sterile solids, for which the test for particulate matter is specified in the individual monograph.

The parenteral product meets the requirements of the test if the average numbers of particles present in the units tested does not exceed the appropriate value listed in the following Table 9.12.

Table 9.12: Light obscuration particle count test		
	Diameter	
	≥10 µm	≥25 µm
SVI	6000	600/container
LVI	25	3/ml

Microscopic Method

This method is performed when some particles are not exactly detected by the light obscuration method. This test enumerates the sub-visible particles essentially solid, particulate matter present in the parenteral preparation. The test sample is collected on a microporous membrane filter.

The USP injection meets the requirements of the test if the average number of particles present in the units tested does not exceed the appropriate value listed in the Table 9.13.

Table 9.13: Microscopic method particle count test		
	Diameter	
	≥10	≥25
SVI	3000	300/container
LVI	12	2/ml

Sterility Test

This is used to test the presence of microorganisms in the test solution. It is done by two methods:
- Membrane filtration method
- Direct inoculation (immersion) method.

Membrane filtration method: In this the test solution is first passed through assize exclusion membrane capable of retaining the microorganisms. The concept is that the microorganisms will collect on the surface of a 0.45 micron pore size filter. The filter is rinsed and then the membrane is transferred to appropriate test medium as specified in the monograph.

Direct inoculation (immersion) method: In this the test article is directly inoculated into the test medium and then the medium is incubated for the growth of microorganisms, if present.

Test media: The test media are fluid thioglycollate medium (FTM) and soybean casein digest medium (SCDM). FTM is selected based upon its ability to support the growth of anaerobic and aerobic microorganisms. SCDM is selected based upon its ability to support a wide range of aerobic bacteria and fungi (i.e. yeasts and molds).

Incubation time: In both the methods the test medium after the transferring of the test solution is to be incubated for 3 days in case of bacteria and 5 days in case of fungi and then the growth is compared with that of standard. If no growth is observed then the sample passes the test and it meets the GMP requirements.

Fluid thioglycollate medium (FTM)	
Gram weight per liter	29.8 gm/l
Pancreatic digest of casein	15.0 gm
Yeast extract	5.0 gm
Dextrose	5.5 gm
Sodium chloride	2.5 gm
Sodium thioglycollate	0.5 gm
L-cystine	0.5 gm
Resazuril	1.0 mg
Final pH 7.1 + /–0.2 at 25°C	
store at room temperature (15–30°C).	

Soybean casein digest medium (SCDM) per liter	
Pancreatic digest of casein	17 g
Soya peptone	3 g
Dextrose	2.5 g
Sodium chloride	5 g
Dipotassium phosphate	2.5 g
Final pH is 7.3 at 25°C.	
Store at room temperature (15–30°C)	

Table 9.14 outlines the requirement for sterility testing as per USP.

Table 9.14: The requirement for sterility testing as per USP

Volume/container	Minimum quantity to test in each media
<1 ml	The entire contents of each container
1–40 ml	Half the contents of each container but not <1 ml
41–100 ml	20 ml
>100 ml	10% of the contents of the container, but not <20 ml

If the average number of particles exceeds this limit, the test article is subjected to microscopic method.

ISOLATED KEY POINTS

- Parenteral (derived from green word, enteron, beside the intestine) dosage forms of drugs are injected directly into body tissue throug om for toxicity and freedom from contamination.
- Parenteral formulation has quick onset of action and 100% bioavailability for IV injection and they are suitable for drugs not absorbed by the gut or those that are too irritant (anti-

Organs	Injection type
Skin	• Intradermal
	• Subcutaneous
Organs	• Intracavernous
	• Intravitreal
	• Transscleral
Central nervous system	• Intracerebral
	• Intrathecal/intraspinal
	• Epidural
	• Intracisternal
Circulatory/musculoskeletal	• Intravenous
	• Intracardiac
	• Intramuscular
	• Intraosseous
	• Intra-articular
	• Intraperitoneal
	• Intra-arterial

cancer) but they need special precautions as they can be fatal if not administered properly.

- They can be classified on the basis of the organs in which they are adminitered and on the basis of the injection volume (SVP and LVP).
- Preformulation studies are critical for product development, where we perform characterization of substance with respect to solubility, stability, particle size, compatibility between the excipients and the drug substance and partition and distribution coefficients.
- The components of the product to be accumulated and selected include vehicles (aqueous vehicle, water miscible and non-aqueous), solute, container and closure.
- "Microbial pyrogen" as opposed to "gram-negative bacterial endotoxin" has become a general descriptive term for many substances. However, some gram-negative bacteria, mycobacteria fungi and also some viruses can produce pyrogenic endotoxins are of singnificance to the pharmaceutical industry.
- Filter integrity test usually is performed as the bubble point test.
- Lyophilization (freeze drying) is the removal of water from frozen material. It is an excellent method for heat-sensitive materials such as proteins, plasma, etc.
- Two areas are defined for parenteral products. The 'critical area' is where the sterilized dosage form, containers, and closures are exposed to the environment. The 'controlled area' is where unsterilized product, in-process materials, and container/closures are prepared.
- Evaluation tests for parenteral preparations are pyrogen test, test for particulate matter (light obstruction particle count test and microscopic particle count tests), and test for sterility of parenteral products and leak tests.
- Prefilled syringes are the latest technology and commercial products available as "PFS" especially insulin administering syringes.

PRACTICE QUESTIONS

1. Define the term parenteral products. Give their advantages and disadvantages.

2. Give classification of parenteral products with the help of suitable examples, based on their route of administration.

3. Give classification of parenteral products with the help of suitable examples on the basis of their injection volumes.

4. Discuss in brief the various factors which can effect solubility of parenteral drugs.

5. Write in detail about the various components of parenteral formulation.

6. Name some common apparatus used for the production of water for injections.

7. Write short notes on:
   a. Non-aqueous vehicles used for parenteral.
   b. Specification for purified water
   c. Water miscible vehicles.
   d. Solutes

8. Write short notes on (Reference to parenteral products).
   a. Antimicrobial agents.
   b. Preservatives
   c. Buffers
   d. Anti-oxidant

9. Describe in detail about the various types of containers used for parenteral formulation.

10. What are the desired characteristics of parenteral container.

11. Write in brief about rubber closure and their criteria of selection for parenteral products.

12. Write in brief about the test done for parenteral closures.

13. Describe the methods used for preparation of parenteral suspension.

14. Describe the methods used for preparation for parenteral solution.

15. Enlist various important operations involved during formulation of parenteral preparation.

16. Give the classification of various methods of sterilization for parenteral products.

17. Write short notes on:
    a. Packaging of parenteral
    b. Labeling of parenteral

18. What is lyophilization? Give basics of lyophilization?
19. Enumerate various factors affecting efficiency of lyophilization.
20. Describe the evaluation test done for parenteral formulations.

OBJECTIVE TYPE QUESTIONS

1. ....dosage forms of drugs are injected directly into body tissue through one or more layer of skin and mucous.
2. The US Pharmacopoeia (USP) defines small volume parenteral (SVPs) which contains................ and large-volume parenterals (LVPs) containing...........
3. .... is the removal of water from frozen material. It is an excellent method for preserving microbes and heat-sensitive materials such as proteins, plasma, etc.
4. The two USP tests for determining glass types are .... and ....
5. Match the following:

S.no.	Parenteral dosage form		Route of administration
1.	Intradermal	a	Inside an eye
2.	Subcutaneous	b	Into the skin
3.	Intravitreal	c	Under the skin
4.	Intracavernous	d	Into the epidural space of the spinal cord
5.	Intrathecal	e	Into the base of the penis
6.	Epidural	f	Through the theca of the spinal cord
7.	Intraosseous infusion	g	Into the bone marrow
8.	Intravenous	h	Into the peritoneum
9.	Intra-articular	i	Within a vein
10.	Intraperitoneal	j	With in joints

6. Match the following:

S. no.	Type of glass		Material used
1.	Type I glass	a	Treated soda lime glass
2.	Type II glass	b	Ordinary soda lime glass
3.	Type III glass	c	Untreated soda lime glass
4.	Type NP glass	d	Highly resistant borosilicate glass

7. Which of the following is the evaluation tests for parenteral preparations?
   a. Pyrogen test and test for particulate matter
   b. Light obstruction particle count test and microscopic particle count test
   c. Test for sterility of ophthalmic products and powder attack test
   d. A and b
   e. All of the above

ANSWERS

1. Parenteral
2. less than 100 ml, more than 100 ml
3. Lyophilization (freeze drying)
4. Powdered glass test, water attack test.
5. 1-b, 2-c, 3-a, 4-e, 5-f, 6-d, 7-g, 8-d, 9-j, 10-h
6. 1-d, 2-a, 3-c, 4-b
7. d

10

Packaging of Pharmaceuticals

After the manufacturing of drugs, it is essential that these should be stored properly. The stability of drug during its storage depends on so many factors are in direct contact with the containers and closures. So improper packing and poor quality of containers may lead to declaration of the products. Pharmaceutical container has been defined as a device that holds the drug and it may or may not be in direct contact with the pharmaceutical preparations. Closures are the devices by means of which containers can be opened and closed. "Packaging is the science, art and technology of enclosing or protecting products for distribution, storage, sale, and use. Packaging also refers to the process of design, evaluation, and production of packages. Packaging can be described as a coordinated system of preparing goods for transport, warehousing, logistics, sale, and end use".

Packaging Types

- Primary packaging is the material that first envelops the product and holds it. This usually is the smallest unit of distribution or use and is the package which is in direct contact with the contents.
- Secondary packaging is outside the primary packaging— perhaps used to group primary packages together.
- Tertiary packaging is used for bulk handling, warehouse storage and transport shipping. The most common form is a palletized unit load that packs tightly into containers.

Functions of Packaging

To efficiently preserve products, and to distribute and market them safely and effectively the functions of packaging are listed below:

1. *To protect the product from the environment:* Majority of the pharmaceutical products have a limited shelf-life, due to interaction with their environment. This may occur during the manufacturing process, manufacturing an intermediate product, the shipping process, storage, marketing by the consumer. Products may need to be protected from many hazards that occur in any or all of these environments. Other environmental considerations are the presence of dust, microbes, yeasts and bacteria in the atmosphere. All of these can have detrimental effects on the products, and packaging is designed to protect the product from their harmful effects.

2. *To protect the environment from the product:* Many products may be harmful to the environment, causing an adverse reaction with the environment.

3. *To maintain the product in its the state in which it was produced:* Many products are manufactured to a degree of consistency that is necessary for their effective use. For example, creams created for skin application on tender skin would be unacceptable if they were allowed to go hard and thus have an abrasive action on application. The manufacturer makes all products with a view to their final use, and any deterioration could render the product unacceptable.

4. *To safely transport the product:* Transportation through a modern transport and storage system, either within a country or via a worldwide distribution network, demands modern packaging. The journey hazards are numerous with palletised storage; movement by fork trucks or conveyor belts; road, sea or air transport and variations in temperature and/or humidity. All potential hazards need to be thought when the product is going to arrive safely to the consumer.

5. *To identify the brand:* The majority of products and companies have a brand identity, the valuation of

companies may differ significantly according to a commercial rating of their brand image. Brand loyalty amongst consumers is highly valued by the brand owners; since advertising is expensive, a strong brand loyalty can minimize the need for advertising.

6. *To sell the product to the consumer:* The pack here serves two vital purposes: to sell the product to the consumer, and to allow the consumer to recognize the product for a repeat purchase.

7. *To inform the consumer of use:* A further function of packs is to inform the consumers of the appropriate ways to use the product and to warn them of the dangers that may exist in use. Packs also provide other information, such as ingredients lists, storage conditions, shelf-life, the name of the manufacturer and a host of other data. Much of the information may be a legal pre-requisite, with restrictions on minimal type size and legibility, depending upon the product.

8. *To warn the consumer of dangers:* Some products, if used incorrectly, are dangerous; thus, the pack can also be used to give warnings. Again, these warnings may be a legal requirement, or they may be placed on the pack by a concerned.

9. *To attain and maintain a cost-effective unit:* Packaging needs to be cost-effective, it must be usable and safe for the consumer, and also efficient to produce and safe to transport.

10. *To protect the consumer:* The packaging may need to have the additional requirements of 'tamper evidence'. In general, it is accepted that ideally, tamper evident features must be seen by the consumer at the time of purchase. Tamper evidence is of no use if the consumer is unaware of the feature and how it works. Thus, any tamper evident feature must be easily seen and easily used. Additional protection for the consumer may be required by law for certain products, such as those that could be dangerous if used incorrectly for example, bleach or other products that may require a child-resistant cap, or warnings for blind consumers.

Desirable Qualities of Good Containers

i. The containers must be neutral towards the material which is stored in it.

ii. The containers must not react physically or chemically with the substance stored in it.

iii. It should help in maintaining the stability of product against the environment factors which cause its deterioration.

iv. It should be made of materials which can withstand wear and tear during normal handling.

v. It should be able to withstand changes in pressure and temperature. This is required in case of sterilization of parenteral products along with its container and closure.

vi. The material used for making the container should be nontoxic.

vii. The container can be labeled easily.

viii. The container must have a pharmaceutically—elegant appearance.

ix. The closure of the container must be easily removable and replaceable.

Types of Containers

Containers are divided into following types on the basis of their utility:

1. *Well-closed containers:* A well-closed containers protects the contents from loss during transportation, handling, storage or sale, etc.

2. *Single-dose containers:* These containers are used to supply only one dose of medicament and hold generally parenteral products, e.g. ampoules and vials.

3. *Multi-dose containers:* These containers allow the withdrawal of dose at various intervals without changing the strength, quality or purity of remaining portion. These containers hold more than one dose and are used for injectables, e.g vials.

4. *Light-resistant containers:* These containers protect the medicament from harmful effects of light. These containers are used to store those medicaments which are photo-sensitive.

5. *Air-tight containers:* These are also called hermetic containers. These containers have air-tight. These containers have air-tight sealing or closing. These containers protect the products from duct, moisture and air. Whereas air-tight sealed containers are used for injectables, air-tight closed containers are meant for the storage of other products.

6. *Aerosol containers:* These containers are used to hold aerosol products. These containers have adequate mechanical strength in order to bear the pressure of aerosol packing.

Materials Used for Containers

The containers used for pharmaceutical products are usually made from the following basis materials:

1. Glass
2. Plastic
3. Metal
4. Paper and board.

Glass

Glass has always been the traditional gold standard for pharmaceutical packaging. Its physical characteristics of clarity and impermeability coupled with its inert chemical nature when exposed to organic or inorganic liquids and solids always made it the standard starting point for package development. Glass is not totally inert. Glass, depending on its composition, can impart hydroxyl ions to a solution; some of the chemicals used in its manufacture are leachable. Glass was and may still be the most widely used material in pharmaceutical packaging worldwide, but plastics and composites are displacing it.

Glass Composition

The chemical materials used to make glass are common materials with layman names of sand, soda ash, and limestone. These materials are readily available and easily obtained from naturally occurring mineral deposits found all over the world. Traces of other materials are added to impart clarity and hardness. Lead (Pb) provides brilliance and clarity but makes glass relatively soft and alumina (Al_2O_3) is a common addition to increase hardness and durability. Other trace materials are used to reduce seeds and blisters in glass, for example, arsenic trioxide (As_2O_3) and sodium sulfate (Na_2SO_4). Glass is recognized as an inert material used to package and contain both strong acid and strong bases (alkaline) along with all types of organic and inorganic liquids and solvents. One problem with glass as a pharmaceutical packaging material is measurable chemical reactions of the material with a number of materials, most commonly water. Glass stored in high temperature and high humidity conditions or high temperature and humidity fluctuations can undergo a physical change called blooming. Blooming, or leaching, is a physical change in which salts in the glass "bleed out" or more properly migrate and accumulate on the surface of the glass.

High-quality glass used for pharmaceutical packaging is designated as type I glass in the United States pharmacopoeia (USP) (1) and is substantially more resistant to surface attack. Normal soda lime glass with surface treatments targeted or designed for specific pharmaceutical applications can and are used for packaging drugs but not in the most demanding applications. The addition of 6 to 10% boron to glass to form borosilicate glass reduces the leaching action of water to 0.5 ppm in a one-year period. Boron, added as an alternative to some of the earth oxides in the form of boron oxide (B_2O_3), reduces the melt viscosity of the material for fabrication to a manageable range, even though this glass still requires the highest processing temperatures for package manufacture. Glass containing boron in the amounts used to produce the most inert glass compositions or chemistries reduces leaching by alkalis while greatly reducing surface leaching by acid solutions. Borosilicate glass is about 10 times more resistant to acids than soda lime glass found in typical consumer packaging. Boron-containing glass is more heat resistant and durable than other forms of glass and displays higher melting point and significantly smaller coefficient of thermal expansion. This is why this material is cited in the USP as the highest quality choice for packaging pharmaceutical solutions, especially acidic solutions that have a potential to interact with the packaging and possibly change in stability or performance because of the interaction. The major drawbacks to this type of glass are cost, difficulties inherent with its fabrication, and a somewhat limited supply because of the small, specialized demand. The reason glass is clear is the material's chemical structure after cooling. Glass remains an amorphous material after cooling. Glass is stabilized to remain clear with the addition of aluminum oxide (Al_2O_3) and lead oxide (PbO_2). These materials help prevent devitrification, a slow crystallization process that can, over time, reduce glass clarity and turn it cloudy. Glass has advantages and disadvantages associated with its choice as a pharmaceutical packaging material. Probably, the two best characteristics of glass are its resistance to chemical attack by almost all liquids except hydrofluoric acid (HF) and strong caustics along with its impermeability. Glass being impermeable prevents any volatile ingredients from escaping and prevents any environmental gases, primarily oxygen, from entering the container. Glass disadvantages include its brittleness and weight. Glass brittleness is a problem that translates into glass breakage and the tendency of glass to break into numerous fragments. Even when care is taken to prepare glass to break by scoring or other techniques that thins the glass, in a container designed to be broken such as an ampule, the glass can shatter into fine fragments that may be ingested with the drug. Glass has a high density (2–2.5 g/cc), which in combination with its brittle nature means that containers must be fabricated with thick walls to achieve adequate durability. The thick walls make the resulting product heavy and increase transportation costs. This is a disadvantage compared with plastic and metal containers. A short list of the advantages and disadvantages of glass as a package is as follows.

Advantages
  i. They are transparent.
  ii. They are available in various shapes and sizes.
  iii. They can withstand the changes in temperature and pressure during sterilization.
  iv. They are cheap and easily available.
  v. Amber colored glass can protect the photosensitive medicaments from light during their storage.
  vi. They are neutral towards the medicament stored.
  vii. They are impermeable to moisture and atmospheric gases.

viii. They provide good protection power.

ix. They can be easily labeled.

x. They can be sealed hermetically or by removable closures.

Disadvantages

i. Glass is fragile, hence easily broken down when dropped or knocked.

ii. Glass containers are heavy, which increase the cost of its transportation from one place to another.

iii. Major problem is glass containers may release alkali to aqueous preparation.

Glass is composed of sand, soda ash, lime stone and cullet is broken glass that is mixed with the batch and acts as a fusion agent for the entire mixture. The composition of glass varies and it depends on the specific purpose for which it is used silicon, aluminum, boron, sodium, potassium, calcium, magnesium, zinc and barium are generally used in the preparation of glass.

Types of glass: Glass of the following types are available commercially for making containers.

1. *Lime-soda glass:* It is composed of SiO_2, MgO and Al_2O_3 lime-soda glass can be manufactured easily. Further, it is not so expensive. It is used for preparing containers which are meant for storage of solid medicaments. It is however not suitable as a container material for storage of parenteral products because:

   • It liberates alkali in aqueous preparations.

   • On repeated use its surface loses some of its brilliance.

   • It is not resistant to sudden loses some of its brilliance.

   • It is not resistant to sudden changes in temperature.

   • Flakes separate more easily as compared to other types of glass.

2. *Borosillicate glass*: It is composed of SiO_2 (80%), B_2O_3 (12%) Al_2O_3 (6%) and mixture of Na_2O, CaO and other oxides (2%). It is chemically more inert than lime-soda glass. It is a highly resistant glass.

3. *Sillicone-treated glass:* Glass is treated with silicon so that it can be used for preparing containers to store alkali sensitive products.

4. *Sulphured glass:* It is a cheaper variety of glass used for construction of containers for parenteral products. The soda-lime glass is exposed to moist SO_2 at about 500°C to get sulphured glass. It does not liberate alkali.

5. *Neutral glass:* It is composed of SiO_2 (72–75%), B_2O_3 (7–10%), Al_2O_3 (4–6%), Na_2O (6–8%), BaO (2–4%) and K_2O (0.5–2%). It is resistant to alkalis, weather and can also withstand autoclaving. It is has the capacity to filter out UV radiations.

6. *Amber colour glass:* Amber colour glass container is used for storage of photosensitive pharmaceutical products because it has the capacity to filter out UV radiations. Some preparation are very sensitive to lead or arsenic. For such preparations only containers made from glass free from lead or arsenic should be used. Containers for injectable preparations must be made from uncoloured glass. However, for substance which are highly sensitive to light coloured glass may be used but it should be transparent to permit visual inspection of its contents. The following two types of glass are used for preparation of containers meant for storage of parenteral preparation.

Types of Glass Used for Pharmaceutical Packaging

There are four types of glass used in pharmaceutical containers. The glass performance grades or "Types" used in pharmaceutical packaging are defined precisely in the USP as type I, type II, type III, and NP glass (1). Type I glass is borosilicate glass. Type II glass is very high-quality soda-lime glass. The last two are lower grades of soda-lime glass and approximate glass found in packaging food and other consumer products. Their performance characteristics are listed in the USP as type III glass and NP or nonparenteral glass. Both type III glass and NP glass are acceptable for food packaging. NP glass has a highest specification for leachable components in USP's standardized test. This difference makes its use and the development of testing to prove its suitability for a drug product more problematic. NP glass must be proven safe and acceptable for use in pharmaceutical packaging but really is closer to a general or generic grade of glass. It is one of the USP standards but not widely used in pharmaceutical packaging. Two limited applications for type NP glass are in packaging oral or topical products. It is not a material normally used in primary drug packaging.

Table 10.1: Glass pigment colors

S. no.	Metal compounds	Colours
1.	Iron oxides	Greens, browns
2.	Manganese oxides	Deep amber, amethyst
3.	Cobalt oxide	Deep blue
4.	Gold chloride	Ruby red
5.	Selenium compounds	Reds
6.	Carbon oxides	Amber/brown
7.	Antimony oxides	White
8.	Sulfur compounds	Amber/brown
9.	Copper compounds	Light blue, red

Table 10.2: Types of glass

S. no.	Type of glass	Material	Test	Size
1.	Type 1	Highly resistant borosilicate glass	Powder glass test	All
2.	Type 2	Treated soda-lime glass	Water attack test	100 ml or less
3.	Type 3	Soda-lime glass	Powder glass test	All
4.	NP	General purpose soda-lime glass	Powder glass test	All

Plastics: Plastics play a large and important role in packaging of pharmaceutical products. Plastic materials can be the primary packaging material, the material that contacts the product being protected often referred to as the primary package, or they can be used in other parts of the package all the way to the pallet and the shrink or stretch wrap film around the pallet. They can be part of a composite structure of materials or an adjunct to another material to improve its properties. They can be used as the sealant, adhesive, or coating material between a wide variety of metal and paper materials. Plastic containers are very commonly used in pharmaceutical packaging because of the following:

Advantages

i. They are light in weight and can be handled easily.
ii. They are poor conductor of heat.
iii. They have sufficient mechanical strength.
iv. They can be transported easily.
v. They are unbreakable.
vi. They are available in various shapes and sizes.
vii. They are resistant to inorganic chemicals.
viii. They have good protection power.
ix. There are no changes of formulation of flakes as it comes in glass containers.

Disadvantages

i. They are permeable to water vapour and atmospheric gases.
ii. They can not withstand heat without softening or distorting.
iii. They may interact with certain chemical to cause softening or distortion.
iv. They may absorb chemical substances, such as preservatives for solution.
v. They are relatively expensive.
vi. Special type of gum or adhesive required for labeling.

Plastic materials vary in use, depending upon the properties that are demanded from the specific packaging requirement. Plastic containers may utilise either plastic or non-plastic closures the following plastic materials are used.

Polyethylene

The basic material of polyethylene (PE) can be classified into several different forms and grades, ranging from the linear-low-density (LLDPE), through to low density (LDPE), medium-density (MDPE) and high-density (HDPE) polyethylene, each having its own specific attributes and manufacturing qualities. LDPE is usually used for closures in the food and beverage markets, since the flexibility of the material gives a good snap and reuse facility. Where tougher materials are required, the preference is for HDPE materials. HDPE materials also have better organoleptic properties and are often chosen for sensitive products.

Polypropylene

This is a common material used for closure applications, because it possesses most of the good properties of the PE range within a single material. Polypropylene (PP) makes very good hinge lids, with a good repeat performance over many closure applications; it is widely used in food, beverage, cosmetic and pharmaceutical products. There are two basic types of materials: homopolymers—which have high rigidity and low impact strength; and copolymers—which are more flexible and perform better at low temperatures.

Due to the high rigidity of PP, due care must be given to the seal integrity when PP is used in the closure and other polymers are used in the container; in these circumstances, the use of a liner material in the cap should be considered.

Polystyrene

Similar to most other plastics materials, polystyrene (PS) is also available in more than one type. General-purpose polystyrene (GP) can be formed with high clarity, and thus it can be used for glass clear' applications. However, in this form it is very brittle and liable to shatter if it is subjected to rough treatment. Another type of polystyrene is *high impact polystyrene* (HIPS), which also has a good gloss and clarity. PS has been used for lidding materials for vacuum-formed trays, where the low oxygen barrier properties can be exploited to retain the red colour for meats. However, because of its brittle nature, it is liable to tearing on closing machines. With the many other materials available, the use of PS is declining in the closure industry.

Other Plastics Materials

Many other materials are available within the palette of the closure designer to give the material the specific properties. For example, there is *acrylonitrile butadiene styrene* (ABS), which has the ability to withstand elevated temperatures without distortion; this is used for steam-sterilisable products.

In addition, one may consider nylon—this comprises a family of products that may be chosen on account of their particular attributes; for example, they are often used for cosmetics closures, since they have good scratch resistance; they may also be used for further finishing operations, such as electroplating. Another such material is *ethylene vinyl acetate* (EVA), which is mainly used as a lining material when the sealing function of the closure is paramount.

Metal: Aluminum, tinplate, and steel are the three primary metals used to make metal cans. Pharmaceutical packaging only uses two of the three primary metals for primary packaging: aluminum and tinplate. Steel is normally not used even when coated with an inert lining of plastic or multiple layers of thermoset organic coatings. It is used for bulk materials in the form of drums, but it is not for primary packages. Tinplate is really a steel composite material that uses a steel core coated with tin.

Aluminum and tinplate are not limited to cans and are materials used to make tubes and pouches. Either these two materials when used for can manufacture require a great deal of processing and manufacturing before they become suitable as a finished package for pharmaceutical or foods products. Almost all metal cans need to coat or paint the metal with an organic lining to separate the product from bare metal. There are few minor exceptions, but almost every can used today requires an inert thermoset coating on the inside to protect the product and metal and a variety of coatings on the outside to label (can makers call it decorating) and protect the can. A wide variety of organic coatings were first to be adapted to seal or insulate the metal from the product. Before coatings, cans relied on zinc or tin surface coating to protect the product from iron in the steel and to prevent or retard corrosion. As more products were sealed in cans and as trial and error knowledge about can performance identified shortcomings, the need for coatings to improve performance became obvious.

Metal are used for the construction of containers. The metals commonly used for this purpose are aluminum, tin plated steel, stainless steel, tin and lead.

Advantages

i. They are sturdy.
ii. They are impermeable to tight, moisture and gases.
iii. They can be made into rigid unbreakable containers by impact extrusion.
iv. They are light in weight as compare to glass containers.
v. Labels can be printed directly on to their surface.

Disadvantages

i. They are expensive.
ii. They may shed metal particles into the pharmaceutical product.
iii. They are not generally used for extemporaneous dispensing.
iv. They react with certain chemicals or drugs.

Aluminum, tin and lead are used for construction of collapsible tubes. The collapsible tubes are available in different sizes. In pharmaceutical industry the collapsible tube made from tin are preferred because they are compatible with a wide range of products. However, they are quite costly. The collapsible tubes made from aluminum are light in weight and are mostly used for toothpastes and creams. These are less costly than collapsible tubes made from tin. Lead tubes are the cheapest among all metal collapsible tubes but are not used for pharmaceutical packing due to the risk of lead poisoning. If the product is not compatible with bare metal, the interior of the collapsible tube can be coated with wax-type formulation or with resin solutions. Wax linings are used as lining material for aluminum tubes. The epoxides and vinyls are used as lining material for aluminum tubes which gives better protection to the product filled in it.

The metal containers are also used for bulk packaging of tablets, capsules, powders and food materials, etc. metal foil may be used for wrapping individual suppositories or pessaries. However, it is mainly used in strip packaging or blister packaging.

Paper and Board

Paper and board are used in various forms for packaging of pharmaceutical products. They are used for preparing outer containers, such as cartons, boxes, envelops and drums, to provide additional mechanical protection to other containers, e.g. strip and blister packs of tablets, capsules, suppositories and pessaries may be packed in an outer paper board carton. Collapsible tubes of ointments, creams and gels as well as liquid medicines in sizes 500 ml and below, may be packed in an other paper board carton, slide paper board boxes suitable lined may be used for extemporaneous dispensed suppositories, pessaries and powders.

Package Validation

The packaging of the medical device must insure the integrity of the device, shield and protect it from mechanical damage, insure the sterile barrier is intact, and in some cases the package must act as a dispenser, a holder, or a fixture for the device. This is why the packaging must meet the same rigorous proof of performance required by a validation procedure. Maintenance of sterility is the primary concern of most agencies and is the most common defect created by exposing a medical device to general conditions found in the distribution chain including handling, dropping, or possible mishandling.

The vibration of packages by over the road vehicles and airplanes can significantly damage the device and the packaging. Common defects created by shipping and handling include slits, cuts, pinholes, tears, fractured thermoform clamshells, crushing, and deformation that may call the integrity of the package or the packaging into question.

1. Distribution Testing

After a package is produced, it must be tested and proven to survive the transportation and distribution environment. This means the package must protect the product through all the drops, vibrations, and other stresses normally associated with transportation and storage testing to answer these questions usually involves the following procedures:

a. Drop Testing

Drop testing is just what the name implies and is carried out from a specified height on all sides of a package and on the corners.

b. Compression Testing

A compression test squeezes the package in a manner similar to it being placed on the bottom of a stack or at the bottom of a pallet.

c. Loose Load Vibration and Shock Testing

Loose load vibration and shock testing subjects the package to being vibrated at a frequency and bounced multiple times. This simulates typical truck shipment.

d. Random Vibration Profile Testing

A random vibration profile subjects the package to the multiple frequencies it would undergo during shipment.

2. Evaluation of Primary Packaging Material

The following test are done for the evaluation of primary packaging:

- Leakage test
- Hydrolytic resistance collapsibility
- Residue on ignition
- Buffering capacity
- Light transmission
- Water vapour permeation
- Heavy metals and non-volatile residue.

3. Evaluation of Secondary Packaging Material

The following test are done for the evaluation of secondary packaging:

- Testing of paper and board
- *Air permeability:* Permeability is the mean air flow through unit area under unit pressure difference in unit time, under specific conditions, expressed in Pa-1s-1.
- *Tensile strength:* Both wet and dry. The maximum tensile force per unit width that a paper or board will withstand before breaking.
- *Cobb test:* This measures the mass of water absorbed by 1cm^2 of the test piece in a specified time under a head of 1 cm of water. It is determined by weighing before and after exposure to the water, and usually quoted in g/m^2
- *Specific tests for cartons compression:* Assessment of the strength of the erected package, thereby estimating the degree of protection that it confers on the contents.
- *Crease stiffness:* Also called the crease recovery test. This involves testing a carton board piece and folding it through 900. It will then try to recover its former position when the bending force is removed. The increase and decrease in the inherent board stiffness after folding is measured.

4. Package Testing

The following test are done:

1. The amount, kind and toxicity of any materials that may be extracted from the package by the product and how this may be avoided.
2. Whether any of the product constituents are being absorbed and how this may be prevented or minimized.
3. The amount size kind of any particulate matter that may appear in the product and the steps necessary to prevent this.
4. The light transmission characteristic if the product is photosensitive.
5. *Closure efficiency:* This is best achieved by placing the product in the proposed package and nothing say, weight changes over a period. An unfilled control will establish weight changes due to the package alone.
6. Any specific interactions, how these aries and how they may be minimized.
7. Whether the package satisfies legal requirement both in the country of origin and in those to which the product may be exported.

5. Filling

Packaging does not finish with the selection of a suitable container for the product. The latter must be filled into the container. This involves further processing and handling producers which themselves may have an effect on the long term stability of the product. If the batch is small, hand filling may be appropriate but on an industrial scale a batch may consist of thousands of product units, requiring for economic filling semi-automatic or automatic equipment. Such equipment would assemble the containers and closures, dispense the medicament into the container, apply the product into a carton. As filling operations are common to many industries, a wide variety of equipment is available to the pharmaceutical manufacturer. Different organization, therefore, are unlikely to adopt the same system for a given operation. Nevertheless, there are problems basis to the filling of liquids, semi-solids, powders and unit-dose products, regardless of the production method and these are briefly discussed here.

6. Liquids

There are obvious problems in filling suspensions, particularly official preparations of kaolin, magnesium trisilicate, etc. which do not contain a suspending agent. If a product of the correct composition is to be packaged, the bulk must be continuously and thoroughly stirred throughout the entire filling operation with particular attention to the corners of the main container where stirring is relatively ineffective and where solid may accumulate. Furthermore the transit time of the product from the bulk to the final container must be short to minimize sedimentation in the filling head. Apart from inaccuracies in the composition of the filling product, accumulating solid may jam the head mechanism. Even solutions present filling problems if the surface tension is low and the foam stability high. The liquid from the filling head jetting into the product already in the bottle cause considerable agitation and build-up of a persistent forth. It is necessary for the vacuum line to suck off to the trap a large volume of forth before the bottle is properly filled with liquid product. A variant of the standard head, that is normally successful in avoiding this problem. The liquid jets into the wall of the container and gently flows as a thin film without frothing. As these types of head fill to a metric accuracy of filling is entirely dependant on the observance of rigid tolerances during manufacturer of the container. Furthermore, it is not easy significantly to vary the filling volume from the nominal value for the container. Machine driven automatic syringes are employed if greater very satility is required, a method which finds considerable use in large scale ampoule filling. The syringe size and plunger stroke determine the volume transferred to the container.

7. Semi-solids

The filling of extract paste, ointments, creams and other semi-solids is sometimes facilitated by warming the product to reduce viscosity. The technique must be applied with care as it may accelerate a degradative chemical reaction or have an effect on physical characteristics or stability. Sedimentation of suspended solids may occur if the viscosity of the vehicle is excessively reduced by heating, while permanent changes on consistency resulting are stirred or heated must be allowed for at the formulation stage. Viscous products, particularly those containing surfactants, are prone to aeration. Apart from the fact that aeration may accelerate oxidation, the entrained air bubbles are highly compressible and interface with pumping when the product is homogenized or filled. Finally it may not be possible to get the required amount of aerated product into the selected container.

8. Powders

It is often possible to resolve a powder filling problem into a powder flow problem. It is worth bearing in mind however, that the filling machine may discuss the powder by stirring, may clause some practical size reduction by attrition in the feed-screw and may expose the powder to atmospheric oxygen or water vapour. If the product is particularly water sensitive, e.g. ampicillin, it may be necessary to provide low humidity filling condition; it is generally accepted that, for stability, 1% represent the water content that may be permitted for penicillin formulation in powder form. There is often a dust hazard associated with the filling of powder and this must be carefully controlled to avoid toxic effects of the operatives and contamination of other products.

9. Unit-dose Product

These are usually packed in sub-multiplies or multiplies of a hundred the tablet or capsule placed in the filling machine each unit separately interrupts a light beam or other machine mechanism that actuates accounting device whereby the product feed is shut of as soon as the correct number of unit have been placed in the container the filling process subjects the product to tumbling action and for the reason tablet should be formulated for high resistance to abrasion, particularly at the edges to minimize abrasion when the tablet is the container to minimize the head space in filled with "necking" material. Formerly, cotton wool was much use but unless thoroughly dried its normal moisture content in sufficient to promoto the degenerate of sensitive products performed polyurethane form is now used for necking it is easier to interest in, has a very low moisture content.

Repacking

After manufacturing a product may undergo one further packing process if perspiration requirement do not match available pack sizes. The repacking process often effects stability and process other problem as well as those specifically associated with the correct choice of dispensing container. It might seam that these difficulty would be mitigated by the shorter period of further storage typical of dispensed item, but the prescribed quantity of drug may be intended to last the patient several months, e.g. tolbutamide or primidone, and this factor must be assessed and taken into account for most official preparation for packing and storage requirements are stated in the relevant monographs. It should be noted that there are now precise meanings attached to such familiar phrases as light-resistance freshly prepared, etc.

Official direction for preparation of cream are intended to minimize microbial contamination of the product, and this must not be increased during the repacking operation. Additional problems are the possible interaction between the new container and the product and the selection of the correct diluent (if required) for the avoidance of incompatibilities and significant change in rheological behaviour. The latter is also a factor to be considered in the provision of dispensing containers for mixtures and lotions. Although the original pack may serve as a guide, it is worth remembering that, even when thinned by shaking thixotropic products such as aluminum, hydroxide gel and mixture of magnesium hydroxide a wide neck. As discussed earlier, some wood flour phenol-formaldehyde screw caps may swell or distort in contact with product with this type. Very through shaking of suspension before dispensing is essential if the original composition is to be maintained in both the dispensed and remaining material. If the product is to be supplied in a diluted foam care must be taken that specific stabilizer and preservative are present in sufficient quantity for the efficient protective action. The oxygen permeability of plastic container may be crucial to the stability of the product if absorption or dilution of the antioxidant has taken placed.

Tablets are often repacked from bulk supply and the danger exist that progressive abrasion will occur as the tablet are tumbled when taken from the bulk container. The latter is frequently an aluminum or tinned—steel container or an amber glass bottle, all of which provide protection against light. The container selected for repacking must also posses this property if the product is photosensitive. A high proportion of the moisture sensitive drug exhibit adequate stability if stored and dispensed in a well-sealed container. More sensitive preparation effervescent potassium tablets, e.g. require in higher level of moisture exclusion. In commercial packs the tablets are sealed in a polythene bag with a desiccant sachet, enveloped in a further polythene bag and than issued in a sealed aluminum screw caped container. Unless this order of moisture protection can be maintained in repackaging it is probably best to obtain the prescribes agreement for the supply of the nearest size commercial pack. It cannot be too strongly stated that thoughtful repackaging may be ruined if appropriate directions for storage and use are not given and explained to the patient.

PRACTICE QUESTIONS

1. Define the term pharmaceutical packaging? What are the various types of packaging?
2. Give function so packaging. What are the desirable qualities of good container?
3. Enlist various types of containers, give there examples.
4. Write short notes on:
   a. Glass
   b. Plastic
   c. Metal
   d. Paper and board
5. What are the various types of glass used for pharmaceutical packaging?
6. Give advantages and disadvantages of plastic as a pharmaceutical packaging material.
7. Give advantages and disadvantages of metal as a pharmaceutical packaging material.
8. Enumerate various package validation methods.
9. Give evaluation methods of primary and secondary package.
10. Discuss in detail about various package testing methods.

Appendix 1: List of Some Commonly Used Additives

ABSORBENTS

Bentonite

Kaolin

Magnesium carbonate

Magnesium oxide

Magnesium silicate

Silica (cab-o-sil, syloid, aerosil)

Starch

Tricalcium phosphate

ANTIADHESIVES

Colloidal silica

Corn starch

DL-leucine

Magnesium stearate

Metallic stearates

Sodium lauryl sulfate

Talc

ANTIFOAMING AGENTS

Ariacel C

Atlas G 1706

Ethylene glycol fatty acid ester

(Emcol EC-50)

GMS

Propylene glycol monostearate

Span 65

Span 85

ANTIOXIDANTS

Acetone

Ascorbic acid

Ascorbyl palmitate

Benzoin

Beta-naphthol

Butylated hydroxytoluene

Butylated hydroxyanisole

Citric acid

Cysteine hydrochloride

Dilauryl thiodipropionate

Distearyl thiodipropionate

Maleic acid

Monoisopropylcitrate

Nordihydroguaiaretic acid

Phenyl alpha naphthlamine

Propyl gallate

Pyrogallol

Pyrocatechol

Sodium bisulfite

Sodium formaldehyde sulfoxylate

Sodium metabisulfite

Sodium sulfite

Ethylgallate
Gallic acid
Glycerin
Guaiac resin
Hydroquinon
Isoascorbic acid
Lecithin

Sodium thiosulfate
Thioglycerol
Thiosolbitol
Thiourea
Thioglycollic acid
Alpha tocopherol
Trihydroxybutyrophenone

COLOURS

1. Natural

Alizarin
Anattenes
Caramel
Beta-carotene
Carbon black
Carmic acid
Chlorophyll
Cochineal
Curcumin
Ferric oxides (red and yellow)

Hesperidin
Indigo
Quercetin
Riboflavin
Rubia tinctorum
Rutin
Saffron
Titanium dioxide
Turmeric
Tyrian purple

2. Synthetic

Alizarin cyanine
Amaranth I N 16785
Brilliant Blue FCS 42090
Carmoisine 14720
Eosine G 45380
Erythrosin 45430
Fast red E 16045
Fast green FCF 42053
Green S 44090
Freen F 61570

Indigo carmine 73015
Napthol blue black 20470
Orange G 16 30
Ponceaux 4 16255
Quinazarine 61565
Quinoline yellow SS 47000
Resoroin brown 20170
Sudan III 26100
Sunset yellow FCF 15185
Tartrazine 19140

EMULSIFYING AGENTS

1. Surfactants forming monomolecular films

Alkylpolyoxyethylene
sulfates

Benzalkonium chloride

Cetrimide

Dioctyl sodium
sulfosuccinate

Polyoxyethylene monolaurate
(Atlas G 2127)

(Polyoxyethylene alkylphenol
(lgepal CA 630)

Polyoxyethylene sorbitan
monolaurate (Tween 20)

Polyoxyethylene sorbitan
monopalmitate (Tween 40)

Lauryldimethylbenzy-
lammonium chloride
Lecithin
N-cetyl N-ethyl
morpholinium ethosulfate
(Atlas G-263)
PEG 400 monostearate
Polyoxyethylene
laurylether (Brij 30)
Polyoxyethylene
monostearate (Myrj 45)
Propylene glycol
monostearate
Propylene glycol
monostearate (Atlas G 917)
Sorbitan monolaurate
(Span 20)
Glyceryl monostearate
(GMS)
Sorbitan sesquioleate
(Alacel C)
Potassium stearate

Polyoxyethylene sorbitan
(Tween 80)
Polyoxyethylene laurylether (Brij 35)
Monostearate (Myrj 52)

Castor oil (Atlas G 1974)
Potassium oleate

Sodium oleate

Sodium lauryl sulfate·

Sorbitan monopalmitate
(span 40)
Sorbitan monostearate
(Arlacel 60)
Sodium laurate

Triethanolamine oleate

Triethanolamine stearate

2. Surfactants forming multimolecular films

Acacia
Agar
Alginates
Atapulgite
Bentonite
Gelatin

Hectorite
Magnesium hydroxide
Pectin
Silica gel
Tragacanth
Veegum

FLAVOURING AGENTS

Almond
Amyl acetate
Anethol
Apricot
Apple
Banana
Benzaldehyde
Black current
Blueberry
Butterscotch
Burgundy
Cherry

Oil of anise
Oil of bergamot
Oil of caraway
Oil of cardamom
Oil of cinnamon
Oil of clove
Oil of coriander
Oil of fennel
Oil of lemon
Oil of lavender
Oil of nutmeg
Oil of orange

Chocolate
Custard
Ethyl acetate
Ethyl vanillin
Eucalyptol
Eugenol
Ginger
Hyacinth
Jasmine
Lemongrass
Liquorice
Mango
Maple
Methyl salicylate
Melon
Narcissus
Neroli
Violet

Oil of narcissus
Oil of peppermint
Oil of rosemary
Oil of rose
Oil of spearmint
Oil of thyme
Orris root
Peach
Pheyl ethyl alcohol
Pineapple
Plum
Raspberry
Samdalwood
Saffron
Strawberry
Thymol
Vanillin

FLOCCULATING AGENTS

Electrolytes like
$KH_2 PO_4$ $AlCl_3$
NaCl, etc.

Ionic and non-ionic surfactants

Hydrocolloids

PRESERVATIVES

Banzalkonium chloride
Benzoic acid and benzoates
Benzylalcohol
Cetylpyridinium chloride
Chlorbutanol
Chlorothymol
p-chlorphenylglyceryl ether
Dichlorometaxylenol
Dehydroacetic acid

Formic acid
Formaldehyde

Boric acid and propyl alcohol
Cetrimide
Dichlorophene
Ortho and parachlorbenzoic acid
Parahydroxybenzoates
Parachlor metacresol
Parachlor metaxylenol
p-chlor phenylpropanediol
Phenyl mercuric nitrate and other
salts of phyenylmercuric acid
Phenol
Phenol hexachlorophene

SOLUBILISING AGENTS

Atlas G 1690
Atlas G 1794
Brij 35
Igepal CA 630

PEG 400 monostearate
Sodium oleate
Triethanolamine oleate
Tween 20

Myrj 45
Myrj 49
Myrj 51
Myrj 52

Tween 40
Tween 60
Tween 80

SUSPENDING AGENTS

Acacia
Agar
Alginates
Attapulgite
Bentonite
Carboxy methyl celluloses
Carbopol
Carbomer
Cellulose powder
Chondorus
Gelatin
Guar gum

Hectorite
Hydroxyethyl cellulose
Hydroxyl propyl cellulose
Methyl celluloses
Microcrystalline cellulose
Polyvinyl alcohol
Povidone
Psyllium seed gum
Pectin
Tragacanth
Veegum

SWEETENING AGENTS

Aspartyl phenylalanine
Cyclamates
Dextrose
Fructose
Glycerin
Glycyrrhizin
Honey
Lactose

Maltose
Mannitol
Neohsperidin dihydrochalone
Saccharin
Sorbitol
Sucrose
Xylitol

WETTING AGENTS

Tween 20
Brij 30

Span 20
Span 40

Appendix 2: Units and Conversion Factors

Length	1 inch	= 0.0254 m
	1 ft	= 0.3048 m
Area	1 ft^2	= 0.0929 m^2
Volume	1 ft^3	= 0.0283 m^3
	1 gal Imp	= 0.004546 m^3
	1 gal US	= 0.003785 m^3 = 3.785 litres
	1 litre	= 0.001 m^3
Mass	1 lb	= 0.4536 kg
	1 mole	molecular weight in kg
Density	1 lb/ft^3	= 16.03 kg m^{-3}
Velocity	1 ft/sec	= 0.3048 m s^{-1}
Pressure	1 lb/m^2	= 6894 Pa
	1 torr	= 133.3 Pa
	1 atm	= 1.013 × 10^5 Pa = 760 mm Hg
	1 Pa	= 1 N m^{-2} = 1 kg m^{-1} s^{-2}
Force	1 Newton1 lb ft s^{-2}	= 1 kg m s$^{-2=\,1.49\ \text{kg m s}{-2}}$
Viscosity	1 cP	= 0.001 N s m^{-2} = 0.001 Pa s
	1 lb/ft sec	= 1.49 N s m^{-2} = 1.49 kg m^{-1} s^{-2}
Energy	1 Btu	= 1055 J
	1 cal	= 4.186 J
Power	1 kW	= 1 kJ s^{-1}
	1 W	= 1 J s^{-1}
	1 horsepower	= 745.7 W = 745.7 J s^{-1}
		= 0.746 kW
	1 ton refrigeration	= 3.519 kW
Temperature units	(°F)	= 5/9 (°C) = 5/9 (K)
Heat-transfer coefficient	1 Btu ft^{-2} h^{-1} °F^{-1}	= 5.678 J m^{-2} s^{-1} °C
Thermal conductivity	1 Btu ft^{-1} h^{-1} °F^{-1}	= 1.731 J m^{-1} s^{-1} °C^{-1}

Constants Π 3.1416

                e (base of   2.7183

                natural logs)

                R   8.314 kJ mole^{-1} K^{-1} or 0.08206 m^3 atm mole^{-1} K^{-1}

(M) Mega = 10^6, (k) kilo = 10^3, (H) Hecto = 10^2, (m) milli = 10^{-3}, (μ) micro = 10^{-6}

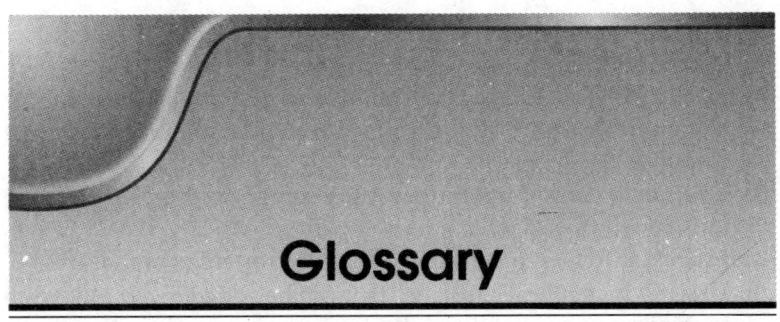

Glossary

Absorption: The assimilation of one substance by another, where the substance being absorbed diffuses into the absorbing material.

Acid: A chemical compound containing a hydrogen atom that dissociates from a molecule to a hydronium ion in water.

Adsorption: The attachment of one substance onto the surface of another by means of a strong interaction between the two substances or materials. This differs from absorption in that the substances are joined only at the surface.

Aerosol: A dispersion of very small (submicron)-sized liquid droplets or solid particles into a gas. The term is used in packaging as a label for all liquid or semisolid solutions or suspensions dispensed under pressure.

Amorphous: Not crystalline when used with plastics, it means molecules arranged in a random order, without structure.

Ampoule: Glass tubing sealed at both ends, containing a drug intended for injection.

Analgesic: A substance that relieves pain.

ANDA: Abbreviated New Drug Application.

Anesthetic: A drug that stops or suppresses sensations such as pain by affecting either the central nervous system (general anesthetic) or the peripheral nerve structures (local anesthetic).

Angina: A heart disease characterized by intermittent chest pain coupled with feelings of suffocation.

Angstrom: A unit of length equal to one hundred millionth of a centimeter.

Annealing: A controlled temperature method of gradually cooling glass containers in ovens to relieve structural stresses and to make the glass less brittle.

Antibiotics: Substances that inhibit the growth of or destroy microorganisms.

Antihistamines: Substances that neutralize or inhibit the effects of histamine released by the body during allergic reactions or in response to a disease.

Anti-inflammatory: Substances that neutralize or inhibit the inflammation of tissue.

Antimicrobial: Refers to substances that destroy microorganisms.

Antioxidant: A chemical substance that can be added to a plastic resin to minimize or prevent the effects of oxygen attack on the plastic (e.g. yellowing or degradation).

Antipruritic: A substance that relieves itching.

Antiseptic: A substance that inhibits the growth of microorganisms.

Antistatic agent: A chemical substance that can be applied to the surface of a plastic bottle or incorporated in the plastic from which the bottle is made. Its function is to render the surface of the plastic article less susceptible to an accumulation of electrostatic charges, which attract and hold fine dust on the surface of the bottle.

API: Active pharmaceutical ingredient—the active ingredient in a pharmaceutical product.

Aseptic: Free from disease-producing microorganisms. In biologic or medical applications, it refers to an operation performed in a presterilized environment that is controlled to prevent contamination through the introduction of microorganisms. Sterile area that is controlled to remain sterile during operation.

Aseptic filling: The process of combining sterilized pharmaceuticals with sterile packaged in a sterile environment.

Assay: The determination of the concentration of the active ingredient in a pharmaceutical.

Astringent: A substance that contracts tissues or canals, reducing the discharge of fluids.

Autoclave: A vessel capable of containing high-pressure steam that is commonly used to sterilize pharmaceuticals, medical instruments, and medical devices.

Bactericide: A substance that kills bacteria.

Bacteriostat: A substance that is added to a drug formulation to control the growth of bacteria.

Base: A chemical compound that when dissolved in water dissociates to form a hydroxyl ion and raises pH above 7. Generally a metal oxide or hydroxide.

Bioavailability: The availability of an administered drug to the circulatory system.

Blank: The mold parts used in all glass container machines for preliminary formation of glass in preparation for completion of the glass containers in the finish mold where the bottles are blown. The blank forms the parison; hence the parison itself is at times referred to as the blank.

Blister package: A package consisting of a cavity thermoformed from a thermoplastic material and a flat lid stock designed to seal each of the cavities to the edges of the trimmed card.

BTU: British thermal unit.

Buccal cavity: The cavity formed by the cheek.

Buffer: A buffer is a substance that when dissolved in water acts to resist changed in pH that would otherwise be caused by environmental factors (e.g. CO_2 in air or alkaline salts in glass containers).

CAD/CAM: Computer-assisted design/computer-assisted manufacturing (or in printing computer-assisted makeup).

Caplet: A tablet-shaped capsule.

Capsule: A transparent or colored gelatin material, hard- or soft-shelled that contains a drug preparation

Catalyst: A chemical compound that accelerates the rate of a chemical reaction without being consumed in the process.

CGMP: Current Good Manufacturing Practice (as written and used outside the FDA).

Coefficient of thermal expansion: A dimensionless number that expresses the degree to which a material will expand when subjected to a known and specified increase in temperature.

Copolymer: A polymer made from at least two different comonomers.

Cosmetic: Formulate products used to decorate, adorn, or beautify but which have no therapeutic effect or purpose.

Cream: A medicated preparation based on an emulsion of oil in water.

Deliquescence: Refers to a substance that readily absorbs moisture. Becoming damp or liquid by absorption of water from the atmosphere and then dissolving in the water taken up. This property is found in salts (e.g. $CaCl_2$).

Demulcent: A substance formulated to soothe the part of the body to which it is applied.

Densitometer: For printing, a reflection densitometer is used to measure and control the density of color inks on a substrate.

Density: Weight per unit of volume of a substance.

Depyrogenation: The elimination of pyrogens by heat or chemical processes.

Dermatological: Pertaining to the skin or diseases of the skin.

Die: Any tool or arrangement of tools designed to cut, shape, or otherwise form materials to a desired configuration.

Distillation: The process in which a liquid is purified by transforming it into a vapor, separating the vapor from the impure liquid and then condensing and collecting it.

Diuretic: A drug formulation that increases urinary discharge.

DMF: Drug Master File, a blinded repository for proprietary information that permits the FDA to review the safety and adequacy of a component.

Dosage form: The form of a drug preparation that determines how the drug is administered (e.g. tablet, oral liquid, suppository, parenteral liquid).

Effervescent: Refers to substances that produce a gas, usually CO_2, upon mixing with water.

Efflorescent: Refers to substances that lose water on exposure to air.

EFPIA: European Federation of Pharmaceutical Industries and Associations.

EHIBCC: Health Industry Business Communication Council (HIBCC) and its affiliate International Organization, the European Health Industry Business Communications Council.

Elastomer: A polymer with the elastic characteristics similar to rubber: the ability to be stretched to at least twice its original length without sustaining permanent deformation.

Elixirs: Syrups containing 20 to 25% alcohol.

EMEA: The European Agency for the evaluation of medicinal products.

Emollients: Substances that soften and relax the tissues when applied locally.

Emulsion: A liquid consisting of a discontinuous, immiscible liquid phase dispersed in a continuous liquid phase.

Enteric: Refers to coatings that delay dissolution until a solid dosage form reaches the intestine.

FD and C: Food, Drug, and Cosmetic Act.

FDA: United States Food and Drug Administration.

FFDCA: Federal Food, Drug, and Cosmetic Act.

Filtration: The process by which solid particles are removed from a liquid by passing the liquid through a porous medium whose pores are so small that the solid particles will not pass through them.

Finish: As applied to bottles and closures, describes the thread design: the size, pitch, profile length, and thickness.

Flint: A term used to describe a glass color that is perfectly clear and transparent.

Fluidized bed: A group of solid particles in a container that are agitated by the upwardflowing stream of gas. The particles appear as a cloud in the bottom of the confining space.

Fluorocarbon: An organic compound containing fluorine.

Flux: A substance or mixture used to promote the fusion of metals or minerals. Can be called a fluxing agent.

Free radical: A highly reactive species formed by the rupture of a chemical bond.

Gastrointestinal: The system of body organs that included the stomach and small intestine.

Gel: A colloidal semisolid consisting of a networked structure of suspended, fine, solid particles surrounded by a liquid. Differs from a colloidal solution, which has no solid particles to confer some rigidity to the structure.

Gelatin: A water soluble substance extracted from animal tissue and bones and used in the manufacturing of capsules.

Generic: Used in the pharmaceutical business to describe any drug that is labeled for sale with its technical name rather than a trade name, and usually manufactured by companies that were not the original developer of the product.

Glass: The USP on the basis of performance in chemical durability tests specifies four types of glass. Type 1, 2, and 3 are intended for packaging parenteral preparations and type NP for nonparenteral products.

HDPE: High-density polyethylene.

Head space: The space between the level of the contents of a container and the closure of the container.

Hermetic seal: Any seal or any container so sealed that is impervious to all gasses under normal conditions of handling and storage.

HIBCC: Health Industry Business Communication Council and its affiliate international organization, the European Health Industry Business Communications Council (EHIBCC).

Hologram: The image formed by a lensless photographic process (holography) that uses laser light to produce three-dimensional images.

Hormone: A substance formed in and secreted by the endocrine glands. May be made synthetically.

Hydrocarbon: An organic compound containing only carbon and hydrogen.

Hydrolysis: Reaction of a compound with water, resulting in destruction of the compound and the formation of at least two new ones.

Hypertonic: Having a greater osmotic pressure than blood plasma, lacrimal fluid, or interstitial fluid. It can be applied more specifically to a fluid in which cells shrink.

Hypoglycemia: An abnormally small concentration of glucose in the circulating blood.

In vitro: Refers to chemical or physical tests of drugs using laboratory procedures and apparatus (in glass).

In vivo: Refers to tests of drugs in laboratory tissue, animals, and humans (in life).

IND: Investigational New Drug.

Induction heating: Heating a metal object by application of an external magnetic field to generate heat-producing eddy currents in the object.

Infusion: Introduction of a fluid other than blood into a vein (e.g. a saline solution drip).

Inhalant: A substance that can be vaporized by mechanical means or by heat and carried into the respiratory tract by inhalation.

Intravenous: Administration of a drug by injection directly into a vein.

Ion: A charged atom or group of atoms formed by the dissociation of a molecule, often in an aqueous medium.

IQ: Installation qualification. This is a review of the equipment that establishes that the equipment meets its design specifications, and was installed in accordance with the design specifications. A term used in validation.

IR: Infrared.

Isotonic: Solutions that have the same osmotic pressure. A more specific definition is a solution in which cells neither swell nor shrink.

Isotonicity: The situation obtained when the colligative or osmotic properties of a pharmaceutical are matched with those of a biological site of administration, frequently mucous membranes.

IV: Intravenous.

Kaolin: A family of clays containing combinations of hydrated alumina and silica.

Keratolytic: A medication used to treat conditions that lead to horny skin growths.

Kpsi: 1000 psi.

Latex: The milky juice of exudation of plants obtained by tapping the trunk (e.g., the fluid from a rubber plant).

LDPE: Low-density polyethylene.

Light-resistant container: A container that protects the contents from the effects of light.

Lipophilic: Having a strong affinity for oily or fatty substances.

LLDPE: Linear low-density polyethylene.

Lot or lot number: A lot refers to all the products made during a single run or manufacturing sequence on a piece of equipment or a complete production line. A run may last for a given quantity, for hours, or days, it normally denotes all products made in one sequence of starting and stopping the equipment when all raw materials are consumed or a given quantity is produced. A lot number is the assigned designation of that specific manufacturing sequence.

Lyophilization: Freeze-drying. The removal of water or solvent from a substance by applying a vacuum to the substance after it has been frozen.

Magma: Highly thickened suspensions for oral administration.

Mandrel: A metal rod or bar used as a core around which metal, glass, etc. is cast molded or shaped.

Mg: Milligram.

Microbial control: Assembly of products in a controlled clean environment, followed by exposure to gamma radiation. This process reduces bioburden load but does not support a "sterile" label claim.

Microencapsulation: The encasement of small particles, either solid or liquid, within a shell that prevents their escape until the shell is ruptured by an external force or dissolved by a solvent.

Micron: One ten-thousandth of a centimeter.

Microorganisms, microbes: Living microscopic entities including bacteria and molds.

Multiple-dose container: A multiple-unit container for parenteral or ophthalmic formulations.

Multiple-unit container: One that permits the withdrawal of part of the contents while containing and protecting the un-withdrawn balance.

NDA: New Drug Application (FDA). Submission of all information necessary for review by the agency prior to approval of a new drug.

NDC: National Drug Code.

NF: National Formulary.

NWDA: The National Wholesale Druggists Association.

OFAS: Office of Food Additive Safety.

Offset: The process of using an intermediate cylinder to transfer an image from the image center to the substrate.

Ointment: A medicated preparation with the oleaginous base. More generally, a semisolid preparation intended for topical administration.

Oleaginous base: A base with the nature or quality of an oil.

ONPLDS: Office of Nutritional Products, Labeling, and Dietary Supplements.

Ophthalmic: Related to the eye.

OPP: Oriented polypropylene.

OTC: Over the counter.

Otic: Related to the ear.

Oxidation: Reaction with oxygen, more generally removal of electrons from an atom or molecule.

Parenteral: Introduction of substances into an organism by subcutaneous, intramuscular, intravenous, or intramedullary injection. Introduction by some other means than through the gastrointestinal tract.

PH: A measure of the hydrogen ion concentration in and the acidity of an aqueous solution.

Pharmaceutical: A manufactured, processed, or compounded form of a drug.

PIM: Product information management.

Plasticizer: A substance mixed into a plastic to decrease its stiffness and increase its softness.

Polymer: A high molecular weight molecule formed by reacting small molecules (monomers) together to form a long chain consisting of many monomer units.

Polyolefin: Any polymer whose monomer units are unsaturated hydrocarbons (olefins) containing only carbon and hydrogen. Polyethylene and polypropylene are the most common polyolefins used in packaging.

PPB: Parts per billion.

Prophylaxis: Prevention of disease or its spread by the administration of drugs and/or procedures.

Protocol: A set of procedures. Test or validation protocols are the set of instructions that govern how a test is run and how the data is to be reported.

PTFE: Polytetrafluoroethylene.

PVC: Polyvinyl chloride.

PVDC: Polyvinylidene chloride.

Pyrogen: Agent that causes a rise in body temperature, especially if injected. The most important pyrogen in sterile drug manufacture is endotoxins, a residue from gram-negative bacteria.

Resin: The term for a polymer in the form of small pellets that is packaged in a bag or in bulk and shipped to a processor. Sometimes a direct reference to the polymer itself.

Reverse osmosis: The process in which the solute in a solution is removed by forcing the solvent, against the normal osmotic pressure to flow through a membrane that is not permeable to the solute. Used to remove salts from seawater.

RH: Relative humidity.

Saturated: When used to describe a type of chemical bond or molecule, the bonding is saturated if no double or triple bonds exist, i.e. each atom is joined within the molecule to other atoms only by single bonds.

Scabacide: A substance that destroys the organism causing scabies.

Secondary package: The package that contains the primary package. It is not in direct contact with the product. Usually a box or carton.

Semipermeable-membrane: A membrane that permits the passage of one or more components of a solution but does not allow the passage of other components. Such membranes are usually permeable only by the solvent.

Shelf life: The time required for the potency of a drug to drop to 90% of its labeled potency.

Single-dose container: A single-unit container for primarily used for parenterals but also for other dosage forms that contains only one dose of product.

Single-unit container: A container that holds the quantity of drug intended for administration as a single dose promptly after the container is opened.

Sol: A colloidal solution or liquid phase of a colloidal solution.

Sterile: The absence of microorganisms.

Sterility testing: Tests performed to determine whether viable microorganisms are present. Commonly, the test involves immersing a component or system or flushing a fluid pathway with sterile microbial growth medium, incubation of the medium under conditions favorable for microbial growth, and observation of turbidity or other indication of microbial growth after a suitable incubation period.

Sterilization: A validated process used to render a product free from viable microorganisms. It is generally accepted that a terminally sterilized unit purporting to be sterile attain a sterility assurance level of 10–6, i.e. probability of less than or equal to one chance in 1 million that a viable microorganism is present in the sterilized unit. Lower SALs may be validated as sterile in some cases.

Steroid: Fat-soluble organic compounds such as sterols, bile acids, and sex hormones.

Stratum corneum: The outermost layer of skin

Strip package: A package made by enclosing an object to be packaged such as a tablet between two webs and then sealing the webs together so that the seal completely surrounds the object being packaged.

Subcutaneous: Beneath the skin.

Sublingual: Under the tongue.

Substrate: Refers to the primary structural material or the surface of the primary material that is applied to other materials designed to alter the characteristics or properties of the original material.

Suppository: The dosage form designed for insertion into the rectum.

Surfactant: Any substance, normally a soap or detergent, that forms a compatibilizing boundary layer between two liquids or a liquid and solid. This layer leads to the staple dispersion one phase in another.

Suspension: Solid particles dispersed in a liquid. If the suspension is stable, it will resist the normal gravitational separation into two phases.

Systemic: Administration of a drug so that it gains access to the circulatory system. Can also refer to the introduction of a drug to all parts of the body to treat only one location.

Tensile strength: The resistance of a specimen to breaking when stressed longitudinally.

Therapeutic: Relating to the treatment of disease.

Thermoplastic: Describes any substance that becomes more pliable as it is heated. In packaging and molding, it refers to a material that can be formed when hot but become rigid after cooling.

Thermoset: Plastics that become rigid when heated or subjected to energy that initiates a chemical reaction at reactive sites linking all the individual polymer strands together permanently.

Tight container: A term defined by the USP that describes a container that protects its contents from contamination by extraneous liquids, solids, or gases from physical loss of the drug and from efflorescence, deliquescence, or evaporating under ordinary or customary conditions of handling, shipment, storage, and distribution.

Tincture: A solution of a drug in alcohol.

Topical: Administration of a drug to the skin surface or the lining of body cavities. Its effectiveness is limited to the localized areas to which it is applied.

Toxin: A noxious or poisonous substance formed during the growth of certain microorganisms.

Toxoid: A toxin that has been treated, e.g. with formaldehyde to destroy its toxic property but retain its antigenicity, i.e. its capability of stimulating the production of antitoxin antibodies and thus engendering immunity.

Transdermal: Administration of drugs through the skin.

Type I glass: Glass composed largely of silica and boric oxide that is very low in water extractable impurities.

Type II glass: Glass containing larger amounts of water-soluble sodium and calcium oxides than type I glass. Soda-lime glass with no boron-containing materials present.

Type III glass: Glass containing even greater quantities of water-extractable oxides than type II glass. A different and lower grade of soda-lime glass.

Unit-dose container: A single-unit container for products for administration by other than parenteral means as a singe dose direct from the container.

Unsaturated: In chemistry, molecules that contain more than one bond between two atoms. In polymers, it is usually referring to double and triple bonds between carbon and another atom.

USP: United States Pharmacopoeia.

USP-NF: United States Pharmacopoeia National Formulary.

UV: Ultraviolet.

Validation: Testing and establishing documented evidence that provides a high degree of assurance that a specific process, component, or piece of equipment will consistently produce a product meeting its predetermined specifications and quality attributes.

Vasoconstrictors: Drugs that reduce the flow of body fluids by constricting the ducts, tubes, and canals through which these fluids flow. Often referred to drugs that constrict the circulatory system.

Vasodilators: Drugs that increase the flow of body fluids by relaxing the muscles surrounding the ducts, tubes, and canals through which those fluids flow.

Wavelength: The distance between identical points in a wave pattern. A measure of the energy content of light, the shorter the wavelength the higher the energy level.

Well-closed container: A USP term. A container that protects its contents from extraneous solids and physical loss under the ordinary and customary conditions of handling, shipment, and distribution.

Index

Adsorbents 93
Ampoule filling 335
Anatomy of ear 280
Angle of repose 6, 84, 85
Antifrictional agents 89
Antioxidant 93
Antiadherents 91
Autoclave 338–340

Base adsorption 21, 22
Binders 81–83
Buffers 93

Capsule 1
  administration 34
  excipients 8, 9
  filling difficulties 16, 17
  ingredients 24
  number 8
  shell filling 9, 11, 13
  shell manufacturer 11
Capsules 1
  packaging 33, 34
  quality control 25
  size 7, 8
  special types 35
  storage 33, 34
Carr's index 84
Coated capsules 36
Coating pan 157
Coating process 64
Coating tablet evaluation 168, 169
Colonic release system 193
Colorants 4, 152
Colour coating 147
Colouring agent 93, 94
Components of parenteral
  formulation 306
Contact lens solution 228, 229
Container type 316

Content uniformity test 125
Controlled release evaluation
  213–217
Copper T 212

Delayed release 174, 186
Depot systems 195–197
Diluents 77–81
Direct compression 109–113
Disintegrant 85–88
Dissolution controlled system
  186–188
Dissolution enhancer 92
Dissolution media 136–138
Dissolution retardants 92
Dissolution test 132–136
Dosage form index 183
Dry granulation 107–109

Empty capsules 6
Enteric coating 153
Evaluation of otic products
  288–295
Eye drop 224–226
Eye-lotion 226–227
Eye ointment 227, 228
Eye physiology 221

FBD 160–163
Film coating 147
Film coating material 148
Film formers 149–151
Flavouring agent 94, 95
Floating capsules 192
Fluidized bed coating 201
Fluidized-bed technology 61
Friability test 130, 131
Function of packaging 363, 364

403

Gelatin 3, 4
Gels 230
Glass 317, 319, 366–371
Glidants 91

Handerson-Hasselbalch
equation 179
Hard gelatin capsules 2
Hardness test 127
Hausner ratio 84
High density pellets 192
Hydrodynamic pressure
controlled system 191

Immersion sword 158
Immersion tube 158
Inserts 235
Intestinal release system 193
Intravaginal and intrauterine
drug delivery systems 212
ISFD 197

LAL test 243
Large volume parenterals 303
305
Liposomes 202–206
Low density pellets 192
Lubricants 89–91
Lyophilization 340–342
Matrix system 187
Metal 374, 375
Metered dose inhaler 262
Microbial quality 310
Microencapsulation 44
applications 45
coating material 44
core material 44
evaluation 65
mechanism 50
techniques 47
Microspheres 200
Mixed monolithic reservoir
devices 210

Monolithic devices 209
Mucoadhesive system 193

Nanoparticles 234
Nasal drops 258
emulsions 260
formulation ingredients 256
gel 260
ointment 260
physiology 251
powders 260
products 250
products evaluation 264–
272
spray 258
Niosomes 236

Opacifier 153
Ophthalmic drug delivery
system 211
Ophthalmic products 220
Oral controlled system 185
Osmotic pressure controlled
system 190
Osmotic pump 191
Otic products 279

Package validation 376–382
Packaging of pharmaceutical 362
Pan coating 63
Paper and board 375
Parenteral routes administration
300–303
Parenteral controlled release
system 194
Parenteral depot system 195
Parenteral products 298
Parenteral suspension 329–334
Penetration enhancer 230
Percentage compressibility 84
Pharmaceutical aids 5
Pharmacodynamics 182, 183

Pharmacokinetics 182
Pharmacosomes 236
Plastic 316, 317
Plastic 371–374
Plasticizers 151
Polishing 147
Preservatives 93
Principle of hearing 281
Prodrugs 230
Progesterone IUD 212
Pyrogen 328
Pyrogen test 242

Rabbit test 243
Rectal capsules 38
Reservoir devices 189, 210
Reverse osmosis 309
Rotary capsule machine 23
Routes of drug administration 181
Rubber closers 319–322

Sealing of vials and bottles 337
Sealing 145
Seamless gelatin capsules 23
Sink condition 195
Small volume parenteral 303, 305
Smoothing 146
Soft contact lenses 236
Soft gelatin capsules 17, 18
Solvent evaporation 62
Specialized coating 155
Sub-coating 146
Sugar coating 145
Super disintegrants 88

Suspensions 207
Sustain release capsules 37
Sustained release 174
Sweetening agent 95–97

Tablet 71
   coating 144
   coating problems 163–168
   disintegration 127–130
   excipients 77
   granulation 102, 103
   manufacturing 97–100
   manufacturing
      problems 115–123
Tablet manufacturing
   stages 102
Tablet manufacturing
   steps 100, 101
   packaging 102
   testing 123–138
   type 73
Targeted drug delivery 174
Test for ophthalmic solutions 240
Test for sterility 241
Thermoplastic pastes 197
Transdermal drug delivery
   system 208
Types of containers 365

Viscosity improver 229

Water for injection 307
Wet granulation 103–106
Wetting agent 92

Reader's Notes